Abridged Nutrition Care Process Reference Terminology (NCPT) Manual

Standardized Terminology for the Nutrition Care Process

2017 EDITION

For Educational Use

 **eat** **right.** Academy of Nutrition and Dietetics

Abridged Nutrition Care Process Terminology (NCPT) Reference Manual:
Standardized Terminology for the Nutrition Care Process, 2017 Edition

ISBN 978-0-88091-969-2

Catalog Number 969218

The views expressed in this publication are those of the authors and do not necessarily reflect policies and/or official positions of the Academy of Nutrition and Dietetics. Mention of product names in this publication does not constitute endorsement by the authors or the Academy of Nutrition and Dietetics. The Academy of Nutrition and Dietetics disclaims responsibility for the application of the information contained herein.

For more information on the Academy of Nutrition and Dietetics, visit www.eatright.org.

10   9   8   7   6   5   4   3   2   1

Contents

Note: The terminology in this publication is based on the electronic Nutrition Care Process Terminology (eNCPT) 2017 edition and is subject to change based on continuing development work. This abridged version does not include all terms in the eNCPT. For the complete eNCPT and suggested references for each step and term, sign in as a subscriber at https://ncpt.webauthor.com. Additional resources are available on the Academy's website (www.eatright.org)—sign in as a member and go to http://www.eatrightpro.org/ncp.

About this Book

This book is about having the best of all worlds in scientific resources: electronic and print. In recent years, we have come to appreciate easy access to information via electronic means but many of us still value a hard-copy book. The complete Nutrition Care Process Terminology (NCPT) has been available from the Academy of Nutrition and Dietetics (Academy) in electronic format for some years now. The NCPT (electronic NCPT: eNCPT) has grown to about 1,500 terms, and continues to evolve as the fields of nutrition and dietetics advance.

This abridged NCPT publication came to life as a complement to the eNCPT due to a rising demand by educators for a selection of NCP terms in print form for student use.

In addition to the selected NCPT terms, the book you are holding contains the Nutrition Assessment Matrix and the Nutrition Diagnosis Etiology Matrix. The Nutrition Assessment Matrix is a resource to cross-reference specific nutrition assessment parameters with associated nutrition diagnoses. The Nutrition Diagnosis Etiology Matrix assists with identifying the etiology category and intent of a chosen Nutrition Diagnosis term.

A great feature of the book is that it comes with an individual 1-year electronic subscription to the eNCPT which can be viewed on a smartphone or tablet. We encourage users to use the book but accessing the eNCPT for complete and current information is essential, as the abridged NCPT book is not a stand-alone resource.

The NCPT has been developed by the Nutrition Care Process Research Outcomes (NCPRO) Committee of the Academy, a committee that has evolved as much as the NCPT itself with significant input from experts within the US and around the world. Also, the NCPT would not have been possible without the dedicated work of Academy staff and consultants who have facilitated the work of the Academy's NCPRO Committee. A comprehensive list of NCPT contributors is available on the eNCPT website (https://ncpt.webauthor.com/)

Constantina (Tina) Papoutsakis, PhD, RD
Senior Director, Data Science Center
Research, International & Scientific Affairs (RISA)
Academy of Nutrition and Dietetics

For more information and questions please write to ncp@eatright.org.
The complete eNCPT is available at https://ncpt.webauthor.com.

SNAPSHOT   NCP Step 1: Nutrition Assessment

Purpose: The purpose of nutrition assessment is to obtain, verify, and interpret data needed to identify nutrition-related problems, their causes, and significance. It is an ongoing, nonlinear, and dynamic process that involves data collection and continual analysis of the patient/client's* status compared to specified criteria. This contrasts with nutrition monitoring and evaluation where nutrition and dietetics practitioners use the same data to determine changes in patient/client behavior, nutritional status, and the efficacy of nutrition intervention.

Finding nutrition assessment data: For individuals, data can come directly from the patient/client through interview, observation and measurements, a medical record, and the referring health care provider. For population groups, data from surveys, administrative data sets, and epidemiological or research studies are used.

Terminology for nutrition assessment is organized in 5 domains (categories):

Food/Nutrition-Related History	Anthropometric Measurements	Biochemical Data, Medical Tests, and Procedures	Nutrition-Focused Physical Findings	Client History
Food and nutrient intake, food and nutrient administration, medication, complementary/alternative medicine use, knowledge/beliefs, food and supplies availability, physical activity, nutrition quality of life	Height, weight, body mass index (BMI), growth pattern indices/percentile ranks, and weight history	Lab data (eg, electrolytes, glucose) and tests (eg, gastric emptying time, resting metabolic rate)	Physical appearance, muscle and subcutaneous fat wasting, swallow function, appetite, and affect	Personal history, medical/health/family history, treatments and complementary/alternative medicine use, and social history

Use of nutrition assessment data: Nutrition assessment data, or indicators, are compared to criteria, or relevant norms and standards. These norms and standards may be national, institutional, or regulatory. Nutrition assessment findings are then documented in nutrition diagnosis statements and nutrition intervention goal setting.

Critical Thinking Skills

- Determining appropriate data to collect
- Determining the need for additional information
- Selecting assessment tools and procedures that match the situation
- Applying assessment tools in valid and reliable ways
- Distinguishing relevant from irrelevant data
- Distinguishing important from unimportant data
- Validating the data

Term selection and organization: The taxonomy or classification system guides the nutrition and dietetics practitioner to logical terminology selection. The terms for nutrition assessment and nutrition monitoring and evaluation are combined because the data points are the same or related; however, the data purpose and use are distinct in these two steps of the Nutrition Care Process.

For more information, sign in as a subscriber at https://ncpt.webauthor.com.

---

*Patient/client refers to individuals, groups, populations, family members, and/or caregivers.

Nutrition Assessment and Monitoring and Evaluation Terminology

This is a combined list of Nutrition Assessment and Monitoring and Evaluation terms. Shaded indicators are used ONLY for nutrition assessment. All of the other indicators are used for both assessment and monitoring and evaluation. Each term is designated with an alphanumeric NCPT hierarchical code, followed by a five-digit (eg, 99999) Academy SNOMED CT/LOINC unique identifier (ANDUID). Neither should be used in nutrition documentation. The ANDUID is for data tracking purposes in electronic health records.

FOOD/NUTRITION-RELATED HISTORY (FH)

Food and nutrient intake, food and nutrient administration, medication and complementary/alternative medicine use, knowledge/beliefs/attitudes, behavior, food and supply availability, physical activity and function, nutrition-related patient/client-centered measures.

Food and Nutrient Intake (1)

Composition and adequacy of food and nutrient intake, meal and snack patterns, current and previous diets and/or food modifications, and eating environment.

Energy Intake (1.1)

Total energy intake from all sources including food, beverages, breastmilk/formula, supplements, and via enteral and parenteral routes.

Energy intake (1.1.1)

	NCPT Code	ANDUID
❑ Total energy intake	FH-1.1.1.1	10005

Food and Beverage Intake (1.2)

Type, amount, and pattern of intake of foods and food groups, indices of diet quality, intake of fluids, breastmilk and infant formula

Fluid/beverage intake (1.2.1)

	NCPT Code	ANDUID
❑ Oral fluids	FH-1.2.1.1	10008
❑ Food-derived fluids	FH-1.2.1.2	10009
❑ Liquid meal replacement or supplement	FH-1.2.1.3	10010

Food intake (1.2.2)

	NCPT Code	ANDUID
❑ Amount of food	FH-1.2.2.1	10012
❑ Types of food/meals	FH-1.2.2.2	10013
❑ Meal/snack pattern	FH-1.2.2.3	10014
❑ Diet quality index	FH-1.2.2.4	10015
❑ Food variety	FH-1.2.2.5	10016

Breastmilk/infant formula intake (1.2.3)

	NCPT Code	ANDUID
❑ Breastmilk intake	FH-1.2.3.1	10018
❑ Infant formula intake	FH-1.2.3.2	10019

Enteral and Parenteral Nutrition Intake (1.3)

Specialized nutrition support intake from all sources, eg, enteral and parenteral routes.

Enteral nutrition intake (1.3.1)

	NCPT Code	ANDUID
❑ Enteral nutrition formula/solution	FH-1.3.1.1	10022
❑ Feeding tube flush	FH-1.3.1.2	10023

Parenteral nutrition intake (1.3.2)

	NCPT Code	ANDUID
❑ Parenteral nutrition formula/solution	FH-1.3.2.1	10025
❑ IV fluids	FH-1.3.2.2	10026

Bioactive Substance Intake (1.4)

Alcohol, plant stanol and sterol esters, soy protein, psyllium and β-glucan, and caffeine intake from all sources, eg, food, beverages, supplements, and via enteral and parenteral routes.

Alcohol intake (1.4.1)

	NCPT Code	ANDUID
❑ Drink size/volume	FH-1.4.1.1	10029
❑ Frequency	FH-1.4.1.2	10030
❑ Pattern of alcohol consumption	FH-1.4.1.3	10031

Bioactive substance intake (1.4.2)

	NCPT Code	ANDUID
❑ Plant stanol ester intake	FH-1.4.2.1	10034
❑ Plant sterol ester intake	FH-1.4.2.2	10807
❑ Soy protein intake	FH-1.4.2.3	10035
❑ Psyllium intake	FH-1.4.2.4	10827
❑ β-glucan intake	FH-1.4.2.5	10037
❑ Food additive intake (specify)	FH-1.4.2.6	10038
❑ Other (specify)	FH-1.4.2.7	10039

Caffeine intake (1.4.3)

	NCPT Code	ANDUID
❑ Total caffeine intake	FH-1.4.3.1	10041

Macronutrient Intake (1.5)

Fat and cholesterol, protein, carbohydrate, and fiber intake from all sources including food, beverages, supplements, and via enteral and parenteral routes.

Fat intake (1.5.1)

	NCPT Code	ANDUID
❑ Total fat intake	FH-1.5.1.1	10044
❑ Saturated fat intake	FH-1.5.1.2	10045
❑ Trans fatty acid intake	FH-1.5.1.3	10046
❑ Polyunsaturated fat intake	FH-1.5.1.4	10047
❑ Linoleic acid intake	FH-1.5.1.4.1	11602
❑ Monounsaturated fat intake	FH-1.5.1.5	10048
❑ Omega 3 fatty acid intake	FH-1.5.1.6	10049
❑ Alpha linolenic acid intake	FH-1.5.1.6.1	11603
❑ Eicosapentaenoic acid intake	FH-1.5.1.6.2	13019
❑ Docosahexaenoic acid intake	FH-1.5.1.6.3	13020
❑ Essential fatty acid intake	FH-1.5.1.7	10051
❑ Medium chain triglyceride intake	FH-1.5.1.8	11606

Cholesterol intake (1.5.2)

	NCPT Code	ANDUID
❑ Dietary cholesterol intake	FH-1.5.2.1	10050

Protein intake (1.5.3)

	NCPT Code	ANDUID
❑ Total protein intake	FH-1.5.3.1	10053

Assessment

	NCPT Code	ANDUID
Protein intake (1.5.3) cont.		
❑ High biological value protein intake	FH-1.5.3.2	10054
❑ Casein intake	FH-1.5.3.3	10055
❑ Whey intake	FH-1.5.3.4	10056
❑ Gluten intake	FH-1.5.3.5	11609
❑ Natural protein intake	FH-1.5.3.6	11610
Carbohydrate intake (1.5.5)		
❑ Total carbohydrate intake	FH-1.5.5.1	10060
❑ Complex carbohydrate intake	FH-1.5.5.2	11627
❑ Simple sugar carbohydrate intake	FH-1.5.5.3	11628
❑ Galactose intake	FH-1.5.5.4	11629
❑ Lactose intake	FH-1.5.5.5	11630
❑ Fructose intake	FH-1.5.5.6	11631
❑ Estimated total daily glycemic index value	FH-1.5.5.7	12013
❑ Estimated total daily glycemic load	FH-1.5.5.8	12142
❑ Total carbohydrate from diet	FH-1.5.5.9	12143
❑ Total carbohydrate from enteral nutrition	FH-1.5.5.10	12014
❑ Total carbohydrate from parenteral nutrition	FH-1.5.5.11	11180
❑ Total carbohydrate from intravenous fluids	FH-1.5.5.12	11240
❑ Insulin-to-carbohydrate ratio	FH-1.5.5.13	10066
Fiber intake (1.5.6)		
❑ Total fiber intake	FH-1.5.6.1	10068
❑ Soluble fiber intake	FH-1.5.6.2	10069
❑ Insoluble fiber intake	FH-1.5.6.3	10070

Micronutrient Intake (1.6)

Vitamin and mineral intake from all sources including food, beverages, supplements, and via enteral and parenteral routes.

	NCPT Code	ANDUID
Vitamin intake (1.6.1)		
❑ A (1)		10073
❑ C (2)		10074
❑ D (3)		10075
❑ E (4)		10076
❑ K (5)		10077
❑ Thiamin (6)		10078
❑ Riboflavin (7)		10079
❑ Niacin (8)		10080
❑ Folate (9)		10081
❑ B6 (10)		10082
❑ B12 (11)		10083

	NCPT Code	ANDUID
Vitamin intake (1.6.1) cont.		
❑ Pantothenic acid (12)		10084
❑ Biotin (13)		10085
❑ Multivitamin (14)		10086
Mineral/element intake (1.6.2)		
❑ Calcium (1)		10089
❑ Chloride (2)		10090
❑ Iron (3)		10091
❑ Magnesium (4)		10092
❑ Potassium (5)		10093
❑ Phosphorus (6)		10094
❑ Sodium (7)		10095
❑ Zinc (8)		10096
❑ Sulfate (9)		10097
❑ Fluoride (10)		10098
❑ Copper (11)		10099
❑ Iodine (12)		10100
❑ Selenium (13)		10101
❑ Manganese (14)		10102
❑ Chromium (15)		10103
❑ Molybdenum (16)		10104
❑ Boron (17)		10105
❑ Cobalt (18)		10106
❑ Multimineral (19)		10107
❑ Multi-trace element (20)		10108

Food and Nutrient Administration (2)

Current and previous diets and/or food modifications, eating environment, and enteral and parenteral nutrition administration.

Diet History (2.1)

Description of food and drink regularly provided or consumed, past diets followed or prescribed and counseling received, and the eating environment.

	NCPT Code	ANDUID
Diet order (2.1.1)		
❑ General, healthful diet order	FH-2.1.1.1	10113
❑ Modified diet order	FH-2.1.1.2	10114
❑ Enteral nutrition order	FH-2.1.1.3	10115
❑ Parenteral nutrition order	FH-2.1.1.4	10116
Diet experience (2.1.2)		
❑ Previously prescribed diets	FH-2.1.2.1	10118
❑ Previous diet/nutrition education/ counseling	FH-2.1.2.2	10119

	NCPT Code	ANDUID
Diet experience (2.1.2) cont.		
❏ Self-selected diet/s followed	FH-2.1.2.3	10120
❏ Dieting attempts	FH-2.1.2.4	10121
❏ Food allergies	FH-2.1.2.5	10805
❏ Food intolerance	FH-2.1.2.6	10806
Eating environment (2.1.3)		
❏ Location	FH-2.1.3.1	10123
❏ Atmosphere	FH-2.1.3.2	10124
❏ Caregiver/companion	FH-2.1.3.3	10125
❏ Appropriate breastfeeding accommodations/facility	FH-2.1.3.4	10126
❏ Eats alone	FH-2.1.3.5	10127
Enteral and parenteral nutrition administration (2.1.4)		
❏ Enteral access	FH-2.1.4.1	10129
❏ Parenteral access	FH-2.1.4.2	10130
❏ Body position, EN	FH-2.1.4.3	10804
Fasting (2.1.5)		
❏ Fasting pattern in one calendar day, reported	FH-2.1.5.1	11633
❏ Fasting pattern in one calendar week, reported	FH-2.1.5.2	11634
❏ Fasting pattern in one calendar month, reported	FH-2.1.5.3	11635
❏ Fasting pattern in one calendar year, reported	FH-2.1.5.4	11636
❏ Fasting tolerance, reported	FH-2.1.5.5	11637

Medication and Complementary/Alternative Medicine Use (3)

Prescription and over-the-counter medications, including herbal preparations and complementary/alternative medicine products used.

	NCPT Code	ANDUID
Medications (3.1)		
❏ Prescription medication use	FH-3.1.1	10820
❏ Insulin sensitivity factor	FH-3.1.1.1	11241
❏ Over-the-counter medication use	FH-3.1.2	10134
❏ Misuse of medication	FH-3.1.3	10135
Complementary/Alternative Medicine (3.2)		
❏ Nutrition-related complementary/ alternative medicine use	FH-3.2.1	10137

Knowledge/Beliefs/Attitudes (4)

Understanding of nutrition-related concepts and conviction of the truth and feelings/emotions toward some nutrition-related statement or phenomenon, along with readiness to change nutrition-related behaviors.

	NCPT Code	ANDUID
Food and nutrition knowledge/skill (4.1)		
❏ Area(s) and level of knowledge/skill	FH-4.1.1	10848

	NCPT Code	ANDUID
Food and nutrition knowledge/skill (4.1) cont.		
❏ Diagnosis specific or global nutrition-related knowledge score	FH-4.1.2	10143
Beliefs and attitudes (4.2)		
❏ Conflict with personal/family value system	FH-4.2.1	10145
❏ Distorted body image	FH-4.2.2	10146
❏ End-of-life decisions	FH-4.2.3	10147
❏ Motivation	FH-4.2.4	10148
❏ Preoccupation with food/nutrients	FH-4.2.5	10149
❏ Preoccupation with weight	FH-4.2.6	10150
❏ Readiness to change nutrition-related behaviors	FH-4.2.7	10151
❏ Self-efficacy	FH-4.2.8	10152
❏ Self-talk/cognitions	FH-4.2.9	10153
❏ Unrealistic nutrition-related goals	FH-4.2.10	10154
❏ Unscientific beliefs/attitudes	FH-4.2.11	10155
❏ Food preferences	FH-4.2.12	10156
❏ Emotions	FH-4.2.13	10157

Behavior (5)

Patient/client activities and actions, which influence achievement of nutrition-related goals.

	NCPT Code	ANDUID
Adherence (5.1)		
❏ Self-reported adherence score	FH-5.1.1	10160
❏ Nutrition visit attendance	FH-5.1.2	10161
❏ Ability to recall nutrition goals	FH-5.1.3	10162
❏ Self-monitoring at agreed upon rate	FH-5.1.4	10163
❏ Self-management as agreed upon	FH-5.1.5	10164
Avoidance behavior (5.2)		
❏ Avoidance	FH-5.2.1	10166
❏ Restrictive eating	FH-5.2.2	10167
❏ Cause of avoidance behavior	FH-5.2.3	10168
Bingeing and purging behavior (5.3)		
❏ Binge eating behavior	FH-5.3.1	10170
❏ Purging behavior	FH-5.3.2	10171
Mealtime behavior (5.4)		
❏ Meal duration	FH-5.4.1	10173
❏ Percent of meal time spent eating	FH-5.4.2	10174
❏ Preference to drink rather than eat	FH-5.4.3	10175
❏ Refusal to eat/chew	FH-5.4.4	10176
❏ Spitting food out	FH-5.4.5	10177
❏ Rumination	FH-5.4.6	10178

	NCPT Code	ANDUID

Mealtime behavior (5.4) cont.

	NCPT Code	ANDUID
❑ Patient/client/caregiver fatigue during feeding process resulting in inadequate intake	FH-5.4.7	10179
❑ Willingness to try new foods	FH-5.4.8	10180
❑ Limited number of accepted foods	FH-5.4.9	10181
❑ Rigid sensory preferences	FH-5.4.10	10182

Social network (5.5)

	NCPT Code	ANDUID
❑ Ability to build and utilize social network	FH-5.5.1	10184

Factors Affecting Access to Food and Food/Nutrition-Related Supplies (6)

Factors that affect intake and availability of a sufficient quantity of safe, healthful food as well as food/nutrition-related supplies.

Food/nutrition program participation (6.1)

	NCPT Code	ANDUID
❑ Eligibility for government programs	FH-6.1.1	10187
❑ Participation in government programs	FH-6.1.2	10188
❑ Eligibility for community programs	FH-6.1.3	10189
❑ Participation in community programs	FH-6.1.4	10190

Safe food/meal availability (6.2)

	NCPT Code	ANDUID
❑ Availability of shopping facilities	FH-6.2.1	10192
❑ Procurement of safe food	FH-6.2.2	10800
❑ Appropriate meal preparation facilities	FH-6.2.3	10194
❑ Availability of safe food storage	FH-6.2.4	10195
❑ Appropriate storage technique	FH-6.2.5	10196
❑ Identification of safe food	FH-6.2.6	10801

Safe water availability (6.3)

	NCPT Code	ANDUID
❑ Availability of potable water	FH-6.3.1	10198
❑ Appropriate water decontamination	FH-6.3.2	10199

Food and nutrition-related supplies availability (6.4)

	NCPT Code	ANDUID
❑ Access to food and nutrition-related supplies	FH-6.4.1	10201
❑ Access to assistive eating devices	FH-6.4.2	10202
❑ Access to assistive food preparation devices	FH-6.4.3	10203

Physical Activity and Function (7)

Physical activity, cognitive and physical ability to engage in specific tasks, eg, breastfeeding and self-feeding.

Breastfeeding (7.1)

	NCPT Code	ANDUID
❑ Initiation of breastfeeding	FH-7.1.1	10206
❑ Duration of breastfeeding	FH-7.1.2	10207
❑ Exclusive breastfeeding	FH-7.1.3	10208
❑ Breastfeeding problems	FH-7.1.4	10209

Nutrition-related ADLs and IADLs (7.2)

	NCPT Code	ANDUID
❑ Physical ability to complete tasks for meal preparation	FH-7.2.1	10211
❑ Physical ability to self-feed	FH-7.2.2	10212
❑ Ability to position self in relation to plate	FH-7.2.3	10213
❑ Receives assistance with intake	FH-7.2.4	10214
❑ Ability to use adaptive eating devices	FH-7.2.5	10215
❑ Cognitive ability to complete tasks for meal preparation	FH-7.2.6	10216
❑ Remembers to eat	FH-7.2.7	10139
❑ Recalls eating	FH-7.2.8	10218
❑ Mini Mental State Examination Score	FH-7.2.9	10219
❑ Nutrition-related activities of daily living (ADL) score	FH-7.2.10	10220
❑ Nutrition-related instrumental activities of daily living (IADL) score	FH-7.2.11	10221

Physical activity (7.3)

	NCPT Code	ANDUID
❑ Physical activity history	FH-7.3.1	10223
❑ Consistency	FH-7.3.2	10224
❑ Frequency	FH-7.3.3	10225
❑ Duration	FH-7.3.4	10226
❑ Intensity	FH-7.3.5	10227
❑ Type of physical activity	FH-7.3.6	10228
❑ Strength	FH-7.3.7	10229
❑ Handgrip Strength	FH-7.3.7.1	11680
❑ TV/screen time	FH-7.3.8	10230
❑ Other sedentary activity time	FH-7.3.9	10231
❑ Involuntary physical movement	FH-7.3.10	10232
❑ Non exercise activity thermogenesis	FH-7.3.11	10233

Factors affecting access to physical activity (7.4)

	NCPT Code	ANDUID
❑ Neighborhood safety	FH-7.4.1	10822
❑ Walkability of neighborhood	FH-7.4.2	10823
❑ Proximity to parks/green space	FH-7.4.3	10824
❑ Access to physical activity facilities/ programs	FH-7.4.4	10825

Nutrition-Related Patient/Client-Centered Measures (8)

Patient/client's perception of his or her nutrition intervention and its impact on life.

Nutrition quality of life (8.1)

	NCPT Code	ANDUID
❑ Nutrition quality of life responses	FH-8.1.1	10236

ANTHROPOMETRIC MEASUREMENTS (AD)

Height, weight, body mass index (BMI), growth pattern indices/percentile ranks, and weight history.

Body composition/growth/weight history (1.1)

	NCPT Code	ANDUID
❑ Height	AD-1.1.1	10239
❑ Measured height	AD-1.1.1.1	11377
❑ Measured length	AD-1.1.1.2	12015
❑ Birth length	AD-1.1.1.3	12016
❑ Pre-amputation measured height	AD-1.1.1.4	12017
❑ Pre-amputation estimated height	AD-1.1.1.5	12018
❑ Estimated height	AD-1.1.1.6	12019
❑ Stated height	AD-1.1.1.7	12020
❑ Measured peak adult height	AD-1.1.1.8	12021
❑ Stated peak adult height	AD-1.1.1.9	12022
❑ Knee height	AD-1.1.1.10	12023
❑ Tibia length	AD-1.1.1.11	12024
❑ Arm span	AD-1.1.1.12	12025
❑ Arm demispan	AD-1.1.1.13	12026
❑ Arm halfspan	AD-1.1.1.14	12027
❑ Height measurement device	AD-1.1.1.15	12028
❑ Weight	AD-1.1.2	10240
❑ Measured weight	AD-1.1.2.1	12029
❑ Stated weight	AD-1.1.2.2	12030
❑ Stated peak weight	AD-1.1.2.3	12031
❑ Measured peak weight	AD-1.1.2.4	12032
❑ Usual stated body weight (UBW)	AD-1.1.2.5	12033
❑ UBW percentage	AD-1.1.2.6	12034
❑ Birth weight	AD-1.1.2.7	12035
❑ Stated pre-pregnancy weight	AD-1.1.2.8	12036
❑ Dosing weight	AD-1.1.2.9	12037
❑ Estimated dry weight	AD-1.1.2.10	12038
❑ Pre-amputation measured weight	AD-1.1.2.11	12039
❑ Pre-amputation estimated weight	AD-1.1.2.12	12040
❑ Post-amputation measured weight	AD-1.1.2.13	12041
❑ Post-amputation estimated weight	AD-1.1.2.14	12042
❑ Pre-dialysis weight	AD-1.1.2.15	12043
❑ Post-dialysis weight	AD-1.1.2.16	12044
❑ Frame	AD-1.1.3	10241
❑ Frame size	AD-1.1.3.1	12045
❑ Wrist circumference	AD-1.1.3.2	12046
❑ Weight change	AD-1.1.4	10242

Body composition/growth/weight history (1.1) cont.

	NCPT Code	ANDUID
❑ Weight gain	AD-1.1.4.1	12047
❑ Weight loss	AD-1.1.4.2	12048
❑ Weight change percentage	AD-1.1.4.3	12049
❑ Measured interdialytic weight gain	AD-1.1.4.4	12050
❑ Measured interdialytic weight loss	AD-1.1.4.5	12051
❑ Measured gestational weight gain	AD-1.1.4.6	12052
❑ Measured gestational weight loss	AD-1.1.4.7	12053
❑ Weight change intent	AD-1.1.4.8	12054
❑ Body mass	AD-1.1.5	10243
❑ Body mass index (BMI)	AD-1.1.5.1	12055
❑ Body mass index prime ratio (BMI prime)	AD-1.1.5.2	12056
❑ Growth pattern indices	AD-1.1.6	10244
❑ BMI-for-age percentile	AD-1.1.6.1	12057
❑ BMI-for-age z score	AD-1.1.6.2	12058
❑ Head circumference	AD-1.1.6.3	12059
❑ Birth head circumference	AD-1.1.6.4	12060
❑ Head circumference-for-age percentile	AD-1.1.6.5	12061
❑ Head circumference-for-age z score	AD-1.1.6.6	12062
❑ Length-for-age percentile	AD-1.1.6.7	12063
❑ Length-for-age z score	AD-1.1.6.8	12064
❑ Stature-for-age percentile	AD-1.1.6.9	12065
❑ Stature-for-age z score	AD-1.1.6.10	12066
❑ Weight-for-length percentile	AD-1.1.6.11	12067
❑ Weight-for-length z score	AD-1.1.6.12	12068
❑ Weight-for-age percentile	AD-1.1.6.13	12069
❑ Weight-for-age z score	AD-1.1.6.14	12070
❑ Weight-for-stature percentile	AD-1.1.6.15	12071
❑ Weight-for-stature z score	AD-1.1.6.16	12072
❑ Mid parental height comparator	AD-1.1.6.17	12073
❑ Body compartment estimates	AD-1.1.7	10245
❑ Body fat percentage	AD-1.1.7.1	12074
❑ Body fat percentage technique	AD-1.1.7.2	12075
❑ Body surface area	AD-1.1.7.3	12076
❑ Calculated body surface area	AD-1.1.7.4	12077
❑ Bone age	AD-1.1.7.5	12078
❑ Bone mineral density t score	AD-1.1.7.6	12079
❑ Bone mineral density z score	AD-1.1.7.7	12080
❑ Bone mineral density technique	AD-1.1.7.8	12081
❑ Mid arm muscle circumference	AD-1.1.7.9	12082

Assessment

	NCPT Code	ANDUID
Body composition/growth/weight history (1.1) cont.		
❑ Mid arm muscle circumference percentile	AD-1.1.7.10	12083
❑ Triceps skinfold thickness	AD-1.1.7.11	12084
❑ Triceps skinfold percentile	AD-1.1.7.12	12085
❑ Triceps skinfold z score	AD-1.1.7.13	12086
❑ Waist circumference	AD-1.1.7.14	12087
❑ Waist circumference narrowest point	AD-1.1.7.15	12088
❑ Waist circumference iliac crest	AD-1.1.7.16	12089
❑ Hip circumference	AD-1.1.7.17	12090
❑ Waist to hip ratio	AD-1.1.7.18	12091
❑ Mid upper arm circumference	AD-1.1.7.19	12092
❑ Mid upper arm circumference left arm	AD-1.1.7.20	12093
❑ Mid upper arm circumference z score	AD-1.1.7.21	12094

BIOCHEMICAL DATA, MEDICAL TESTS AND PROCEDURES (BD)

Laboratory data, (eg, electrolytes, glucose, and lipid panel) and tests (eg, gastric emptying time, resting metabolic rate).

Acid-base balance (1.1)		
❑ Arterial pH	BD-1.1.1	10248
❑ Arterial bicarbonate	BD-1.1.2	10249
❑ Partial pressure of carbon dioxide in arterial blood ($PaCO_2$)	BD-1.1.3	10250
❑ Partial pressure of oxygen in arterial blood (PaO_2)	BD-1.1.4	10251
❑ Venous pH	BD-1.1.5	10252
❑ Venous bicarbonate	BD-1.1.6	10253
Electrolyte and renal profile (1.2)		
❑ BUN	BD-1.2.1	10255
❑ Creatinine	BD-1.2.2	10256
❑ BUN:creatinine ratio	BD-1.2.3	10257
❑ Glomerular filtration rate	BD-1.2.4	10258
❑ Sodium	BD-1.2.5	10259
❑ Chloride	BD-1.2.6	10260
❑ Potassium	BD-1.2.7	10261
❑ Magnesium	BD-1.2.8	10262
❑ Calcium, serum	BD-1.2.9	10263
❑ Calcium, ionized	BD-1.2.10	10264
❑ Phosphorus	BD-1.2.11	10265
❑ Serum osmolality	BD-1.2.12	10266
❑ Parathyroid hormone	BD-1.2.13	10267
Essential fatty acid profile (1.3)		
❑ Triene:tetraene ratio	BD-1.3.1	10269

	NCPT Code	ANDUID
Gastrointestinal profile (1.4)		
❑ Alkaline phosphatase	BD-1.4.1	10271
❑ Alanine aminotransferase (ALT)	BD-1.4.2	10272
❑ Aspartate aminotransferase (AST)	BD-1.4.3	10273
❑ Gamma glutamyl transferase (GGT)	BD-1.4.4	10274
❑ Gastric residual volume	BD-1.4.5	10275
❑ Bilirubin, total	BD-1.4.6	10276
❑ Ammonia, serum	BD-1.4.7	10277
❑ Toxicology report, including alcohol	BD-1.4.8	10278
❑ Prothrombin time (PT)	BD-1.4.9	10279
❑ Partial thromboplastin time (PTT)	BD-1.4.10	10280
❑ INR ratio	BD-1.4.11	10281
❑ Amylase	BD-1.4.12	10283
❑ Lipase	BD-1.4.13	10284
❑ Fecal fat, 24 hour	BD-1.4.14	11242
❑ Fecal fat, 72 hour	BD-1.4.15	11243
❑ Fecal fat, qualitative	BD-1.4.16	11244
❑ Fecal calprotectin	BD-1.4.17	11245
❑ Fecal lactoferrin	BD-1.4.18	11246
❑ Pancreatic elastase	BD-1.4.19	11150
❑ 5'nucleotidase	BD-1.4.20	11247
❑ D-xylose	BD-1.4.21	10286
❑ Lactulose hydrogen breath test	BD-1.4.22	11248
❑ Lactose hydrogen breath test	BD-1.4.23	11249
❑ Fructose hydrogen breath test	BD-1.4.24	11250
❑ Glucose hydrogen breath test	BD-1.4.25	11251
❑ Urea hydrogen breath test	BD-1.4.26	11252
❑ Intestinal biopsy	BD-1.4.27	10288
❑ Stool culture	BD-1.4.28	10289
❑ Gastric emptying time	BD-1.4.29	10290
❑ Small bowel transit time	BD-1.4.30	10291
❑ Abdominal X-ray	BD-1.4.31	11253
❑ Abdominal CT (computed tomography)	BD-1.4.32	11254
❑ Abdominal ultrasound	BD-1.4.33	11255
❑ Endoscopic ultrasound	BD-1.4.34	11256
❑ Pelvic CT (computed tomography)	BD-1.4.35	11257
❑ Modified barium swallow	BD-1.4.36	11258
❑ Barium swallow	BD-1.4.37	11259
❑ Esophagogastroduodenoscopy	BD-1.4.38	11260
❑ Endoscopic retrograde cholangiopancreatography (ERCP)	BD-1.4.39	11261
❑ Capsule endoscopy	BD-1.4.40	11262

Nutrition Assessment and Monitoring and Evaluation Terminology

	NCPT Code	ANDUID
Gastrointestinal profile (1.4) cont.		
❑ Esophageal manometry	BD-1.4.41	13121
❑ Esophageal pH test	BD-1.4.42	11264
❑ Gastroesophageal reflux monitoring	BD-1.4.43	11265
❑ Gastrointestinal sphincter monitoring	BD-1.4.44	11266
❑ Urate	BD-1.4.45	11638
Glucose/endocrine profile (1.5)		
❑ Glucose, fasting	BD-1.5.1	10295
❑ Glucose, casual	BD-1.5.2	10296
❑ Hemoglobin A1c	BD-1.5.3	10297
❑ Preprandial capillary plasma glucose	BD-1.5.4	10298
❑ Peak postprandial capillary plasma glucose	BD-1.5.5	10299
❑ Glucose tolerance test	BD-1.5.6	10300
❑ Cortisol level	BD-1.5.7	10301
❑ IGF-binding protein	BD-1.5.8	10302
❑ Thyroid stimulating hormone	BD-1.5.9	11639
❑ Thyroxine test	BD-1.5.10	11640
❑ Triiodothyronine	BD-1.5.11	11641
❑ Adrenocorticotropic hormone	BD-1.5.12	11642
❑ Follicle stimulating hormone	BD-1.5.13	11643
❑ Growth hormone	BD-1.5.14	11644
❑ Luteinizing hormone	BD-1.5.15	11645
Inflammatory profile (1.6)		
❑ C-reactive protein	BD-1.6.1	10305
Lipid profile (1.7)		
❑ Cholesterol, serum	BD-1.7.1	10307
❑ Cholesterol, HDL	BD-1.7.2	10308
❑ Cholesterol, LDL	BD-1.7.3	10309
❑ Cholesterol, non-HDL	BD-1.7.4	10310
❑ Total cholesterol:HDL cholesterol ratio	BD-1.7.5	10311
❑ LDL:HDL ratio	BD-1.7.6	10312
❑ Triglycerides, serum	BD-1.7.7	10313
Metabolic rate profile (1.8)		
❑ Resting metabolic rate, measured	BD-1.8.1	10315
❑ Respiratory quotient, measured	BD-1.8.2	10316
Mineral profile (1.9)		
❑ Copper, serum or plasma	BD-1.9.1	10318
❑ Iodine, urinary excretion	BD-1.9.2	10319
❑ Zinc, serum or plasma	BD-1.9.3	10320
❑ Boron, serum or plasma	BD-1.9.4	10841
❑ Chromium, serum or urinary	BD-1.9.5	10842

	NCPT Code	ANDUID
Mineral profile (1.9) cont.		
❑ Fluoride, plasma	BD-1.9.6	10843
❑ Manganese, urinary, blood, plasma	BD-1.9.7	10844
❑ Molybdenum, serum	BD-1.9.8	10845
❑ Selenium, serum or urinary	BD-1.9.9	10846
Nutritional anemia profile (1.10)		
❑ Hemoglobin	BD-1.10.1	10323
❑ Hematocrit	BD-1.10.2	10324
❑ Mean corpuscular volume	BD-1.10.3	10325
❑ Red blood cell folate	BD-1.10.4	10326
❑ Red cell distribution width	BD-1.10.5	10327
❑ B12, serum	BD-1.10.6	10328
❑ Methylmalonic acid, serum	BD-1.10.7	10329
❑ Folate, serum	BD-1.10.8	10330
❑ Homocysteine, serum	BD-1.10.9	10331
❑ Ferritin, serum	BD-1.10.10	10332
❑ Iron, serum	BD-1.10.11	10333
❑ Total iron-binding capacity	BD-1.10.12	10334
❑ Transferrin saturation	BD-1.10.13	10335
Protein profile (1.11)		
❑ Albumin	BD-1.11.1	10337
❑ Prealbumin	BD-1.11.2	10338
❑ Transferrin	BD-1.11.3	10339
❑ Phenylalanine, plasma	BD-1.11.4	10340
❑ Tyrosine, plasma	BD-1.11.5	10341
❑ Amino acid panel	BD-1.11.6	10342
Urine profile (1.12)		
❑ Urine color	BD-1.12.1	10345
❑ Urine osmolality	BD-1.12.2	10346
❑ Urine specific gravity	BD-1.12.3	10347
❑ Urine volume	BD-1.12.4	10349
Vitamin profile (1.13)		
❑ Vitamin A, serum or plasma retinol	BD-1.13.1	10351
❑ Vitamin C, plasma or serum	BD-1.13.2	10352
❑ Vitamin D, 25-hydroxy	BD-1.13.3	10353
❑ Vitamin E, plasma alpha tocopherol	BD-1.13.4	10354

Assessment

	NCPT Code	ANDUID

NUTRITION-FOCUSED PHYSICAL FINDINGS (PD)

Findings from a nutrition-focused physical exam, interview, or the medical record including muscle and subcutaneous fat, oral health, suck/swallow/breathe ability, appetite, and affect.

Nutrition-focused physical findings (1.1)

❑ Overall findings (1)

	NCPT Code	ANDUID
❑ Asthenia	PD-1.1.1.1	11646
❑ Buffalo hump	PD-1.1.1.2	11647
❑ Cachexia	PD-1.1.1.3	11648
❑ Cushingoid appearance	PD-1.1.1.4	11649
❑ Ectomorph	PD-1.1.1.5	11650
❑ Endomorph	PD-1.1.1.6	11651
❑ Lethargic	PD-1.1.1.7	11652
❑ Mesomorph	PD-1.1.1.8	11653
❑ Neglect of personal hygiene	PD-1.1.1.9	11654
❑ Obese	PD-1.1.1.10	11655
❑ Short stature for age	PD-1.1.1.11	11656
❑ Tall stature	PD-1.1.1.12	11657

CLIENT HISTORY (CH)

Current and past information related to personal, medical, family, and social history.

Personal History (1)

General patient/client information such as age, gender, sex, race, ethnicity, language, education, and role in family.

Personal data (1.1)

	NCPT Code	ANDUID
❑ Age	CH-1.1.1	10374
❑ Gender	CH-1.1.2	10375
❑ Sex	CH-1.1.3	11138
❑ Race	CH-1.1.4	11139
❑ Ethnicity	CH-1.1.5	11140
❑ Language	CH-1.1.6	10377
❑ Literacy factors	CH-1.1.7	10378
❑ Education	CH-1.1.8	10379
❑ Role in family	CH-1.1.9	10380
❑ Tobacco use	CH-1.1.10	10381
❑ Physical disability	CH-1.1.11	10382
❑ Mobility	CH-1.1.12	10383

	NCPT Code	ANDUID

Patient/Client/Family Medical/Health History (2)

Patient/client or family disease states, conditions, and illnesses that may have nutritional impact.

Patient/Client OR Family Nutrition-Oriented Medical/Health History (2.1)

Specify issue(s) and whether it is patient/client history (P) or family history (F)

	NCPT Code	ANDUID
❑ Patient/client chief nutrition complaint	CH-2.1.1	10386
(specify) _____ P or F		
❑ Cardiovascular	CH-2.1.2	10387
(specify) _____ P or F		
❑ Endocrine/metabolism	CH-2.1.3	10388
(specify) _____ P or F		
❑ Excretory	CH-2.1.4	10389
(specify) _____ P or F		
❑ Gastrointestinal	CH-2.1.5	10390
(specify) _____ P or F		
❑ Gynecological	CH-2.1.6	10391
(specify) _____ P or F		
❑ Hematology/oncology	CH-2.1.7	10392
(specify) _____ P or F		
❑ Immune (eg, food allergies)	CH-2.1.8	10393
(specify) _____ P or F		
❑ Integumentary	CH-2.1.9	10394
(specify) _____ P or F		
❑ Musculoskeletal	CH-2.1.10	10395
(specify) _____ P or F		
❑ Neurological	CH-2.1.11	10396
(specify) _____ P or F		
❑ Psychological	CH-2.1.12	10397
(specify) _____ P or F		
❑ Respiratory	CH-2.1.13	10398
(specify) _____ P or F		
❑ Other	CH-2.1.14	10399
(specify) _____ P or F		

Treatments/therapy (2.2)

Documented medical or surgical treatments that may impact nutritional status of the patient.

	NCPT Code	ANDUID
❑ Medical treatment/therapy	CH-2.2.1	10401
(specify) _____		
❑ Surgical treatment	CH-2.2.2	10402
(specify) _____		

	NCPT Code	ANDUID

Treatments/therapy (2.2) cont.

☐ Palliative/end-of-life care — CH-2.2.3 — 10404

(specify) _____

Social History (3)

Patient/client socioeconomic status, housing situation, medical support, and involvement in social groups.

Social history (3.1)

☐ Socioeconomic factors — CH-3.1.1 — 10407

(specify) _____

☐ Living/housing situation — CH-3.1.2 — 10408

(specify) _____

☐ Domestic issues — CH-3.1.3 — 10409

(specify) _____

☐ Social and medical support — CH-3.1.4 — 10410

(specify) _____

☐ Geographic location of home — CH-3.1.5 — 10411

(specify) _____

☐ Occupation — CH-3.1.6 — 10412

(specify) _____

☐ Religion — CH-3.1.7 — 10413

(specify) _____

☐ History of recent crisis — CH-3.1.8 — 10414

(specify) _____

☐ Daily stress level — CH-3.1.9 — 10415

(specify) _____

COMPARATIVE STANDARDS (CS)

Energy Needs (1)

Estimated energy needs (1.1)

☐ Total energy estimated needs in 24 hours — CS-1.1.1 — 12029

☐ Method for estimating total energy needs — CS-1.1.2 — 10420

☐ Total energy estimated needs per kg body weight — CS-1.1.3 — 12022

Macronutrient Needs (2)

Estimated fat needs (2.1)

☐ Total fat estimated needs in 24 hours — CS-2.1.1 — 12030

☐ Total fat estimated needs per kg body weight — CS-2.1.2 — 12024

☐ Method for estimating total fat needs — CS-2.1.3 — 10425

☐ Proportion of energy needs from fat in 24 hours — CS-2.1.4 — 12023

Estimated protein needs (2.2)

☐ Total protein estimated needs in 24 hours — CS-2.2.1 — 12031

☐ Total protein estimated needs per kg body weight — CS-2.2.2 — 12025

☐ Method for estimating total protein needs — CS-2.2.3 — 10429

☐ Proportion of energy needs from protein in 24 hours — CS-2.2.4 — 12026

Estimated carbohydrate needs (2.3)

☐ Total carbohydrate estimated needs in 24 hours — CS-2.3.1 — 12032

☐ Total carbohydate estimated needs per kg body weight — CS-2.3.2 — 12027

☐ Method for estimating total carbohydate needs — CS-2.3.3 — 10433

☐ Proportion of energy needs from carbohydrate in 24 hours — CS-2.3.4 — 12028

Estimated fiber needs (2.4)

☐ Total fiber estimated needs in 24 hours — CS-2.4.1 — 12033

☐ Method for estimating total fiber needs — CS-2.4.2 — 10437

Fluid Needs (3)

Estimated fluid needs (3.1)

☐ Total fluid estimated needs — CS-3.1.1 — 10440

☐ Method for estimating needs — CS-3.1.2 — 10441

Micronutrient Needs (4)

Estimated vitamin needs (4.1)

☐ A (1) — 10444
☐ C (2) — 10445
☐ D (3) — 10446
☐ E (4) — 10447
☐ K (5) — 10448
☐ Thiamin (6) — 10449
☐ Riboflavin (7) — 10450
☐ Niacin (8) — 10451
☐ Folate (9) — 10452
☐ B6 (10) — 10453
☐ B12 (11) — 10454
☐ Pantothenic acid (12) — 10455
☐ Biotin (13) — 10456
☐ Method for estimating needs (14) — 10458

	NCPT Code	ANDUID

Estimated mineral needs (4.2)

- ☐ Calcium (1) — 10460
- ☐ Chloride (2) — 10461
- ☐ Iron (3) — 10462
- ☐ Magnesium (4) — 10463
- ☐ Potassium (5) — 10464
- ☐ Phosphorus (6) — 10465
- ☐ Sodium (7) — 10466
- ☐ Zinc (8) — 10467
- ☐ Sulfate (9) — 10469
- ☐ Fluoride (10) — 10470
- ☐ Copper (11) — 10471
- ☐ Iodine (12) — 10473
- ☐ Selenium (13) — 10474
- ☐ Manganese (14) — 10475
- ☐ Chromium (15) — 10476
- ☐ Molybdenum (16) — 10477
- ☐ Boron (17) — 10478
- ☐ Cobalt (18) — 10479
- ☐ Method for estimating needs (19) — 10480

Weight and Growth Recommendation (5)

Recommended body weight/body mass Index/growth (5.1)

	NCPT Code	ANDUID
☐ Ideal/reference body weight (IBW)	CS-5.1.1	10483
☐ Recommended body mass index (BMI)	CS-5.1.2	10484
☐ Goal weight	CS-5.1.3	12144
☐ Goal weight gain/day	CS-5.1.4	12145
☐ Goal weight-for-length z score	CS-5.1.5	12146
☐ Goal mid upper arm circumference z score	CS-5.1.6	12147
☐ Goal BMI-for-age z score	CS-5.1.7	12148
☐ Percent median BMI	CS-5.1.8	12149

Energy Intake (FH-1.1.1)

Definition

Amount of energy intake from all sources including food, beverages, breastmilk/formula, supplements, and via enteral and parenteral routes

Note: Whenever possible, nutrient intake data should be considered in combination with clinical, biochemical, anthropometric information, medical diagnosis, clinical status, and/or other factors as well as diet to provide a valid assessment of nutritional status based on a totality of the evidence (Institute of Medicine. Dietary Reference Intakes: Applications in Dietary Assessment. Washington, DC: National Academies Press; 2000).

Nutrition Assessment and Monitoring and Evaluation

Indicators

- Total energy intake (specify, eg, calories, kcal or kJ/day, calories, kcal or kJ/kg/day)

Note: Weight and weight change can be found on the Body Composition/Growth/Weight History reference sheet.

Examples of the measurement methods or data sources for these indicators: Food intake records, 24-hour recalls, 3 to 5 day food diary, food frequency questionnaire, caretaker intake records, menu analysis, intake and output records

Typically used with the following domains of nutrition interventions: Food and/or nutrient delivery, nutrition education, nutrition counseling, coordination of nutrition care by nutrition professional

Typically used to determine and to monitor and evaluate change in the following nutrition diagnoses: Inadequate energy intake, excessive energy intake, malnutrition (undernutrition), inadequate protein-energy intake, underweight, unintended weight loss, overweight/obesity, unintended weight gain, swallowing difficulty, breastfeeding difficulty, altered GI function, limited adherence to nutrition-related recommendations

Note: Clinical judgment must be used to select indicators and determine the appropriate measurement techniques and reference standards for a given patient population and setting. Once identified, these indicators, measurement techniques, and reference standards should be identified in policies and procedures or other documents for use in patient/client records, quality or performance improvement, or in formal research projects.

Evaluation

Criteria for Evaluation

Comparison to Goal or Reference Standard:

1. Goal (tailored to individual's needs)

   OR

2. Reference Standard (estimated or measured energy requirement)

Energy Intake (FH-1.1.1)

Assessment

Patient/Client Example

Indicator(s) Selected

Total energy intake

Criteria for Evaluation

Comparison to Goal or Reference Standard:

1. Goal: Food diary indicates patient/client consumes approximately 2600 calories/kcal (10,885 kJ) per day. Patient/client's target calorie intake level is 1800 calories/ kcal (7540 kJ) per day.

   OR

2. Reference Standard: Patient/client's I & O indicates patient/client's intake at approximately 2000 calories/kcal (8375kJ) per day, 80% of goal based on an estimated energy requirement of 2500 calories/kcal (10465 kJ) per day.

Sample Nutrition Assessment	Monitoring and Evaluation Documentation
Initial encounter with patient/client	Based on patient/client food diary, patient/client consuming approximately 2600 calories/kcal (10,885 kJ) per day, 144% of recommended level of 1800 calories/kcal (7540 kJ) per day. Will evaluate calorie intake at next encounter in two weeks.
Reassessment after nutrition intervention	Significant progress toward meeting goal. Based on patient/client food diary, patient/client consuming approximately 2100 calories/kcal (8790 kJ) per day, 117% of recommended level of 1800 calories/ kcal (7540 kJ) per day. Will evaluate calorie intake at next encounter in two weeks.

Fluid/Beverage Intake (FH-1.2.1)

Definition

Amount and type of fluid/beverage intake consumed orally

Note: Whenever possible, nutrient intake data should be considered in combination with clinical, biochemical, anthropometric information, medical diagnosis, clinical status, and/or other factors as well as diet to provide a valid assessment of nutritional status based on a totality of the evidence (Institute of Medicine. Dietary Reference Intakes: Applications in Dietary Assessment. Washington, DC: National Academies Press; 2000).

Nutrition Assessment and Monitoring and Evaluation

Indicators

- Oral fluid (specify, eg, oz or mL or cups/day and type)
  - Water
  - Coffee and tea
  - Juice
  - Milk
  - Soda (specify regular or artificially sweetened)
- Food-derived fluids (eg, 3 oz (90 mL) fluid in 4 oz (120 mL) apple sauce) (mL/day)
- Liquid meal replacement or supplement (eg, oz, or mL/day and name/description)

Note: Biochemical measures of hydration status are found on the Electrolyte and Renal Profile and the Urine Profile reference sheets.

Examples of the measurement methods or data sources for these indicators: Food intake records, 24-hour recalls, food frequency questionnaire, intake and output data, observation

Typically used with the following domains of nutrition interventions: Food and/or nutrient delivery, nutrition education, nutrition counseling, coordination of nutrition care by nutrition professional

Typically used to determine and to monitor and evaluate change in the following nutrition diagnoses: Excessive or inadequate oral intake, food—medication interaction, underweight, overweight/obesity, unintended weight loss, unintended weight gain, disordered eating pattern, undesirable food choices, limited adherence to nutrition-related recommendations, inability to manage self-care, swallowing difficulty, breastfeeding difficulty, altered GI function

Note: Clinical judgment must be used to select indicators and determine the appropriate measurement techniques and reference standards for a given patient population and setting. Once identified, these indicators, measurement techniques, and reference standards should be identified in policies and procedures or other documents for use in patient/client records, quality or performance improvement, or in formal research projects.

Fluid/Beverage Intake (FH-1.2.1)

Assessment

Evaluation

Criteria for Evaluation

Comparison to Goal or Reference Standard:

1. Goal (tailored to patient/client's needs)

   OR

2. Reference Standard

Patient/Client Example(s)

Example(s) of one or two of the Nutrition Care Indicators (includes sample initial and reassessment documentation for one of the indicators)

Indicator(s) Selected

Oral fluid amounts

Criteria for Evaluation

Comparison to Goal or Reference Standard:

1. Goal: Patient/client currently drinks 33 oz (1000 mL) of fluid per day and has a personal goal of consuming 64 oz (1920 mL) of fluid per day.

   OR

2. Reference Standard: No validated standard exists.

Sample Nutrition Assessment	Monitoring and Evaluation Documentation
Initial nutrition assessment with patient/client	Based on patient/client food diary, patient/client consuming approximately 1000 mL fluid per day. Goal is to consume approximately 3000 mL/day. Will monitor fluid intake at next encounter.
Reassessment after nutrition intervention	Significant progress toward recommended fluid intake. Based on fluid intake records, patient/client increased consumption of fluids from 1000 mL to 2600 mL per day.

Food Intake (FH-1.2.2)

Definition

Amount, type, and pattern of food consumed and quality of diet

Note: Whenever possible, nutrient intake data should be considered in combination with clinical, biochemical, anthropometric information, medical diagnosis, clinical status, and/or other factors as well as diet to provide a valid assessment of nutritional status based on a totality of the evidence (Institute of Medicine. Dietary Reference Intakes: Applications in Dietary Assessment. Washington, DC: National Academies Press; 2000).

Nutrition Assessment and Monitoring and Evaluation

Indicators

- Amount of food
  - Grains (servings, cups/dL/mL, oz/g)
  - Fruits (servings/piece, cups/dL, oz/g)
  - Vegetables (servings/piece, cups/dL, oz/g)
  - Fruit and vegetable (servings/piece, cups/dL, oz/g)
  - Milk/milk products (servings, cups/dL/mL, oz/g)
  - Meat, poultry, fish, eggs, beans, nut products (servings/piece, cups/dL, oz/g, teaspoon/tablespoon/mL)
  - Fat and oils (servings, teaspoons/mL/g)
  - Concentrated sweets (servings, oz/g)
  - Percent total meal eaten (percent)
- Types of food/meals
  - Fortified/enriched foods (specify, eg, amount or servings of calcium-fortified orange juice)
  - Special dietary products or foods (specify, eg, servings/day or week, and type, eg, non-nutritive sweeteners, lactose-free, gluten-free)
  - Ready-to-eat food selections (eg, type and number/day or week)
  - Convenience frozen meals (eg, type and number/day or week)
  - Self-prepared foods/snacks (specify type, eg, low or high in sodium, fat, fiber)
- Meal/snack* pattern
  - Number of meals (number/day)
  - Number of snack(s) (number/day)
- Diet (food and beverages) quality index
  - Healthy Eating Index (HEI)
  - Children's Diet Quality Index (C-DQI)
  - Revised Children's Diet Quality Index (RC-DQI)
  - Other (specify)
- Food variety (present/absent)

Note: Liquid meal replacements/supplements are found on the Fluid Intake reference sheet.

---

*Snack is defined as food served between regular meals.

Food Intake (FH-1.2.2)

Examples of the measurement methods or data sources for these indicators: Food intake records, 24-hour recalls, food frequency questionnaire, menu analysis, dietary and physical activity assessment tool (eg, MyPlate Super-Tracker), diet quality index (eg, Healthy Eating Index, C-DQI, RC-DQI) or other reference intake standard tool

Typically used with the following domains of nutrition interventions: Food and/or nutrient delivery, nutrition education, nutrition counseling, coordination of nutrition care by nutrition professional

Typically used to determine and to monitor and evaluate change in the following nutrition diagnoses: Excessive or inadequate oral food/beverage intake, food—medication interaction, underweight, overweight/obesity, disordered eating pattern, involuntary weight gain, involuntary weight loss, undesirable food choices, limited adherence to nutrition-related recommendations, inability or lack of desire to manage self-care, limited access to food, intake of unsafe food, inadequate or excessive energy, macronutrient or micronutrient intake

Note: Clinical judgment must be used to select indicators and determine the appropriate measurement techniques and reference standards for a given patient population and setting. Once identified, these indicators, measurement techniques, and reference standards should be identified in policies and procedures or other documents for use in patient/client records, quality or performance improvement, or in formal research projects.

Evaluation

Criteria for Evaluation

Comparison to Goal or Reference Standard:

1. Goal (tailored to patient/client's needs)

   OR

2. Reference Standard

Patient/Client Example(s)

Example(s) of one or two of the Nutrition Care Indicators (includes sample initial and reassessment documentation for one of the indicators)

Indicator(s) Selected

Amount of food

Criteria for Evaluation

Comparison to Goal or Reference Standard:

1. Goal: Patient/client currently eats approximately 1 to 2 servings of fruits and vegetables per day. Goal is to increase fruit and vegetable intake to 5 servings per day.

   OR

2. Reference Standard: Patient/client's current intake of 1 to 2 servings of fruits and vegetables per day is below the DASH Eating Plan recommendation of 9 servings of fruits and vegetables per day.

Food Intake (FH-1.2.2)

Sample Nutrition Assessment	Monitoring and Evaluation Documentation
Initial nutrition assessment with patient/client	Based on patient/client recalls, patient/client consuming approximately 1 to 2 servings of fruits and vegetables per day. Will monitor fruit and vegetable intake at next encounter.
Reassessment after nutrition intervention	Some progress toward goal of 9 servings of fruits and vegetables per day. Based on food records, patient/client increased consumption of fruits and vegetables from approximately 1 to 4 servings per day.

Breastmilk*/Infant Formula Intake (FH-1.2.3)

Assessment

Definition

Amount of breastmilk, and/or the amount, type, and concentration of infant formula consumed orally

Nutrition Assessment and Monitoring and Evaluation

Indicators

- Breastmilk intake (adequacy or oz or mL/day, mL/kg, percent recommended intake)
  - Number of feedings (feedings/24-hour period)
  - Duration of feedings (number of minutes)
  - Modifier/supplement (specify, eg, thickener, lipid, formula, protein)
- Infant formula intake (oz or mL/day)
  - Type (specify, eg, brand, cow's milk-based, soy-based, preterm formula, or other specialty with or without DHA and ARA)
  - Concentration (specify, eg, calorie, kcal or kJ/oz or calorie, kcal or kJ/mL)
  - Number of feedings (number/day)
  - Volume of formula per feeding (oz or mL; amount prepared – amount left in bottle)
  - Number and volume or weight of cans of formula used per week (powder, liquid concentrate, or ready- to-feed)
  - Modifier/supplement (specify, eg, thickener, lipid, formula, protein)

Note: Initiation, duration, exclusivity of breastfeeding and breastfeeding problems can be found on the Breastfeeding reference sheet.

Weight change is found on the Body Composition/Growth/Weight History reference sheet. Number of wet diapers per day is found on the Urine Profile reference sheet. Number/consistency of bowel movements is found on the Nutrition-Focused Physical Exam reference sheet.

If provided via tube use the Enteral and Parenteral Nutrition Intake reference sheet.

Examples of the measurement methods or data sources for these indicators: Intake records, 24-hour recalls, usual intake recalls, observation of feeding (bottle or breast)

Typically used with the following domains of nutrition interventions: Food and/or nutrient delivery, nutrition education, nutrition counseling, coordination of nutrition care by nutrition professional

Typically used to determine and to monitor and evaluate change in the following nutrition diagnoses: Underweight, overweight, unintended weight gain, unintended weight loss, limited adherence to nutrition-related recommendations, inadequate or excessive energy intake, inadequate or excessive oral or fluid intake

Note: Clinical judgment must be used to select indicators and determine the appropriate measurement techniques and reference standards for a given patient population and setting. Once identified, these indicators, measurement techniques, and reference standards should be identified in policies and procedures or other documents for use in patient/client records, quality or performance improvement, or formal research projects.

---

*If a synonym for the term "breastmilk" is helpful or needed, an approved alternative is "human milk."

Breastmilk*/Infant Formula Intake (FH-1.2.3)

Evaluation

Criteria for Evaluation

Comparison to Goal or Reference Standard:

1. Goal (tailored to patient/client needs)

    OR

2. Reference Standard

Patient/Client Example(s)

Example(s) of one or two of the Nutrition Care Indicators (includes sample initial and reassessment documentation for one of the indicators)

Indicator(s) Selected

Infant formula intake

Criteria for Evaluation

Comparison to Goal or Reference Standard:

1. Goal: Patient/client currently consumes approximately 100 mL/kg body weight of infant formula per day. Goal is to increase intake to 150 mL/kg/day.

    OR

2. Reference Standard: Patient/client's current intake of 100 mL/kg/day is below the recommended intake of 150 mL/kg/day to support adequate growth.

Sample Nutrition Assessment	Monitoring and Evaluation Documentation
Initial nutrition assessment with patient/client	Based on mother's recalls, patient/client consuming approximately 100 mL/kg/day of infant formula per day, 33% below the recommended level of 150 mL/kg/day. Will monitor formula intake at next encounter.
Reassessment after nutrition intervention	Significant progress toward goal of consuming 150 mL/kg/day. Based on mother's records, patient/client increased consumption of infant formula to approximately 140 mL/kg/day over the past 7 days.

*If a synonym for the term "breastmilk" is helpful or needed, an approved alternative is "human milk."

Enteral Nutrition Intake (FH-1.3.1)

Assessment

Definition

Amount or type of enteral nutrition provided via a tube

Note: Whenever possible, nutrient intake data should be considered in combination with clinical, biochemical, anthropometric information, medical diagnosis, clinical status, and/or other factors as well as diet to provide a valid assessment of nutritional status based on a totality of the evidence (Institute of Medicine. Dietary Reference Intakes: Applications in Dietary Assessment. Washington, DC: National Academies Press; 2000).

Nutrition Assessment and Monitoring and Evaluation

Indicators

- Enteral nutrition formula/solution (specify)
  - Composition (formula name or description; special additives including supplemental fat, carbohydrate, protein fiber, or other [specify])
  - Concentration (eg, calories/kcal/kJ in each mL)
  - Rate (eg, mL/hour)
  - Volume (eg, mL/day, mL/h, mL/feeding)
  - Schedule (eg, number of hours per 24 hours, continuous, intermittent, bolus)
- Feeding tube flush (eg, type, volume, mL/flush, frequency)

Note: Enteral nutrition tolerance can be accomplished with the Physical Exam reference sheet and/or the pertinent biochemical sign or symptom reference sheet.

Examples of the measurement methods or data sources for these indicators: Patient/client report/recalls, patient/client record, home evaluation, intake and output record

Typically used with the following domains of nutrition interventions: Food and/or nutrient delivery, nutrition education, coordination of nutrition care by nutrition professional

Typically used to determine and to monitor and evaluate change in the following nutrition diagnoses: Inadequate or excessive intake of enteral nutrition, inadequate fluid intake, food—medication interaction, unintended weight loss or gain

Note: Clinical judgment must be used to select indicators and determine the appropriate measurement techniques and reference standards for a given patient population and setting. Once identified, these indicators, measurement techniques, and reference standards should be identified in policies and procedures or other documents for use in patient/client records, quality or performance improvement, or in formal research projects.

Enteral Nutrition Intake (FH-1.3.1)

Evaluation

Criteria for Evaluation

Comparison to Goal or Reference Standard:

1. Goal (tailored to patient/client needs)

   OR

2. Reference Standard

Patient/Client Example

Example(s) of one or two of the Nutrition Care Indicators (includes sample initial and reassessment documentation for one of the indicators)

Indicator(s) Selected

Rate/schedule (mL/hour × number of hours)

Criteria for Evaluation

Comparison to Goal or Reference Standard:

1. Goal: Patient/client's enteral nutrition formula is at a rate of 50 mL per hour × 24 hours of 1 calorie or kcal per mL compared to the nutrition prescription of 80 mL/hour × 24 hours to meet estimated nutrition requirements.

   OR

2. Reference Standard: There is no reference standard for this outcome because the provision of EN/PN is individualized.

Sample Nutrition Assessment	Monitoring and Evaluation Documentation
Initial nutrition assessment with patient/client	Enteral nutrition formula rate of 25 mL per hour × 24 hours of 1 calorie or kcal per mL compared to the nutrition prescription of 80 mL/hour to meet estimated nutrition requirements. Monitor enteral nutrition initiation and rate advancement.
Reassessment after nutrition intervention	Enteral nutrition formula at 70 mL per hour × 24 hours. Significant progress toward nutrition prescription of 1 calorie or kcal per mL at 80 mL per hour × 24 hours.

Parenteral Nutrition Intake (FH-1.3.2)

Assessment

Definition

Amount or type of parenteral nutrition and/or fluids provided intravenously.

Note: Whenever possible, nutrient intake data should be considered in combination with clinical, biochemical, anthropometric information, medical diagnosis, clinical status, and/or other factors as well as diet to provide a valid assessment of nutritional status based on a totality of the evidence (Institute of Medicine. Dietary Reference Intakes: Applications in Dietary Assessment. Washington, DC: National Academies Press; 2000).

Nutrition Assessment and Monitoring and Evaluation

Indicators

- Parenteral nutrition formula/solution (specify)
  - Composition (formula or description)
  - Concentration (eg, percent, grams of solute per mL)
  - Rate (eg, mL/hour)
  - Schedule (eg, hours, timing, taper schedule)
- Intravenous fluids (eg, type; amount [mL/day, mL/h, mL with medications])

Note: Parenteral nutrition tolerance can be accomplished with the Physical Exam Reference sheet and/or the pertinent biochemical sign or symptom reference sheet.

Examples of the measurement methods or data sources for these indicators: Patient/client report/recalls, patient/client record, home evaluation, intake and output record

Typically used with the following domains of nutrition interventions: Food and/or nutrient delivery, nutrition education, coordination of nutrition care by nutrition professional

Typically used to determine and to monitor and evaluate change in the following nutrition diagnoses: Inadequate or excessive intake of parenteral nutrition, inadequate fluid intake, food—medication interaction, unintended weight loss or gain

Note: Clinical judgment must be used to select indicators and determine the appropriate measurement techniques and reference standards for a given patient population and setting. Once identified, these indicators, measurement techniques, and reference standards should be identified in policies and procedures or other documents for use in patient/client records, quality or performance improvement, or in formal research projects.

Evaluation

Criteria for Evaluation

Comparison to Goal or Reference Standard:

1. Goal (tailored to patient/client needs)

   OR

2. Reference Standard

Parenteral Nutrition Intake (FH-1.3.2)

Patient/Client Example

Example(s) of one or two of the Nutrition Care Indicators (includes sample initial and reassessment documentation for one of the indicators)

Indicator(s) Selected

Rate/schedule (mL/hour × number of hours)

Criteria for Evaluation

Comparison to Goal or Reference Standard:

1. Goal: Patient/client's parenteral nutrition formula is at a rate of 50 mL per hour × 24 hours of standard solution compared to the nutrition prescription of 80 mL/hour × 24 hours to meet estimated nutrition requirements.
   OR
2. Reference Standard: There is no reference standard for this outcome as the provision of EN/PN is individualized.

Sample Nutrition Assessment	Monitoring and Evaluation Documentation
Initial nutrition assessment with patient/client	Parenteral nutrition formula rate of 25 mL per hour × 24 hours of standard solution compared to the nutrition prescription of 80 mL/hour to meet estimated nutrition requirements. Monitor nutrition initiation and rate advancement.
Reassessment after nutrition intervention	Parenteral nutrition formula at 70 mL per hour × 24 hours. Significant progress toward nutrition prescription of 80 mL per hour × 24 hours.

Alcohol Intake (FH-1.4.1)

Assessment

Definition

Amount and pattern of alcohol consumption

Nutrition Assessment and Monitoring and Evaluation

Indicators

- Drink size/volume (oz or mL)
- Frequency (drinks/day and/or number of drinking days per week)
- Pattern of alcohol consumption (number/size of drinks on drinking days)

> **Note:** 1 drink = 5 oz (150 mL) wine, 12 oz (350 mL) beer, 1.5 oz (45 mL) distilled alcohol

Examples of the measurement methods or data sources for these indicators: Patient/client report/recalls, self-monitoring log

Typically used with the following domains of nutrition interventions: Nutrition education, nutrition counseling

Typically used to determine and to monitor and evaluate change in the following nutrition diagnoses: Excessive intake of alcohol, excessive or inadequate intake of energy, altered nutrition-related laboratory values, impaired nutrient utilization, overweight/obesity

> **Note:** Clinical judgment must be used to select indicators and determine the appropriate measurement techniques and reference standards for a given patient population and setting. Once identified, these indicators, measurement techniques, and reference standards should be identified in policies and procedures or other documents for use in patient/client records, quality or performance improvement, or in formal research projects.

Evaluation

Criteria for Evaluation

Comparison to Goal or Reference Standard:

1. Goal (tailored to patient/client needs)

   OR

2. Reference Standard

Alcohol Intake (FH-1.4.1)

Patient/Client Example

Example(s) of one or two of the Nutrition Care Indicators (includes sample initial and reassessment documentation for one of the indicators)

Indicator(s) Selected

Pattern of alcohol consumption (number/size of drinks on drinking days)

Criteria for Evaluation

Comparison to Goal or Reference Standard:

1. Goal: Patient/client's intake of one 5 oz (150 mL) glass of wine 2 to 3 times per week is significantly above and noncompliant with the goal to abstain from alcohol during pregnancy.

   OR

2. Reference Standard: Patient/client's intake of three to four, 5 oz (150 mL) glasses of wine on drinking days is significantly above the recommendation of one 5 oz (150 mL) glass of wine per day for adult females.

Sample Nutrition Assessment	Monitoring and Evaluation Documentation
Initial nutrition assessment with patient/client	Based on recalls, patient/client consuming three to four 5 oz (150 mL) glasses of wine on drinking days, which is above the recommended amount for adult females. Will monitor change in alcohol intake at next encounter.
Reassessment after nutrition intervention	Progress toward reference standard of up to one 5 oz (150 mL) glass of wine per day. Based on 7-day record, patient/client consuming 3 oz (90 mL) of wine on drinking days.

Bioactive Substance Intake (FH-1.4.2)

Assessment

Definition

Amount and type of bioactive substances consumed

> **Note:** Bioactive substances are not part of the Dietary Reference Intakes, and therefore there are no established minimum requirements or Tolerable Upper Intake Levels. However, nutrition and dietetics practitioners can assess whether estimated intakes are adequate or excessive using the patient/client goal or nutrition prescription for comparison.
>
> Working definition of bioactive substances—physiologically active components of foods that may have an effect on health. There is no scientific consensus about a definition for bioactive substances/components.

Nutrition Assessment and Monitoring and Evaluation

Indicators

- Plant stanol esters (g/day)
- Plant sterol esters (g/day)
- Soy protein (g/day)
- Psyllium (g/day)
- ß-glucan (g/day)
- Food additives (those thought to have an impact on a patient/client's health) (specify)
- Other (specify)

Examples of the measurement methods or data sources for these indicators: Patient/client report/recalls, self-monitoring log

Typically used with the following domains of nutrition interventions: Nutrition education, nutrition counseling

Typically used to determine and to monitor and evaluate change in the following nutrition diagnoses: Inadequate or excessive intake of bioactive substances, food—medication interaction

> **Note:** Clinical judgment must be used to select indicators and determine the appropriate measurement techniques and reference standards for a given patient population and setting. Once identified, these indicators, measurement techniques, and reference standards should be identified in policies and procedures or other documents for use in patient/client records, quality or performance improvement, or in formal research projects.

Evaluation

Criteria for Evaluation

Comparison to Goal or Reference Standard:

1. Goal (tailored to patient/client needs)

   OR

2. Reference Standard

Bioactive Substance Intake (FH-1.4.2)

Patient/Client Example

Example(s) of one or two of the Nutrition Care Indicators (includes sample initial and reassessment documentation for one of the indicators)

Indicator(s) Selected

- Plant sterol and/or stanol esters (g/day)

Criteria for Evaluation

Comparison to Goal or Reference Standard:

1. Goal: The patient/client does not consume plant sterol or stanol esters compared to the goal intake of 2 to 3 g/day.

   OR

2. Reference Standard: No validated standard exists.

Sample Nutrition Assessment	Monitoring and Evaluation Documentation
Initial assessment with patient/client	Based on recalls, patient/client not consuming (0 g) stanol and/or sterol esters per day, which is below the goal intake of 2 to 3 g/day. Will monitor change in stanol/sterol ester intake at next encounter.
Reassessment after nutrition intervention	Good progress toward the goal of 2 to 3 g/day of stanol and/or sterol ester. Based on 7-day diet record, patient/client consuming 2 to 3 g/day of stanol/sterol ester per day 2 to 3 days per week.

Caffeine Intake (FH-1.4.3)

Definition

Amount of caffeine intake from all sources including food, beverages, supplements, medications, and via enteral and parenteral routes

Nutrition Assessment and Monitoring and Evaluation

Indicators

- Total caffeine intake (mg/day, eg, naturally occurring caffeine in leaves, seeds, fruits of plants and sources with added caffeine such as water/beverages, medications)

Examples of the measurement methods or data sources for these indicators: Patient/client report/recalls, self-monitoring log

Typically used with the following domains of nutrition interventions: Nutrition education, nutrition counseling

Typically used to determine and to monitor and evaluate change in the following nutrition diagnoses: Food and nutrition-related knowledge deficit

Note: Clinical judgment must be used to select indicators and determine the appropriate measurement techniques and reference standards for a given patient population and setting. Once identified, these indicators, measurement techniques, and reference standards should be identified in policies and procedures or other documents for use in patient/client records, quality or performance improvement, or in formal research projects.

Evaluation

Criteria for Evaluation

Comparison to Goal or Reference Standard:

1. Goal (tailored to patient/client needs)

   OR

2. Reference Standard

Patient/Client Example

Example(s) of one or two of the Nutrition Care Indicators (includes sample initial and reassessment documentation for one of the indicators)

Indicator(s) Selected

Total caffeine intake (mg/day)

Criteria for Evaluation

Comparison to Goal or Reference Standard:

1. Goal: The patient/client's intake is 600 mg of caffeine per day, which is above the goal of < 300 mg caffeine/day.

   OR

2. Reference Standard: The patient/client's intake is approximately 600 mg of caffeine per day, which is above the reference standard of 400 mg caffeine/day.

Caffeine Intake (FH-1.4.3)

Sample Nutrition Assessment	Monitoring and Evaluation Documentation
Initial assessment with patient/client	Based on recalls, patient/client consuming approximately 600 mg of caffeine per day, which is above the reference standard of 400 mg/day. Will monitor change in caffeine intake at next encounter.
Reassessment after nutrition intervention	No progress toward the reference standard of 400 mg of caffeine per day. Based on 3-day diet record, patient/client still consuming 600 mg of caffeine per day.

Assessment

Fat Intake (FH-1.5.1)

Definition

Fat and cholesterol consumption from all sources including food, beverages, supplements, and via enteral and parenteral routes

Note: Whenever possible, nutrient intake data should be considered in combination with clinical, biochemical, anthropometric information, medical diagnosis, clinical status, and/or other factors as well as diet to provide a valid assessment of nutritional status based on a totality of the evidence (Institute of Medicine. Dietary Reference Intakes: Applications in Dietary Assessment. Washington, DC: National Academies Press; 2000).

Nutrition Assessment and Monitoring and Evaluation

Indicators

- Total fat intake (specify, eg, g/day, g/kg/day, percentage of calories, kcal or kJ; dietary source portion size, frequency)
- Saturated fat intake—defined as intake of a fat that has no double bonds between carbon molecules (specify, eg, g/day or percentage of calories, kcal or kJ/day; dietary source portion size, frequency)
- Trans fatty acid intake—defined as intake of an unsaturated fatty acid that is hydrogenated with the trans arrangement of the hydrogen atoms adjacent to its double bonds (specify, eg, g/day or percentage of calories, kcal or kJ/day; dietary source portion size, frequency)
- Polyunsaturated fat intake—defined as intake of a fatty acid that contains more than one double bond (specify, eg, g/day or percentage of calories, kcal or kJ/day; dietary source portion size, frequency)
  - Linoleic acid (LA) intake—defined as intake of a polyunsaturated, omega 6, and essential fatty acid with an 18 carbon chain length and two cis double bonds (18:2) (specify, eg, mg/day or g/day or percentage of calories, kcal or kJ/day; dietary source portion size, frequency)
- Monounsaturated fat intake—defined as intake of a fatty acid with one unsaturated (double) carbon bond (specify, eg, g/day or percentage of calories, kcal or kJ/day; dietary source portion size, frequency)
- Omega 3 fatty acid intake—defined as intake of a polyunsaturated fatty acid with a double bond at the third carbon atom from the methyl end of the carbon chain (specify, eg, mg/day or g/day or percentage of calories, kcal or kJ/day; dietary source portion size, frequency)
  - Alpha linolenic acid intake—defined as intake of a polyunsaturated and essential omega 3 fatty acid with an 18-carbon chain and three cis double bonds (18:3) (specify, eg, mg/day or g/day or percentage of calories, kcal or kJ/day; dietary source portion size, frequency)
  - Eicosapentaenoic acid (EPA) intake—defined as intake of a polyunsaturated, omega 3 fatty acid with a 20-carbon chain and five cis double bonds (specify, eg, mg/day or g/day or percentage of calories, kcal or kJ/day; dietary source portion size, frequency)
  - Docosahexaenoic acid (DHA) intake—defined as intake of a polyunsaturated, omega 3 fatty acid with a 22-carbon chain and six cis double bonds (specify, eg, mg/day or g/day or percentage of calories, kcal or kJ/day; dietary source portion size, frequency)
- Essential fatty acid intake—defined as intake of a fatty acid (linoleic acid [18:2] and alpha linolenic acid [18:3]) that must be provided in the diet or enteral or parenteral nutrition because the human body cannot synthesize it (specify, eg, mg/day or g/day or percentage of calories, kcal or kJ/day; dietary source portion size, frequency)
- Medium chain triglyceride intake—defined as intake of a triglyceride molecule with fatty acids having a carbon chain length of 6-12 (specify, eg, g/day or percentage of calories, kcal or kJ/day; dietary source portion size, frequency)

Fat Intake (FH-1.5.1)

- Total fat from diet (g/day)—defined as the estimated intake of fat in grams per day derived from oral dietary intake
- Total fat from enteral nutrition (g/day)—defined as the estimated intake of fat in grams per day derived from enteral nutrition infusion
- Total fat from parenteral nutrition (g/day)—defined as the estimated intake of fat in grams per day derived from parenteral nutrition infusion
- Total fat from intravenous fluids (g/day)—defined as the estimated intake of fat in grams per day derived from intravenous fluid (IV) infusion

Note: Plant sterol and stanol esters can be found on the Bioactive Substance Intake reference sheet.

Examples of the measurement methods or data sources for these indicators: Food intake records, 24-hour recalls, food frequency questionnaires, qualitative intake assessment, menu analysis, fat and cholesterol targeted questionnaires and monitoring devices

Typically used with the following domains of nutrition interventions: Food and/or nutrient delivery, nutrition education, nutrition counseling

Typically used to determine and to monitor and evaluate change in the following nutrition diagnoses: Inadequate and excessive fat intake, intake of types of fats inconsistent with needs, overweight/obesity, altered nutrition-related lab values, altered food and nutrition-related knowledge deficit

Note: Clinical judgment must be used to select indicators and determine the appropriate measurement techniques and reference standards for a given patient population and setting. Once identified, these indicators, measurement techniques, and reference standards should be identified in policies and procedures or other documents for use in patient/client records, quality or performance improvement, or in formal research projects.

Evaluation

Criteria for Evaluation

Comparison to Goal or Reference Standard:

1. Goal (tailored to patient/client's needs)

   OR

2. Reference Standard

Fat Intake (FH-1.5.1)

Patient/Client Example(s)

Example(s) of one or two of the Nutrition Care Indicators (includes sample initial and reassessment documentation for one of the indicators)

Indicator(s) Selected

Total fat (percentage of calories, kcal or kJ from fat)

Criteria for Evaluation

Comparison to Goal or Reference Standard:

1. Goal: Patient/client currently consumes 40% of calories, kcal or kJ from fat. Goal is to decrease fat intake to 25% to 35% of calories, kcal or kJ.

   OR

2. Reference Standard

Sample Nutrition Assessment	Monitoring and Evaluation Documentation
Initial nutritional assessment with patient/client	Based on a three-day food diary, patient/client is consuming approximately 40% of calories, kcal or kJ from fat. Patient/client goal is to reduce total fat intake to 25% to 35% of calories, kcal or kJ. Will monitor fat and calorie intake at next appointment.
Reassessment after nutrition intervention	Significant progress toward the goal intake of 25% to 35% calories, kcal or kJ from fat. Based on a three-day food diary patient/client's total fat intake decreased from approximately 40% to 38% calories, kcal or kJ from fat/day. Will continue to monitor progress at next encounter in 6 weeks.

Cholesterol Intake (FH-1.5.2)

Definition

Dietary cholesterol consumption from all sources including food, beverages, supplements, and via enteral and parenteral routes

Note: Whenever possible, nutrient intake data should be considered in combination with clinical, biochemical, anthropometric information, medical diagnosis, clinical status, and/or other factors as well as diet to provide a valid assessment of nutritional status based on a totality of the evidence (Institute of Medicine. Dietary Reference Intakes: Applications in Dietary Assessment. Washington, DC: National Academies Press; 2000).

Nutrition Assessment and Monitoring and Evaluation

Indicators

- Dietary cholesterol intake (specify, eg, mg/day, dietary source portion size, frequency)

Note: Plant sterol and stanol esters can be found on the Bioactive Substance Intake Reference sheet.

Examples of the measurement methods or data sources for these indicators: Food intake records, 24-hour recalls, food frequency questionnaires, qualitative intake assessment, menu analysis, fat and cholesterol targeted questionnaires and monitoring devices

Typically used with the following domains of nutrition interventions: Food and/or nutrient delivery, nutrition education, nutrition counseling

Typically used to determine and to monitor and evaluate change in the following nutrition diagnoses: Excessive fat intake, excessive cholesterol intake, overweight/obesity, altered nutrition-related lab values, altered food and nutrition-related knowledge deficit

Note: Clinical judgment must be used to select indicators and determine the appropriate measurement techniques and reference standards for a given patient population and setting. Once identified, these indicators, measurement techniques, and reference standards should be identified in policies and procedures or other documents for use in patient/client records, quality or performance improvement, or in formal research projects.

Evaluation

Criteria for Evaluation

Comparison to Goal or Reference Standard:

1. Goal (tailored to patient/client's needs)

   OR

2. Reference Standard

Cholesterol Intake (FH-1.5.2)

Assessment

Patient/Client Example(s)

Example(s) of one or two of the Nutrition Care Indicators (includes sample initial and reassessment documentation for one of the indicators)

Indicator(s) Selected

Dietary cholesterol (mg/day)

Criteria for Evaluation

Comparison to Goal or Reference Standard:

1. Goal: Patient/client currently consumes approximately 350 mg/day of dietary cholesterol. Goal is to decrease intake to <300 mg/day of dietary cholesterol.

   OR

2. Reference Standard: NA

Sample Nutrition Assessment	Monitoring and Evaluation Documentation
Initial nutritional assessment with patient/client	Based on a three-day food diary, patient/client is consuming approximately 350 mg/day of dietary cholesterol. Patient/client goal is to reduce dietary cholesterol intake to <300 mg/day. Will monitor fat and calorie intake at next appointment.
Reassessment after nutrition intervention	Progress toward the goal intake of <300 mg dietary cholesterol. Based on a three-day food diary, patient/client's total dietary cholesterol intake decreased from approximately 350 mg/day to approximately 250 mg/day. Will continue to monitor progress at next encounter in 6 weeks.

Protein Intake (FH-1.5.3)

Definition

Protein intake from all sources including food, beverages, supplements, and via enteral and parenteral routes

Note: Whenever possible, nutrient intake data should be considered in combination with clinical, biochemical, anthropometric information, medical diagnosis, clinical status, and/or other factors as well as diet to provide a valid assessment of nutritional status based on a totality of the evidence (Institute of Medicine. Dietary Reference Intakes: Applications in Dietary Assessment. Washington, DC: National Academies Press, 2000).

Nutrition Assessment and Monitoring and Evaluation

Indicators

- Total protein intake (specify, eg, grams/day, g/kg/day, percentage of calories, kcal or kJ; dietary source portion size, frequency)
- High biological value protein intake—defined as intake from proteins which contain a ratio of essential amino acids that are needed for humans (specify, eg, g/day, percentage of calories, kcal or kJ; dietary source portion size, frequency)
- Casein intake—defined as intake from the phosphoprotein component in milk and milk products that can also be an ingredient in food (specify, eg, g/day, dietary source portion size, frequency)
- Whey intake—defined as intake of the complete protein component in milk and milk products that can also be an ingredient in food (specify, eg, g/day, dietary source portion size, frequency)
- Gluten intake—defined as intake of the protein found primarily in cereal grains and contains gliadin and a glutenin (specify, eg, g/day, dietary source portion size, frequency)
- Natural protein intake—defined as intake of the portion of total protein that comes from food sources (specify, eg, g/day, dietary source portion size, frequency)
- Total protein from diet (g/day)—defined as the estimated intake of protein in grams per day derived from oral dietary intake
- Total protein from enteral nutrition (g/day)—defined as the estimated intake of protein in grams per day derived from intact or semi-elemental protein enteral nutrition infusion

Note: Soy protein can be found on the Bioactive Substance Intake reference sheet. Amino acid intake from elemental enteral nutrition, parenteral nutrition, or intravenous (IV) fluids can be documented using terms on the Amino Acid Intake (FH-1.5.4) reference sheet; however, this has been omitted from this publication for brevity.

Examples of the measurement methods or data sources for these indicators: Food intake records, 24-hour recalls, food frequency questionnaires, qualitative protein intake collection tools, nutrition fact labels, other product information, nutrient composition tables

Typically used with the following domains of nutrition interventions: Food and/or nutrient delivery, nutrition education, nutrition counseling, coordination of nutrition care by nutrition professional

Typically used to determine and to monitor and evaluate change in the following nutrition diagnoses: Inadequate and excessive protein intake, intake of types of proteins or amino acids inconsistent with needs, malnutrition, inadequate protein-energy intake, altered GI function, limited adherence to nutrition-related recommendations

Protein Intake (FH-1.5.3)

Note: Clinical judgment must be used to select indicators and determine the appropriate measurement techniques and reference standards for a given patient population and setting. Once identified, these indicators, measurement techniques, and reference standards should be identified in policies and procedures or other documents for use in patient/client records, quality or performance improvement, or in formal research projects.

Evaluation

Criteria for Evaluation

Comparison to Goal or Reference Standard:

1. Goal (tailored to patient/client's needs)

   OR

2. Reference Standard

Patient/Client Example(s)

Example(s) of one or two of the Nutrition Care Indicators (includes sample initial and reassessment documentation for one of the indicators)

Indicator(s) Selected

Total protein

Criteria for Evaluation

Comparison to Goal or Reference Standard:

1. Goal: Patient/client's current intake of 25 g of protein per day is below the recommended level of 55 to 65 g/day.

   OR

2. Reference Standard: (Used when patient goal is based on the population standard) Patient/client's intake of 12 g protein/day is less than the DRI of 53 g/day (0.8 g/kg body weight). Patient/client's goal is to increase protein intake to approximately 55 g/day.

Sample Nutrition Assessment	Monitoring and Evaluation Documentation
Initial nutrition assessment with patient/client	Enteral feeding currently providing 25 g protein/day, well below the recommended level of 55 to 65 g/day (1 to 1.2 g/kg BW). Will continue to monitor protein intake daily.
Reassessment after nutrition intervention	Some progress toward goal intake of 55 to 65 g protein/day. Current intake approximately 30 g of protein/day, 25 g protein below desired level. Will continue to monitor protein intake daily.

Carbohydrate Intake (FH-1.5.5)

Definition

Carbohydrate consumption from all sources including food, beverages, supplements, and via enteral and parenteral routes, including relative measures of the quantity and/or type of carbohydrate consumed.

Note: Whenever possible, nutrient intake data should be considered in combination with clinical, biochemical, anthropometric information, medical diagnosis, clinical status, and/or other factors as well as diet to provide a valid assessment of nutritional status based on a totality of the evidence (Institute of Medicine. Dietary Reference Intakes: Applications in Dietary Assessment. Washington, DC: National Academies Press; 2000).

Nutrition Assessment and Monitoring and Evaluation

Indicators

- Total carbohydrate intake—defined as intake of total carbohydrate (specify, eg, g/day, grams per meal, g/kg/min, percent of calories, kcal or kJ; dietary source portion size, frequency)
- Complex carbohydrate intake—defined as intake of a polysaccharide that is comprised of three or more sugars; also called starch (specify, eg, g/day, percentage of calories, kcal or kJ; dietary source portion size, frequency)
- Simple sugar (sucrose) intake—defined as intake of a disaccharide of glucose and fructose; also called table sugar (specify, eg, g/day or percentage of calories, kcal or kJ; dietary source portion size, frequency)
- Galactose intake—defined as intake of a monosaccharide which is a common component of lactose (specify, eg, g/day, percentage of calories, kcal or kJ; dietary source portion size, frequency)
- Lactose intake—defined as intake of a disaccharide sugar of galactose and glucose present in milk (specify, eg, g/day or percentage of calories, kcal or kJ; dietary source portion size, frequency)
- Estimated total daily index value (number)—defined as the estimated measure per day reflecting the consumption of all carbohydrate
- Estimated daily glycemic load (number)—defined as the estimated measure per day reflecting the quantity and type of all carbohydrate consumed
- Total carbohydrate from diet (g/day)—defined as the estimated intake of carbohydrate in grams per day derived from dietary intake
- Total carbohydrate from enteral nutrition (g/day)—defined as the estimated intake of carbohydrate in grams per day derived from enteral nutrition infusion
- Total carbohydrate from parenteral nutrition (g/day)—defined as the estimated intake of carbohydrate in grams per day derived from parenteral nutrition infusion
- Total carbohydrate from intravenous fluids (g/day)—defined as the estimated intake of carbohydrate in grams per day derived from intravenous (IV) infusion
- Insulin-to-carbohydrate ratio (ratio)—defined as the estimated number of grams of carbohydrate covered by one unit of rapid-acting (or short-acting) insulin

Note: Fiber intake is listed on the Fiber Intake reference sheet.

Psyllium and ß-glucan can be found on the Bioactive Substance Intake reference sheet.

Carbohydrate Intake (FH-1.5.5)

Examples of the measurement methods or data sources for these indicators: Food intake records, 24-hour or typical day's recalls, food frequency questionnaires, qualitative intake assessment, menu analysis, carbohydrate counting tools, intake/output sheets (for tube feeding or parenteral nutrition)

Typically used with the following domains of nutrition interventions: Food and/or nutrient delivery, nutrition education, nutrition counseling, coordination of nutrition care by nutrition professional

Typically used to determine and to monitor and evaluate change in the following nutrition diagnoses: Inadequate and excessive carbohydrate intake, intake of types of carbohydrate inconsistent with needs, inconsistent carbohydrate intake, altered nutrition-related laboratory values, food medication interaction

Note: Clinical judgment must be used to select indicators and determine the appropriate measurement techniques and reference standards for a given patient population and setting. Once identified, these indicators, measurement techniques, and reference standards should be identified in policies and procedures or other documents for use in patient/client records, quality or performance improvement, or in formal research projects.

Evaluation

Criteria for Evaluation

Comparison to Goal or Reference Standard:

1. Goal (tailored to patient/client's needs)

   OR

2. Reference Standard

Patient/Client Example(s)

Example(s) of one or two of the Nutrition Care Indicators (includes sample initial and reassessment documentation for one of the indicators)

Indicator(s) Selected

Total carbohydrate (distribution by meal)

Criteria for Evaluation

Comparison to Goal or Reference Standard:

1. Goal: Patient/client's current carbohydrate intake in the morning ranges from 0 to 95 g. The goal is for the patient/client to consume approximately 30 g of carbohydrate at breakfast 6 days per week.

   OR

2. Reference Standard: No validated standard exists.

Carbohydrate Intake (FH-1.5.5)

Sample Nutrition Assessment	Monitoring and Evaluation Documentation
Initial nutrition assessment with patient/client	Based on carbohydrate counting tools, patient/client consumed 30 g carbohydrate at breakfast 2 days/week. Goal is to consume 30 g carbohydrate for breakfast 6 days per week.
Reassessment after nutrition intervention	Some progress made toward goal. Based on carbohydrate counting tools, patient/client consumed 30 g carbohydrate at breakfast 2 days/week. Will monitor breakfast carbohydrate intake at next encounter.

Assessment

Fiber Intake (FH-1.5.6)

Assessment

Definition

Amount and/or type of plant source matter consumed that is not completely digested but may be at least partially fermented in the distal bowel and is derived from all sources including food, beverages, supplements, and via enteral routes

Note: Whenever possible, nutrient intake data should be considered in combination with clinical, biochemical, anthropometric information, medical diagnosis, clinical status, and/or other factors as well as diet to provide a valid assessment of nutritional status based on a totality of the evidence (Institute of Medicine. Dietary Reference Intakes: Applications in Dietary Assessment. Washington, DC: National Academies Press; 2000).

Nutrition Assessment and Monitoring and Evaluation

Indicators

- Total fiber (g/day, dietary source portion size, frequency)
- Soluble fiber (g/day, dietary source portion size, frequency)
- Insoluble fiber (g/day, dietary source portion size, frequency)
  - Fructooligosaccharides (g/day, dietary source portion size, frequency)

Note: Psyllium and ß-glucan can be found on the Bioactive Substance Intake reference sheet.

Examples of the measurement methods or data sources for these indicators: Food intake records, 24-hour recalls, food frequency questionnaires, qualitative intake assessment, menu analysis, fiber counting tools, nutrition fact labels, other product information, nutrient composition tables

Typically used with the following domains of nutrition interventions: Food and/or nutrient delivery, nutrition education, nutrition counseling, coordination of nutrition care by nutrition professional

Typically used to determine and to monitor and evaluate change in the following nutrition diagnoses: Inadequate and excessive fiber intake, altered GI function, disordered eating pattern, inadequate bioactive substance intake

Note: Clinical judgment must be used to select indicators and determine the appropriate measurement techniques and reference standards for a given patient population and setting. Once identified, these indicators, measurement techniques, and reference standards should be identified in policies and procedures or other documents for use in patient/client records, quality or performance improvement, or in formal research projects.

Evaluation

Criteria for Evaluation

Comparison to Goal or Reference Standard:

1. Goal (tailored to patient/client's needs)

   OR

2. Reference Standard

Fiber Intake (FH-1.5.6)

Patient/Client Example(s)

Example(s) of one or two of the Nutrition Care Indicators (includes sample initial and reassessment documentation for one of the indicators)

Indicator(s) Selected

Total dietary fiber intake, including those from foods and dietary fiber supplements

Criteria for Evaluation

Comparison to Goal or Reference Standard:

1. Goal: Patient/client has current fiber intake of 15 g/day. Goal is to increase fiber intake to approximately 25 g/day. OR

2. Reference Standard: Patient/client's current intake of 15 g of dietary fiber per day is below the DRI of 25 g/day for a 40-year-old woman.

Sample Nutrition Assessment	Monitoring and Evaluation Documentation
Initial nutrition assessment with patient/client	Based on patient/client's food diary, patient/client is consuming approximately 15 g of fiber/day. Will monitor fiber intake at next encounter in three weeks.
Reassessment after nutrition intervention	Goal achieved. Patient/client's intake of 27 g fiber exceeded goal intake of 25 g/day. Will continue to monitor to ensure success is sustained.

Vitamin Intake (FH-1.6.1)

Assessment

Definition

Vitamin intake from all sources including food, beverages, supplements, and via enteral and parenteral routes

Note: Whenever possible, nutrient intake data should be considered in combination with clinical, biochemical, anthropometric information, medical diagnosis, clinical status, and/or other factors as well as diet to provide a valid assessment of nutritional status based on a totality of the evidence (Institute of Medicine. Dietary Reference Intakes: Applications in Dietary Assessment. Washington, DC: National Academies Press; 2000).

Nutrition Assessment and Monitoring and Evaluation

Indicators

- Vitamin A (specify form, µg or RE, dietary source portion size, frequency)
- Vitamin C (specify form, mg, dietary source portion size, frequency)
- Vitamin D (specify form, µg or IU, dietary source portion size, frequency)
- Vitamin E (specify form, mg or IU, dietary source portion size, frequency)
- Vitamin K (specify form, µg, dietary source portion size, frequency)
- Thiamin (specify form, mg, dietary source portion size, frequency)
- Riboflavin (specify form, mg, dietary source portion size, frequency)
- Niacin (specify form, mg, dietary source portion size, frequency)
- Folate (specify form, µg, dietary source portion size, frequency)
- Vitamin B6 (specify form, mg, dietary source portion size, frequency)
- Vitamin B12 (specify form, µg, dietary source portion size, frequency)
- Pantothenic acid (specify form, mg, dietary source portion size, frequency)
- Biotin (specify form, µg, frequency)
- Multivitamin (yes/no, specify form, dose, frequency)

Note: Laboratory measures associated with body vitamin status can be found on the Vitamin Profile reference sheet.

Examples of the measurement methods or data sources for these indicators: Patient/client report or recalls, food frequency, qualitative intake assessment, home evaluation, supplement use questionnaire

Typically used with the following domains of nutrition interventions: Food and/or nutrient delivery, nutrition education, nutrition counseling, coordination of nutrition care by nutrition professional

Typically used to determine and to monitor and evaluate change in the following nutrition diagnoses: Excessive or inadequate intake of vitamins, parenteral, or enteral nutrition

Note: Clinical judgment must be used to select indicators and determine the appropriate measurement techniques and reference standards for a given patient population and setting. Once identified, these indicators, measurement techniques, and reference standards should be identified in policies and procedures or other documents for use in patient/client records, quality or performance improvement, or in formal research projects.

Vitamin Intake (FH-1.6.1)

Evaluation

Criteria for Evaluation

Comparison to Goal or Reference Standard:

1. Nutrition prescription or goal (tailored to patient/client needs)

   OR

2. Reference Standard

Patient/Client Example

Example(s) of one or two of the Nutrition Care Indicators (includes sample initial and reassessment documentation for one of the indicators)

Indicator(s) Selected

Vitamin D (specify form, µg or IU, dietary source portion size, frequency)

Criteria for Evaluation

Comparison to Goal or Reference Standard:

1. Nutrition Prescription or Goal: Use if patient/client's nutrition prescription/goal is different from the reference standard.

   OR

2. Reference Standard: The patient/client's intake of 4 µg (160 IU) per day of vitamin D is below (above, below, consistent with) the estimated average requirement of 10 µg (400 IU) and the recommended dietary allowance of 15 µg (600 IU) (EAR and RDA in the reference intake standard [eg, DRIs]) for males ages 14 to 18.

Vitamin Intake (FH-1.6.1)

Sample Nutrition Assessment	Monitoring and Evaluation Documentation
Initial nutrition assessment with patient/client	Based on recalls, patient/client with cystic fibrosis consuming approximately 4 µg of vitamin D per day, which is below the estimated average requirement of 10 µg (400 IU) and the recommended dietary allowance of 15 ug (600 IU) per day for vitamin D for a 15-year-old male. Patient/client has also discontinued fat-soluble vitamin supplement. Will monitor vitamin D intake at next encounter and monitor intake of fat-soluble vitamin supplement; will also request 25-hydroxy vitamin D level (Vitamin Profile reference sheet).
Reassessment after nutrition intervention	25-hydroxy vitamin D level below expected range (from Vitamin Profile reference sheet). Progress toward the estimated average requirement of 10 µg (400 IU) and the recommended dietary allowance of 15 ug (600 IU) for vitamin D. Based on 3-day diet record, patient/client has increased consumption of vitamin D from food sources to 5–7 µg (200–280 IU) for vitamin D and is taking fat-soluble vitamin supplement 5 days per week on average. Despite progress, because patient/client has cystic fibrosis, will need to continue fat-soluble vitamin supplementation in addition to food sources. Repeat lab in 3 months.

Assessment

Mineral/Element Intake (FH-1.6.2)

Definition

Mineral/element intake from all sources including food, beverages, supplements, and via enteral and parenteral routes

Note: Whenever possible, nutrient intake data should be considered in combination with clinical, biochemical, anthropometric information, medical diagnosis, clinical status, and/or other factors as well as diet to provide a valid assessment of nutritional status based on a totality of the evidence (Institute of Medicine. Dietary Reference Intakes: Applications in Dietary Assessment. Washington, DC: National Academies Press; 2000).

Nutrition Assessment and Monitoring and Evaluation

Indicators

- Calcium (specify form, mg, dietary source portion size, frequency)
- Chloride (specify form, mg, dietary source portion size, frequency)
- Iron (specify form, mg, dietary source portion size, frequency)
- Magnesium (specify form, mg, dietary source portion size, frequency)
- Potassium (specify form, g or mg, dietary source portion size, frequency)
- Phosphorus (specify form, mg, dietary source portion size, frequency)
- Sodium (specify form, mg or g, dietary source portion size, frequency)
- Zinc (specify form, mg, dietary source portion size, frequency)
- Sulfate (specify form, g or mmol, dietary source portion size, frequency)
- Fluoride (specify form, mg, dietary source portion size, frequency)
- Copper (specify form, μg or mg, dietary source portion size, frequency)
- Iodine (specify form, μg, dietary source portion size, frequency)
- Selenium (specify form, μg, dietary source portion size, frequency)
- Manganese (specify form, mg, dietary source portion size, frequency)
- Chromium (specify form, μg, dietary source portion size, frequency)
- Molybdenum (specify form, μg, dietary source portion size, frequency)
- Boron (specify form, mg, dietary source portion size, frequency)
- Cobalt (specify form, μg, frequency)
- Multimineral (yes/no, specify dose, frequency)
- Multi-trace element (yes/no, specify dose, frequency)

Examples of the measurement methods or data sources for these indicators: Patient/client report or recalls, food frequency, qualitative intake assessment, home evaluation, home care or pharmacy report, supplement use questionnaire

Typically used with the following domains of nutrition interventions: Food and/or nutrient delivery, nutrition education, nutrition counseling, coordination of nutrition care by nutrition professional

Mineral/Element Intake (FH-1.6.2)

Typically used to determine and to monitor and evaluate change in the following nutrition diagnoses:
Excessive or inadequate intake of minerals, food–medication interaction, altered nutrition-related laboratory values, impaired nutrient utilization, undesirable food choices, limited adherence to nutrition-related recommendations

Note: Clinical judgment must be used to select indicators and determine the appropriate measurement techniques and reference standards for a given patient population and setting. Once identified, these indicators, measurement techniques, and reference standards should be identified in policies and procedures or other documents for use in patient/client records, quality or performance improvement, or in formal research projects.

Evaluation

Criteria for Evaluation

Comparison to Goal or Reference Standard:

1. Nutrition Prescription or Goal (tailored to individual's needs)

    OR

2. Reference Standard

Patient/Client Example

Example(s) of one or two of the Nutrition Care Indicators (includes sample initial and reassessment documentation for one of the indicators)

Indicator(s) Selected

Sodium (specify form, mg or g, dietary source portion size, frequency)

Calcium (specify form, mg, dietary source portion size, frequency)

Criteria for Evaluation

Comparison to Goal or Reference Standard:

1. Nutrition Prescription or Goal: The patient/client's intake of sodium is approximately 6000 mg/day, which is above the nutrition prescription of 4000 mg/day.

    OR

2. Reference Standard: The patient/client's intake of calcium is 500 mg/day, which is 50% of the recommended dietary allowance (RDA in the reference intake standard [eg, DRIs]) for adult females 31 to 50 years of age.

Sample Nutrition Assessment	Monitoring and Evaluation Documentation
Initial nutrition assessment with patient/client	Based on recalls, patient/client consuming approximately 500 mg/day, which is below the recommended dietary allowance for calcium per day for adult females 31 to 50 years of age. Will monitor calcium intake at next encounter.
Reassessment after nutrition intervention	Significant progress toward the recommended dietary allowance. Based on 3-day diet record, patient/client has increased consumption from 500 mg/day to 750 mg/day of the recommended dietary allowance for calcium.

Diet Order (FH-2.1.1)

Definition

A general or modified diet prescribed and documented in a patient/client medical record by a credentialed provider as part of a medical treatment plan

Nutrition Assessment

Indicators

- General, healthful diet order
- Modified diet order (eg, type, amount of energy and/or nutrients per day, distribution, texture)
- Enteral nutrition order (eg, formula, rate/schedule, access)
- Parenteral nutrition order (eg, solution, access, rate)

Examples of the measurement methods or data sources for these indicators: Medical record, referring health care provider or agency, resident/client history

Typically used with the following domains of nutrition interventions: Food and/or nutrient delivery, nutrition education, nutrition counseling, coordination of nutrition care by nutrition professional

Typically used with the following nutrition diagnoses: Inadequate or excessive energy, macronutrient or micronutrient intake, inadequate or excessive oral intake, swallowing difficulty

Note: Clinical judgment must be used to select indicators and determine the appropriate measurement techniques and reference standards for a given patient population and setting. Once identified, these indicators, measurement techniques, and reference standards should be identified in policies and procedures or other documents for use in patient/client records, quality or performance improvement, or formal research projects.

Evaluation

Criteria for Evaluation

Comparison to Goal or Reference Standard:

1. Goal (tailored to patient/client needs)

   OR

2. Reference Standard

Diet Order (FH-2.1.1)

Assessment

Patient/Client Example(s)

Example(s) of one or two of the Nutrition Care Indicators (includes sample initial assessment documentation for one of the indicators)

Indicator(s) Selected

Modified diet order

Criteria for Evaluation

Comparison to Goal or Reference Standard:

1. Goal: Not generally used

   OR

2. Reference Standard: No validated standard exists.

Sample Nutrition Assessment	Monitoring and Evaluation Documentation
Initial nutrition assessment with patient/client	Patient/client prescribed a 2,400 calorie or kcal (10,050 kJ) diet.

Diet Experience (FH-2.1.2)

Definition

Previous nutrition/diet orders, diet education/counseling, and diet characteristics that influence patient/client's dietary intake

Nutrition Assessment

Indicators

- Previously prescribed diets
  - Previous modified diet (specify, eg, type, amount of energy and/or nutrients per day, distribution, texture)
  - Enteral nutrition order (specify)
  - Parenteral nutrition order (specify)
- Previous diet/nutrition education/counseling (specify, eg, type, year)
- Self-selected diets followed (specify, eg, commercial diets, diet books, culturally directed)
- Dieting attempts
  - Number of past diet attempts (number)
  - Results (specify, eg, successful/unsuccessful, pounds or kg lost)
  - Successful strategies (specify, eg, no snacking, self-monitoring)
- Food allergies
  - Previous modified diet (specify, eg, type and/or foods/food group) followed as a result of diagnosed or reported food allergy
- Food intolerance
  - Previous modified diet (specify, eg, type and/or foods/food group) followed as a result of diagnosed or reported food intolerance

Examples of the measurement methods or data sources for these indicators: Patient/client report, medical record, patient/client history, food and nutrition delivery coordination of care

Typically used with the following domains of nutrition interventions: Nutrition education, nutrition counseling

Typically used with the following nutrition diagnoses: Disordered eating pattern, not ready for diet/lifestyle change, excessive oral intake, food- and nutrition-related knowledge deficit, unsupported beliefs/attitudes about food- or nutrition-related topics, undesirable food choices, swallowing difficulty, intake of unsafe food

Note: Clinical judgment must be used to select indicators and determine the appropriate measurement techniques and reference standards for a given patient population and setting. Once identified, these indicators, measurement techniques, and reference standards should be identified in policies and procedures or other documents for use in patient/client records, quality or performance improvement, or in formal research projects.

Diet Experience (FH-2.1.2)

Assessment

Evaluation

Criteria for Evaluation

Comparison to Goal or Reference Standard:

1. Goal (tailored to patient/client needs)

   OR

2. Reference Standard

Patient/Client Example(s)

Example(s) of one or two of the Nutrition Care Indicators (includes sample initial assessment documentation for one of the indicators)

Indicator(s) Selected

Previous diet/nutrition education/counseling

Criteria for Evaluation

Comparison to Goal or Reference Standard:

1. Goal: Not generally used

   OR

2. Reference Standard: No validated standard exists.

Sample Nutrition Assessment	Monitoring and Evaluation Documentation
Initial nutrition assessment with patient/client	Patient/client completed a 6-week diabetic education class two years ago.

Eating Environment (FH-2.1.3)

Definition

The aggregate of surrounding things, conditions, or influences that affect food intake

Nutrition Assessment and Monitoring and Evaluation

Indicators

- Location (specify, eg, home, school, day care, restaurant, nursing home, senior center)
  - Atmosphere
  - Acceptable noise level (yes/no)
  - Appropriate lighting (yes/no)
  - Appropriate room temperature (yes/no)
  - Appropriate table height (yes/no)
  - Appropriate table service (eg, plates, napkins)/meal service (type of service, eg, table service, buffet)/setup (make food accessible for consumption) (yes/no)
  - Eats at designated eating location (does not wander) (yes/no)
  - Eats without distractions (eg, watching TV/reading) (yes/no)
  - No unpleasant odors (yes/no)
- Caregiver/companion
  - Allowed to select foods (often, sometimes, never)
  - Caregiver influences/controls what client eats (eg, encourages, forces) (yes/no)
  - Caregiver models expected eating behavior (yes/no)
  - Caretaker presence (present/not present)
  - Favorite food is offered or withheld to influence behavior (reward/punishment) (yes/no)
  - Has companionship while eating (another or others present) (yes/no)
  - Meal/snacks offered at consistent times ("grazing" discouraged) (yes/no)
- Appropriate breastfeeding accommodations/facility (yes/no)
- Eats alone (specify reason, frequency)

Examples of the measurement methods or data sources for these indicators: Patient/client report, medical record, referring health care provider or agency, observation

Typically used with the following domains of nutrition interventions: Food and/or nutrient delivery, nutrition education, nutrition counseling, coordination of nutrition care by nutrition professional

Typically used to determine and to monitor and evaluate change in the following nutrition diagnoses: Inadequate oral intake, self-feeding difficulty, poor nutrition quality of life, limited access to food

Note: Clinical judgment must be used to select indicators and determine the appropriate measurement techniques and reference standards for a given patient population and setting. Once identified, these indicators, measurement techniques, and reference standards should be identified in policies and procedures or other documents for use in patient/client records, quality or performance improvement, or in formal research projects.

Eating Environment (FH-2.1.3)

Evaluation

Criteria for Evaluation

Comparison to Goal or Reference Standard:

1. Goal (tailored to patient/client needs)

   OR

2. Reference Standard

Patient/Client Example(s)

Example(s) of one or two of the Nutrition Care Indicators (includes sample initial and reassessment documentation for one of the indicators)

Indicator(s) Selected

Eats at designated eating location

Criteria for Evaluation

Comparison to Goal or Reference Standard:

1. Goal: Two-year-old child with inadequate intake of calories/kcal/kJ and/or nutrients. Goal is to improve intake through modifications in feeding environment and meal pattern.

   OR

2. Reference Standard: No validated standard exists.

Sample Nutrition Assessment	Monitoring and Evaluation Documentation
Initial nutrition assessment with patient/client	Caregiver completed 3-day food record indicating multiple (10) feeding opportunities throughout the day. Child consumes mostly juice, dry cereal, and chips. Prefers foods that can be consumed from bottle or finger foods. Child does not sit at the table to eat but wanders the house and is allowed to request and receive snacks ad lib. Energy and nutrient intake is less than 75% of standard. Referral to behavioral specialist offered.
Reassessment after nutrition intervention	Caregiver completed follow-up 3-day food record indicating reduced number of feeding opportunities throughout the day (6 to 7). States child resisted at first but now eats at table at regular meal/snack times. Caregiver is continuing to work with behavioral specialist for both mealtime and other behavior issues. Energy and nutrient intake have improved to 85% to 90% of standard.

Enteral and Parenteral Nutrition Administration (FH-2.1.4)

Definition

Delivery of enteral and/or parenteral nutrition

Nutrition Assessment and Monitoring and Evaluation

Indicators

- Enteral access (specify, eg, nasoenteric, oroenteric, percutaneous, or surgical access with gastric, duodenal, or jejunal placement)
- Parenteral access (specify, eg, peripheral, central, and/or type of catheter)
- Body position, enteral nutrition (EN), specify, eg, degree angle

Examples of the measurement methods or data sources for these indicators: Patient/client report/recalls, patient/client record, patient/client nutrition-focused physical exam, provider referral

Typically used with following domains of nutrition interventions: Food and/or nutrient delivery, nutrition education, coordination of nutrition care by nutrition professional

Typically used to determine the following nutrition diagnoses: Inadequate or excessive enteral or parenteral nutrition infusion, inadequate fluid intake, predicted food—medication interaction

> **Note:** Clinical judgment must be used to select indicators and determine the appropriate measurement techniques and reference standards for a given patient population and setting. Once identified, these indicators, measurement techniques, and reference standards should be identified in policies and procedures or other documents for use in patient/client records, quality or performance improvement, or in formal research projects.

Evaluation

Criteria for Evaluation

Comparison to Goal or Reference Standard:

1. Goal (tailored to patient/client's needs)

   OR

2. Reference Standard

Enteral and Parenteral Nutrition Administration (FH-2.1.4)

Assessment

Patient/Client Example(s)

Example(s) of one or two of the Nutrition Care Indicators (includes sample initial and reassessment documentation for one of the indicators)

Indicator(s) Selected

Enteral access (nasocenteric)

Criteria for Evaluation

Comparison to Goal or Reference Standard:

1. Goal: Patient/client's enteral nutrition is delivered via nasoenteric feeding tube that will remain patent so patient/client can receive feeding to meet estimated nutrition requirements.

   OR

2. Reference Standard: There is no reference standard for this outcome.

Sample Nutrition Assessment	Monitoring and Evaluation Documentation
Initial nutrition assessment with patient/client	Patient/client's enteral nutrition is delivered via nasoenteric feeding tube that will remain patent so patient/client can receive feeding to meet estimated nutrition requirements. Monitor enteral nutrition feeding access for patency.
Reassessment after nutrition intervention	Enteral nutrition via nasoenteric feeding tube is blocked requiring replacement of feeding tube.

Fasting (FH-2.1.5)

Definition

Absence of nutrient administration from all sources.

Nutrition Assessment and Monitoring and Evaluation

Indicators

- Fasting pattern in one calendar day, reported—defined as the timing within one calendar day when the patient/client does not take in or infuse nutrients (eg, overnight fast, fast between meals)
- Fasting pattern in one calendar week, reported—defined as the timing within one calendar week when the patient/client does not take in or infuse nutrients (eg, Friday evening)
- Fasting pattern in one calendar month, reported—defined as the timing within one calendar month when the patient/client does not take in or infuse nutrients (eg, every Sabbath)
- Fasting pattern in one calendar year, reported—defined as the timing within one calendar year when the patient/client does not take in or infuse nutrients (eg, Lent, Passover, Ramadan, occasional fasting)
- Fasting tolerance, reported—defined as the length of time a patient/client can endure a lack of nutrient intake or nutrient infusion without physiological consequence (specify in hours)

Examples of the measurement methods or data sources for these indicators: Patient/client report, medical record, patient/client history, food and nutrition delivery coordination of care

Typically used with the following domains of nutrition interventions: Nutrition education, nutrition counseling

Typically used to determine and to monitor and evaluate change in the following nutrition diagnoses: Inadequate oral intake, inadequate carbohydrate intake, food- and nutrition-related knowledge deficit, unsupported beliefs/attitudes about food- or nutrition-related topics

Note: Clinical judgment must be used to select indicators and determine the appropriate measurement techniques and reference standards for a given patient population and setting. Once identified, these indicators, measurement techniques, and reference standards should be identified in policies and procedures or other documents for use in patient/client records, quality or performance improvement, or formal research projects.

Evaluation

Criteria for Evaluation

Comparison to Goal or Reference Standard:

1. Goal (tailored to patient/client's needs)

   OR

2. Reference Standard

Fasting (FH-2.1.5)

Assessment

Patient/Client Example(s)

Example(s) of one or two of the Nutrition Care Indicators (includes sample initial assessment documentation for one of the indicators)

Indicator(s) Selected

Fasting tolerance, reported

Criteria for Evaluation

Comparison to Goal or Reference Standard:

1. Goal: Limit or avoid fasting longer than five hours because longer periods result in physiological consequence.
   OR
2. Reference Standard: No validated standard exists.

Sample Nutrition Assessment	Monitoring and Evaluation Documentation
Initial nutritional assessment with patient/client	The patient/client's (with an inborn error of metabolism) reported fasting tolerance is approximately 5 h, at which time the patient/client must take in nutrients to avoid hypoglycemia. Goal established to fast no longer than 4 h on 7 of 7 nights per week.
Reassessment after nutrition intervention	Meeting goal. Patient/client limiting fasts to no longer than 4 h on 7 of 7 nights per week.

Medications (FH-3.1)

Definition

Prescription and over-the-counter (OTC) medications that may impact nutritional status

Nutrition Assessment and Monitoring and Evaluation

Indicators

- Prescription medication use
  - Current prescriptions with nutrient/food–medication interactions (specify)
  - Insulin or insulin secretagogues (specify)
    - Insulin sensitivity factor (mg/dL)—defined as the estimated reduction in blood glucose in mg/dL per unit of rapid-acting (or short-acting) insulin, referred to as the correction insulin
  - Medication, alter blood pressure (specify)
  - Medication, alter breastmilk production (specify)
  - Medication, lipid lowering (specify)
  - Medications, alter glucose levels (specify)
  - Other (specify)
- Over-the-counter (OTC) medication use
  - Current OTC products with nutrient/food–medication implications (specify)
  - Medication, alter blood pressure (specify)
  - Medication, alter breastmilk production (specify)
  - Medication, lipid lowering (specify)
  - Medications, alter glucose levels (specify)
  - Other (specify)
- Misuse of medications (eg, accidental overdose, illegal drugs, laxatives, diuretics, drug use during pregnancy [specify])

Note: Vitamin and mineral supplements can be found on the vitamin and mineral intake reference sheets. Alcohol can be found on the Alcohol Intake reference sheet.

Examples of the measurement methods or data sources for these indicators: Patient/client report, medical record, referring health care provider or agency

Typically used with the following domains of nutrition interventions: Food and/or nutrient delivery, nutrition education, nutrition counseling, coordination of nutrition care by nutrition professional

Typically used to determine the following nutrition diagnoses: Food–medication interaction; increased energy expenditure; malnutrition (undernutrition); inadequate or excessive energy; oral, fluid, carbohydrate, protein, fat, vitamin, and mineral intake; unintended weight gain or loss; overweight/obesity; underweight; disordered eating pattern

Note: Clinical judgment must be used to select indicators and determine the appropriate measurement techniques and reference standards for a given patient population and setting. Once identified, these indicators, measurement techniques, and reference standards should be identified in policies and procedures or other documents for use in patient/client records, quality or performance improvement, or in formal research projects.

Medications (FH-3.1)

Assessment

Evaluation

Criteria for Evaluation

Comparison to Goal or Reference Standard:

1. Goal (tailored to patient/client's needs)

   OR

2. Reference Standard

Patient/Client Example(s)

Example(s) of one or two of the Nutrition Care Indicators (includes sample initial and reassessment documentation for one of the indicators)

Indicator(s) Selected

Prescription medication with nutrient/food–medication interactions—Prednisone

Criteria for Evaluation

Comparison to Goal or Reference Standard:

1. Goal: Patient/client with prescription for 50 mg/d of prednisone and concerned about concurrent weight gain caused by increased appetite and fluid retention. Goal is to minimize weight gain and maintain good nutritional status during prednisone therapy.

   OR

2. Reference Standard: Not applicable

Sample Nutrition Assessment	Monitoring and Evaluation Documentation
Initial nutrition assessment with patient/client	Patient/client's prescription medication is 50 mg/d prednisone for rheumatoid arthritis. Current weight is 182 lb (83 kg). Long-term therapy may result in a need for protein; calcium; potassium; phosphorus; folate; and vitamin A, C, and D supplementation. Patient/client currently taking a vitamin/mineral supplement and concerned about weight gain caused by increased appetite and fluid retention.
Reassessment after nutrition intervention	Patient/client's prescription medication prednisone dose reduced to 25 mg/day. Currently taking a one-a-day multivitamin/multimineral and snacking on raw vegetables between meals. Weight stable.

Complementary/Alternative Medicine (FH-3.2)

Definition

Complementary and alternative medicine products, including herbal preparations that may impact nutritional status

Nutrition Assessment and Monitoring and Evaluation

Indicators

- Nutrition-related complementary/alternative medicine use (eg, gingko, St John's wort, elderberry, garlic, ephedra)

Note: Vitamin and mineral supplements can be found on the vitamin and mineral intake reference sheets. Alcohol can be found on the Alcohol Intake reference sheet.

Examples of the measurement methods or data sources for these indicators: Patient/client report, medical record, referring health care provider or agency

Typically used with the following domains of nutrition interventions: Food and/or nutrient delivery, nutrition education, nutrition counseling, coordination of nutrition care by nutrition professional

Typically used to determine the following nutrition diagnoses: Food–medication interaction, increased energy expenditure, malnutrition (undernutrition), unintended weight gain or loss, overweight/obesity, intake of unsafe foods, disordered eating pattern

Note: Clinical judgment must be used to select indicators and determine the appropriate measurement techniques and reference standards for a given patient population and setting. Once identified, these indicators, measurement techniques, and reference standards should be identified in policies and procedures or other documents for use in patient/client records, quality or performance improvement, or in formal research projects.

Evaluation

Criteria for Evaluation

Comparison to Goal or Reference Standard:

1. Goal (tailored to patient/client's needs)

   OR

2. Reference Standard

Complementary/Alternative Medicine (FH-3.2)

Patient/Client Example(s)

Example(s) of one or two of the Nutrition Care Indicators (includes sample initial and reassessment documentation for one of the indicators)

Indicator(s) Selected

Complementary/alternative medicine use—ephedra

Criteria for Evaluation

Comparison to Goal or Reference Standard:

1. Goal: Patient/client taking ephedra with the hope that it will promote weight loss. Goal is to have patient/client eliminate ephedra for safety reasons and engage in nutrition counseling for weight management.

   OR

2. Reference Standard: Not applicable

Sample Nutrition Assessment	Monitoring and Evaluation Documentation
Initial nutrition assessment with patient/client	Patient/client's complementary/alternative medicine use of ephedra is for weight loss. Patient/client reports being unaware of safety concerns.
Reassessment after nutrition intervention	Patient/client's complementary/alternative medicine use of ephedra has stopped and success with weight loss as a result of nutrition counseling.

Assessment

Food and Nutrition Knowledge/Skill (FH-4.1)

Definition

Content areas and level of understanding about food, nutrition, and health or nutrition-related information and guidelines relevant to patient/client needs

Nutrition Assessment and Monitoring and Evaluation

Indicators

- Use the following terms to specify level of knowledge/skill by each area of concern:
  ○ Inadequate
  ○ Basic (survival, identify facts, little application)
  ○ Moderate (some application in typical situations)
  ○ Comprehensive (synthesize and evaluate for application in new situations)

Area(s) and level of knowledge/skill	
Breastfeeding (eg, signs of infant satiety)	Nutrition recommendations
Consequences of food behavior	Physiological functions
Disease/condition	Self-management parameters
Goal-setting techniques	Control food portions
Food label	Food preparation/cooking
Food products	Manage behavior in response to stimuli (eg, identify triggers/cues, develop a plan, modify environment or behavior)
Food/nutrient requirements	
Health knowledge gap (eg, understanding of health or health guidance versus true health)	Plan meals/snacks
Health care literacy	Select healthful foods/meals
Laboratory results compared to desirable	Self-monitor
Level of physical conditioning	Other (specify topic and level of knowledge)

Diagnosis specific or global nutrition-related knowledge score (specify instrument used, eg, Type 2 Diabetes BASICS Pre/Post Knowledge Test and score)

Examples of the measurement methods or data sources for this indicator: Pre- and/or post-tests administered orally, on paper, or by computer; scenario discussions; patient/client restates key information; review of food records; practical demonstration/test; survey; nutrition quotient; nutrition questionnaire; nutrition assessment inventory

Typically used to determine and monitor and evaluate change in the following domains of nutrition interventions: Nutrition education, nutrition counseling

Typically used to determine and to monitor and evaluate change in the following nutrition diagnoses: Food- and nutrition-related knowledge deficit, limited adherence to nutrition-related recommendations, undesirable food choices, breastfeeding difficulty, overweight/obesity, intake domain nutrition diagnoses

FOOD/NUTRITION-RELATED HISTORY DOMAIN—KNOWLEDGE/BELIEFS/ATTITUDES

Food and Nutrition Knowledge/Skill (FH-4.1)

Evaluation

Criteria for Evaluation

Comparison to Goal or Reference Standard:

1. Goal (tailored to individual's needs)

   OR

2. Reference Standard

Patient/Client Example(s)

Example(s) of one or two of the Nutrition Care Indicators (includes sample initial and reassessment documentation for one of the indicators)

Indicator(s) Selected

Area and level of knowledge (carbohydrate counting)

Criteria for Evaluation

Comparison to Goal or Reference Standard:

1. Goal: Patient/client will be able to accurately read a food label and identify the total number of grams of carbohydrate per serving.

   OR

2. Reference Standard: No validated standard exists.

Sample Nutrition Assessment	Monitoring and Evaluation Documentation
Initial nutrition assessment with patient/client	Patient/client with newly diagnosed diabetes with inadequate knowledge regarding carbohydrate counting.
Reassessment after nutrition intervention	Patient/client with basic knowledge regarding carbohydrate counting. Able to apply knowledge to common scenarios but not consistently able to apply knowledge to own diet. Will continue to monitor at next encounter in one week.

Beliefs and Attitudes (FH-4.2)

Definition

Conviction of the truth of some nutrition-related statement or phenomenon and feelings or emotions toward that truth or phenomenon, along with a patient/client's readiness to change food, nutrition, or nutrition-related behaviors

Nutrition Assessment and Monitoring and Evaluation

Indicators

- Conflict with personal/family value system (specify)
- Distorted body image (yes/no)
- End-of-life decisions (specify)
- Motivation
  - Perceived susceptibility to nutrition-related health problems (eg, patient/client believes he or she is diabetic or at high risk for developing diabetes) (yes/no)
  - Understanding of severity of risk to health/lifestyle (perceived severity) (yes/no)
  - Belief that benefits of diet change outweigh barriers (benefits are worth the sacrifice and effort) (yes/no)
  - Verbalizes desire to change diet and nutrition-related behaviors (yes/no)
- Preoccupation with food (yes/no)
- Preoccupation with weight (yes/no)
- Readiness to change nutrition-related behaviors
  - Precontemplation (yes/no)
  - Contemplation (yes/no)
  - Preparation (yes/no)
  - Action (yes/no)
  - Maintenance (yes/no)
- Self-efficacy
  - Breastfeeding self-efficacy (specify, eg, high, low)
  - Eating self-efficacy (specify, eg, high, low)
  - Weight loss self-efficacy (specify, eg, high, low)
  - Other (specify)
- Self-talk/cognitions (documented cognitions related to food/nutrition activity) (positive/negative)
- Unrealistic nutrition-related goals (specify, eg, current weight loss goal of 20 lb (9 kg)/month is unrealistic)
- Unscientific beliefs/attitudes (specify, eg, specific food with unsubstantiated curative power)
- Food preferences (specify)
- Emotions (specify, eg, anger, guilt, sad, lonely, nervous)

Beliefs and Attitudes (FH-4.2)

Examples of the measurement methods or data sources for these outcome indicators: Patient/client report, patient/client assessment questionnaire or interview, medical record, referring health care provider or agency

Typically used to monitor and evaluate change in the following domains of nutrition interventions: Nutrition education, nutrition counseling

Typically used to determine and to monitor and evaluate change in the following nutrition diagnoses: Unsupported beliefs/attitudes about food- or nutrition-related topics; not ready for diet/lifestyle change; inability to manage self-care; self-monitoring deficit; excessive or inadequate oral, energy, macronutrient, micronutrient, or bioactive substance intake; imbalance of nutrients; intake of types of fats inconsistent with needs; intake of types of proteins inconsistent with needs; underweight; overweight/obesity; disordered eating pattern; physical inactivity; excess physical activity; limited access to food or water

Note: Clinical judgment must be used to select indicators and determine the appropriate measurement techniques and reference standards for a given patient population and setting. Once identified, these indicators, measurement techniques, and reference standards should be identified in policies and procedures or other documents for use in patient/client records, quality or performance improvement, or formal research projects.

Evaluation

Criteria for Evaluation

Comparison to Goal or Reference Standard:

1. Goal (tailored to individual's needs)

   OR

2. Reference Standard

Patient/Client Example(s)

Example(s) of one or two of the Nutrition Care Indicators (includes sample initial and reassessment documentation for one of the indicators)

Indicator(s) Selected

Readiness to change nutrition-related behaviors

Criteria for Evaluation

Comparison to Goal or Reference Standard:

1. Goal: Patient/client is currently in the precontemplation stage of change. Patient/client goal is to move to the preparation stage of change within 3 months.

   OR

2. Reference Standard: No validated standard exists.

Beliefs and Attitudes (FH-4.2)

Sample Nutrition Assessment	Monitoring and Evaluation Documentation
Initial nutrition assessment with patient/client	Assessment results indicate patient/client is currently in the precontemplation stage of change related to need for DASH diet adherence. Will initiate motivational interviewing and reassess in two weeks.
Reassessment after nutrition intervention	Significant progress toward goal. Reassessment indicates that patient/client has moved from the precontemplation stage to the contemplation stage related to need for DASH diet adherence. Will reassess in two weeks.

Assessment

Adherence (FH-5.1)

Assessment

Definition

Level of compliance or adherence with nutrition-related recommendations or behavioral changes agreed upon by patient/client to achieve nutrition-related goals

Nutrition Assessment and Monitoring and Evaluation

Indicators

- Self-reported adherence score (rated on scale of 1 to 10; 1 = not adherent, 10 = completely adherent)
- Nutrition visit attendance (ratio, number attended:total)
- Ability to recall nutrition goals (full, partial, none)
- Self-monitoring at agreed upon rate (rated on scale of 1 to 10; 1 = not adherent, 10 = completely adherent)
- Self-management based on details agreed upon (within the nutrition plan) (rated on scale of 1 to 10; 1 = not adherent, 10 = completely adherent)

Note: Use in conjunction with appropriate Food and Nutrition Intake, Anthropometric Data, and Biochemical Data reference sheets.

May be useful in relapse prevention treatment (analyze and control factors that caused the lapse).

Examples of the measurement methods or data sources for these indicators: Nutrition visit attendance, self-monitoring records (eg, to evaluate fat, sodium, calories/kcal/kJ, diet quality), patient/client report, adherence tools or questionnaires, provider assessment

Typically used with the following domains of nutrition interventions: Food and/or nutrient delivery, nutrition education, nutrition counseling

Typically used to determine and to monitor and evaluate change in the following nutrition diagnoses: Limited adherence to nutrition-related recommendations

Note: Clinical judgment must be used to select indicators and determine the appropriate measurement techniques and reference standards for a given patient population and setting. Once identified, these indicators, measurement techniques, and reference standards should be identified in policies and procedures or other documents for use in patient/client records, quality or performance improvement, or in formal research projects.

Evaluation

Criteria for Evaluation

Comparison to Goal or Reference Standard:

1. Goal (tailored to individual's needs)

   OR

2. Reference Standard

Adherence (FH-5.1)

Patient/Client Example(s)

Example(s) of one or two of the Nutrition Care Indicators (includes sample initial and reassessment documentation for one of the indicators)

Indicator(s) Selected

Self-reported adherence score

Criteria for Evaluation

Comparison to Goal or Reference Standard:

1. Goal: Patient/client rates herself a 4 on a scale of 1 to 10 (1 = not adherent, 10 = completely adherent) on her level of adherence to nutrition-related goals. Patient/client desires to move to a rating of 8.

   OR

2. Reference Standard: No validated standard exists.

Sample Nutrition Assessment	Monitoring and Evaluation Documentation
Initial nutrition assessment with patient/client	Patient/client rates herself a 4 on a scale of 1 to 10 on her ability to adhere to her meal plan. Patient/client set a goal to adhere to her meal plan 5 days per week. Will evaluate adherence at the next encounter.
Reassessment after nutrition intervention	Some progress toward goal. Patient/client rated herself a 6 on a scale of 1 to 10 on her ability to meet her adherence goal of following her meal plan 5 days per week. Is doing well on weekdays but states she must improve on weekends. Discussed ways to improve adherence to meal plan on the weekends. Will monitor at next encounter in two weeks.

Avoidance Behavior (FH-5.2)

Assessment

Definition

Keeping away from something or someone to postpone an outcome or perceived consequence

Nutrition Assessment and Monitoring and Evaluation

Indicators

- Avoidance
  - Specific foods (specify, eg, grapefruit, seeds)
  - Food groups (specify, eg, milk/milk products)
  - Fluids (specify)
  - Textures (specify)
  - Social situations (specify)
  - Other (specify)
  - Restrictive eating (yes/no)
- Cause of avoidance behavior (eg, personal choice, prescribed dietary restriction, GI distress, suspected allergy, eating disorder, cancer treatment side effects, medications, mental illness, Parkinson's disease)

Examples of the measurement methods or data sources for these indicators: Self-monitoring records, patient/client interview

Typically used with the following domains of nutrition interventions: Nutrition counseling

Typically used to determine and to monitor and evaluate change in the following nutrition diagnoses: Disordered eating pattern, overweight/obesity, underweight, altered GI function

Note: Clinical judgment must be used to select indicators and determine the appropriate measurement techniques and reference standards for a given patient population and setting. Once identified, these indicators, measurement techniques, and reference standards should be identified in policies and procedures or other documents for use in patient/client records, quality or performance improvement, or formal research projects.

Evaluation

Criteria for Evaluation

Comparison to Goal or Reference Standard:

1. Goal (tailored to patient/client needs)

   OR

2. Reference Standard

Avoidance Behavior (FH-5.2)

Patient/Client Example(s)

Example(s) of one or two of the Nutrition Care Indicators (includes sample initial and reassessment documentation for one of the indicators)

Indicator(s) Selected

Avoidance of social situations

Criteria for Evaluation

Comparison to Goal or Reference Standard:

1. Goal: Patient/client avoiding social situations in an effort to avoid overeating. Goal is to learn strategies to control eating in social situations.

   OR

2. Reference Standard: No validated standard exists.

Sample Nutrition Assessment	Monitoring and Evaluation Documentation
Initial nutrition assessment with patient/client	Patient/client avoids social situations because she is afraid she will overeat. Reviewed client's food diary and client brainstormed strategies that may help her control eating in social situations. Patient/client will preplan food intake on days she has social engagements, will have a piece of fruit before going to help curb her appetite, and will maintain a food diary.
Reassessment after nutrition intervention	Patient/client made some progress toward goal. Attended 2 of 4 social engagements where food was served and successfully controlled food intake both times. Patient/client will continue to use strategies. Will reevaluate avoidance behavior at next encounter.

Bingeing and Purging Behavior (FH-5.3)

Assessment

Definition

Eating a larger amount of food than normal for the individual during a short period of time (within any two-hour period) accompanied by a lack of control over eating during the binge episode (ie, the feeling that one cannot stop eating). This may be followed by compensatory behavior to make up for the excessive eating, referred to as purging.

Nutrition Assessment and Monitoring and Evaluation

Indicators

- Binge eating behavior (present/absent)
  - Number of binge episodes (eg, number per day, number per week, number per month)
- Purging behavior (present/absent)
  - Self-induced vomiting (eg, number per day, number per week, number per month)
  - Fasting (yes/no)
  - Other (specify)

Note: Misuse of laxatives, diuretics, or other drugs is found on the Medication and Complementary/Alternative Medicine reference sheets. Amount and type of physical activity is found on the Physical Activity reference sheet.

Examples of the measurement methods or data sources for these indicators: Patient/client interview, medical record, referring health care provider or agency, self-monitoring records

Typically used with following domains of nutrition interventions: Nutrition counseling

Typically used to determine and to monitor and evaluate change in the following nutrition diagnoses: Excessive oral intake, disordered eating pattern, overweight/obesity

Note: Clinical judgment must be used to select indicators and determine the appropriate measurement techniques and reference standards for a given patient population and setting. Once identified, these indicators, measurement techniques, and reference standards should be identified in policies and procedures or other documents for use in patient/client records, quality or performance improvement, or in formal research projects.

Evaluation

Criteria for Evaluation

Comparison to Goal or Reference Standard:

1. Goal (tailored to patient/client needs)

   OR

2. Reference Standard

Bingeing and Purging Behavior (FH-5.3)

Patient/Client Example(s)

Example(s) of one or two of the Nutrition Care Indicators (includes sample initial and reassessment documentation for one of the indicators)

Indicator(s) Selected

Number of binge episodes

Criteria for Evaluation

Comparison to Goal or Reference Standard:

1. Goal: Patient/client reports 3 binge eating episodes per week. Goal is to reduce binge eating to one episode per week.

   OR

2. Reference Standard: No validated standard exists.

Sample Nutrition Assessment	Monitoring and Evaluation Documentation
Initial encounter with patient/client	Patient/client reports 3 binge eating episodes this week.
Reassessment after nutrition intervention	Some progress toward goal. Patient/client reported 2 binge eating episodes this week. Will continue to monitor at next encounter.

Mealtime Behavior (FH-5.4)

Assessment

Definition

Manner of acting, participating, or behaving at mealtime which influences patient/client's food and beverage intake

Nutrition Assessment and Monitoring and Evaluation

Indicators

- Meal duration (minutes)
- Percent of meal time spent eating (percent)
- Preference to drink rather than eat (yes/no)
- Refusal to eat/chew (specify, eg, meal, food type)
- Spitting food out (specify, eg, food type, frequency)
- Rumination (yes/no)
- Patient/client/caregiver fatigue during feeding process, resulting in inadequate intake (yes/no)
- Willingness to try new foods (yes/no)
- Limited number of accepted foods (specify)
- Rigid sensory preferences (flavor, temperature, texture)

Examples of the measurement methods or data sources for these indicators: Observation, medical record, referring health care provider or agency, caregiver observation, patient/client interview

Typically used with following domains of nutrition interventions: Food and/or nutrient delivery, coordination of nutrition care by nutrition professional

Typically used to determine and to monitor and evaluate change in the following nutrition diagnoses: Self-feeding difficulty, inadequate and excessive oral intake

Note: Clinical judgment must be used to select indicators and determine the appropriate measurement techniques and reference standards for a given patient population and setting. Once identified, these indicators, measurement techniques, and reference standards should be identified in policies and procedures or other documents for use in patient/client records, quality or performance improvement, or in formal research projects.

Evaluation

Criteria for Evaluation

Comparison to Goal or Reference Standard:

1. Goal (tailored to patient/client needs)

    OR

2. Reference Standard

Mealtime Behavior (FH-5.4)

Patient/Client Example(s)

Example(s) of one or two of the Nutrition Care Indicators (includes sample initial and reassessment documentation for one of the indicators)

Indicator(s) Selected

Percent of meal spent eating (percentage)

Criteria for Evaluation

Comparison to Goal or Reference Standard:

1. Goal: Four-year-old patient/client with inadequate food/beverage intake. Lunch meal observation revealed less than 10% of meal time was spent eating. Goal is to reduce environmental distractions and increase percent of meal spent eating to 55%.

   OR

2. Reference Standard: No validated standard exists.

Sample Nutrition Assessment	Monitoring and Evaluation Documentation
Initial nutrition assessment with patient/client	Lunch meal observation revealed that patient/client is highly distracted and spends less than 10% of the meal time eating.
Reassessment after nutrition intervention	Significant progress toward goal. Environmental distractions were minimized, and caregiver eats meals with patient/client. Observation reveals that approximately 40% of meal time is spent eating. Will monitor at next encounter.

Social Network (FH-5.5)

Assessment

Definition

Ability to build and utilize a network of family, friends, colleagues, health professionals, and community resources for encouragement, emotional support, and to enhance one's environment to support behavior change

Nutrition Assessment and Monitoring and Evaluation

Indicators

- Ability to build and utilize social networks (eg, may include perceived social support, social integration, and assertiveness)

Examples of the measurement methods used or data sources for these indicators: Self-monitoring records, patient/client report, goal-tracking tools

Typically used with the following domains of nutrition interventions: Nutrition counseling

Typically used to determine and to monitor and evaluate change in the following nutrition diagnoses: Intake domain nutrition diagnoses, underweight, overweight/obesity, disordered eating pattern, undesirable food choices, inability to manage self-care, breastfeeding difficulty, not ready for diet/lifestyle change, limited adherence to nutrition-related recommendations

Note: Clinical judgment must be used to select indicators and determine the appropriate measurement techniques and reference standards for a given patient population and setting. Once identified, these indicators, measurement techniques, and reference standards should be identified in policies and procedures or other documents for use in patient/client records, quality or performance improvement, or in formal research projects.

Evaluation

Criteria for Evaluation

Comparison to Goal or Reference Standard:

1. Goal (tailored to individual's needs)

   OR

2. Reference Standard

Social Network (FH-5.5)

Patient/Client Example

Example(s) of one or two of the Nutrition Care Indicators (includes sample initial and reassessment documentation for one of the indicators)

Indicator(s) Selected

Ability to build and utilize social support (eg, may include perceived social support, social integration, and assertiveness)

Criteria for Evaluation

Comparison to Goal or Reference Standard:

1. Goal: Overweight patient/client's wife adds fat to all foods prepared at home. Goal is to reduce the amount of fat in meals prepared at home by asking wife to not dress the salad or add fat seasoning to vegetables before serving.

   OR

2. Reference Standard: No validated standard exists.

Sample Nutrition Assessment	Monitoring and Evaluation Documentation
Initial encounter with patient/client	Patient/client states that he rarely verbalizes his nutrition-related desires/needs in family or social situations and rates his ability to elicit social support a 3 on a scale of 1 to 10. Will evaluate at the next encounter.
Reassessment after nutrition intervention	Some progress toward goal. Patient/client rated himself a 5 on a scale of 1 to 10 on his ability to elicit social support. Has begun to verbalize his needs and plans to research restaurants that meet his needs that others will enjoy. Will monitor at next encounter in two weeks.

Food/Nutrition Program Participation (FH-6.1)

Assessment

Definition

Patient/client eligibility for and participation in food assistance programs

Nutrition Assessment and Monitoring and Evaluation

Indicators

- Eligibility for government programs (specify, eg, qualification for federal programs [eg, WIC, supplemental nutrition assistance program—refer to state for title of program]; school breakfast/lunch program; food distribution program on US Indian Reservations; or state assistance programs, such as emergency food assistance programs)
- Participation in government programs (specify patient/client or family/caregiver influence)
- Eligibility for community programs (specify, eg, qualification for community programs such as food pantries, meal sites, and meal delivery programs)
- Participation in community programs (specify patient/client or family/caregiver influence)

Examples of the measurement methods or data sources for these indicators: Patient/client report of eligibility/participation, referral information, home evaluation

Typically used with the following domains of nutrition interventions: Nutrition education, nutrition counseling, coordination of nutrition care by nutrition professional

Typically used to determine and to monitor and evaluate change in the following nutrition diagnoses: Limited access to food, inadequate or excessive energy intake

Note: Clinical judgment must be used to select indicators and determine the appropriate measurement techniques and reference standards for a given patient population and setting. Once identified, these indicators, measurement techniques, and reference standards should be identified in policies and procedures or other documents for use in patient/client records, quality or performance improvement, or in formal research projects.

Evaluation

Criteria for Evaluation

Comparison to Goal or Reference Standard:

1. Goal (tailored to patient/client needs)

   OR

2. Reference Standard

Food/Nutrition Program Participation (FH-6.1)

Patient/Client Example(s)

Example(s) of one or two of the Nutrition Care Indicators (includes sample initial and reassessment documentation for one of the indicators)

Indicator(s) Selected

Participation in government programs

Criteria for Evaluation

Comparison to Goal or Reference Standard:

1. Goal: Patient/client is not participating in federal school lunch program, as parent has not completed required forms.

   OR

2. Reference Standard: No validated standard exists.

Sample Nutrition Assessment	Monitoring and Evaluation Documentation
Initial nutrition assessment with patient/client	The patient/client not participating in federal school lunch program, as the required forms are not complete. Will follow up with family/guardian and monitor change in school lunch program participation at next appointment.
Reassessment after nutrition intervention	Progress toward goal, as patient/client's family/guardian has completed school lunch program forms.

Safe Food/Meal Availability (FH-6.2)

Assessment

Definition

Availability of enough healthful, safe food

Nutrition Assessment and Monitoring and Evaluation

Indicators

- Availability of shopping facilities (specify, eg, access to facilities with a wide variety of healthful food choices)
- Procurement of safe food (specify, eg, financial resources for obtaining food, community gardens, growing own food, hunting and fishing)
- Appropriate meal preparation facilities (specify, eg, access to cooking apparatus and supplies used in preparation, sanitary conditions and supplies for meal preparation, appropriate temperatures of hot/cold food)
- Availability of safe food storage (specify, eg, refrigerator/freezer, dry storage, designated containers)
- Appropriate storage techniques (specify, eg, appropriate refrigeration/freezer temperatures, canning/preservation, length of storage, sanitary conditions)
- Identification of safe food (specify, eg, identification of spoilage, expiration dates, identification of foods containing poisons such as specific berries, mushrooms, etc)

Examples of the measurement methods or data sources for these indicators: Patient/client report of overall food availability/food consumed during the week, referral information, home evaluation

Typically used with the following domains of nutrition interventions: Nutrition education, nutrition counseling, coordination of nutrition care by nutrition professional

Typically used to determine and to monitor and evaluate change in the following nutrition diagnoses: Limited access to food, intake of unsafe food, inadequate or excessive energy intake

Note: Clinical judgment must be used to select indicators and determine the appropriate measurement techniques and reference standards for a given patient population and setting. Once identified, these indicators, measurement techniques, and reference standards should be identified in policies and procedures or other documents for use in patient/client records, quality or performance improvement, or in formal research projects.

Evaluation

Criteria for Evaluation

Comparison to Goal or Reference Standard:

1. Goal (tailored to patient/client needs)

   OR

2. Reference Standard

Safe Food/Meal Availability (FH-6.2)

Patient/Client Example(s)

Example(s) of one or two of the Nutrition Care Indicators (includes sample initial and reassessment documentation for one of the indicators)

Indicator(s) Selected

Availability of meal preparation facilities

Criteria for Evaluation

Comparison to Goal or Reference Standard:

1. Goal: Patient/client has no access to meal preparation facilities when extensive access to meal preparation facilities is the goal.

   OR

2. Reference Standard: No validated standard exists.

Sample Nutrition Assessment	Monitoring and Evaluation Documentation
Initial nutrition assessment with patient/client	The patient/client has no access to meal preparation facilities. Will monitor change in access at next appointment after coordination of nutrition care with social work.
Reassessment after nutrition intervention	Substantial progress toward goal, as patient/client has consistent access to meal preparation facility with repair of stove.

Safe Water Availability (FH-6.3)

Assessment

Definition

Availability of potable water

Nutrition Assessment and Monitoring and Evaluation

Indicators

- Availability of potable water (specify, eg, functioning well, access to treated public water supply)
- Appropriate water decontamination (specify, eg, awareness of and compliance with public health warnings; use of strategies such as boiling or chemical or filtration treatment)

Examples of the measurement methods or data sources for these indicators: Patient/client report of water availability and/or decontamination strategies, referral information, home evaluation

Typically used with the following domains of nutrition interventions: Nutrition education, nutrition counseling, coordination of nutrition care by nutrition professional

Typically used to determine and to monitor and evaluate change in the following nutrition diagnoses: Inadequate fluid intake, intake of unsafe food

Note: Clinical judgment must be used to select indicators and determine the appropriate measurement techniques and reference standards for a given patient population and setting. Once identified, these indicators, measurement techniques, and reference standards should be identified in policies and procedures or other documents for use in patient/client records, quality or performance improvement, or in formal research projects.

Evaluation

Criteria for Evaluation

Comparison to Goal or Reference Standard:

1. Goal (tailored to patient/client needs)

   OR

2. Reference Standard

Safe Water Availability (FH-6.3)

Patient/Client Example(s)

Example(s) of one or two of the Nutrition Care Indicators (includes sample initial and reassessment documentation for one of the indicators)

Indicator(s) Selected

Appropriate water decontamination

Criteria for Evaluation

Comparison to Goal or Reference Standard:

1. Goal: Patient/client has limited awareness and no compliance with water decontamination recommendations when extensive awareness and compliance with the decontamination guidelines is the goal.

   OR

2. Reference Standard: No validated standard exists.

Sample Nutrition Assessment	Monitoring and Evaluation Documentation
Initial nutrition assessment with patient/client	The patient/client has limited awareness and no compliance with water decontamination recommendations (eg, community has a boil water alert for water used for drinking and cooking) when extensive awareness and compliance with the decontamination guidelines is the goal. Will monitor change in compliance at next appointment.
Reassessment after nutrition intervention	Substantial progress toward goal, as patient/client is complying with water decontamination guidelines.

Food/Nutrition-Related Supplies Availability (FH-6.4)

Assessment

Definition

Access to necessary food/nutrition-related supplies

Nutrition Assessment and Monitoring and Evaluation

Indicators

- Access to food/nutrition-related supplies (specify, eg, glucose monitor, monitoring strips, lancets, pedometer, PN/EN supplies, thickeners, blood pressure–related devices)
- Access to assistive eating devices (specify, eg, modified utensils, plates, bowls, gavage feeding supplies)
- Access to assistive food preparation devices (specify, eg, modified utensils for food preparation, electric can openers, rocking knives, one-handed devices)

Examples of the measurement methods or data sources for these indicators: Patient/client report, referral information, home evaluation

Typically used with the following domains of nutrition interventions: Nutrition education, nutrition counseling, coordination of nutrition care by nutrition professional

Typically used to determine and to monitor and evaluate change in the following nutrition diagnoses: Inability to manage self-care, inadequate oral intake, self-feeding difficulty, limited adherence to nutrition-related recommendations

Note: Clinical judgment must be used to select indicators and determine the appropriate measurement techniques and reference standards for a given patient population and setting. Once identified, these indicators, measurement techniques, and reference standards should be identified in policies and procedures or other documents for use in patient/client records, quality or performance improvement, or in formal research projects.

Evaluation

Criteria for Evaluation

Comparison to Goal or Reference Standard:

1. Goal (tailored to patient/client needs)

   OR

2. Reference Standard

Food/Nutrition-Related Supplies Availability (FH-6.4)

Patient/Client Example(s)

Example(s) of one or two of the Nutrition Care Indicators (includes sample initial and reassessment documentation for one of the indicators)

Indicator(s) Selected

Access to food/nutrition-related supplies

Criteria for Evaluation

Comparison to Goal or Reference Standard:

1. Goal: Patient/client has limited access to a sufficient quantity of glucose monitoring strips when extensive access is the goal.

   OR

2. Reference Standard: No validated standard exists.

Sample Nutrition Assessment	Monitoring and Evaluation Documentation
Initial nutrition assessment with patient/client	The patient/client has limited access to a sufficient quantity of glucose monitoring strips. Will monitor change in access to glucose monitoring strips at next appointment.
Reassessment after nutrition intervention	Some progress toward goal, as patient/client has moderate access to a sufficient supply of glucose monitoring strips.

Breastfeeding (FH-7.1)

Assessment

Definition

Degree to which breastfeeding plans and experience meet nutritional and other needs of the infant and mother

Nutrition Assessment and Monitoring and Evaluation

Indicators

- Initiation of breastfeeding
  - Breastfeeding attempts (number)
- Duration of breastfeeding (specify, eg, weeks, months, years)
- Exclusive breastfeeding (yes/no)
- Breastfeeding problems
  - Evaluation of latch (correct/incorrect)
  - Evaluation of mother's nipples (not irritated/irritated)
  - Evaluation of sucking (minutes of rhythmic sucking per feeding)
  - Presence of breastmilk* in baby's mouth when unlatched from breast (yes/no)
  - Evaluation of mother's breasts (specify, eg, full/firm prior to feeding, soft after feeding)
  - Mother's evaluation of baby's satisfaction after feeding (specify, eg, still hungry/satisfied)
  - Other (specify)

> **Note:** Infant/child growth can be found on the Body Composition/Growth/Weight History reference sheet.
>
> Breastfeeding self-efficacy and intention to breastfeed can be found on the Beliefs and Attitudes reference sheet.

Examples of the measurement methods or data sources for this indicator: Patient/client report, practitioner observation of breastfeeding, self-monitoring records, infant weight trends

Typically used to determine and monitor and evaluate change in the following domains of nutrition interventions: Nutrition education, nutrition counseling, coordination of nutrition care by nutrition professional

Typically used to determine and to monitor and evaluate change in the following nutrition diagnoses: Breastfeeding difficulty, food- and nutrition-related knowledge deficit, unsupported beliefs/attitudes about food- or nutrition-related topics, unintended weight loss, inadequate fluid intake

> **Note:** Clinical judgment must be used to select indicators and determine the appropriate measurement techniques and reference standards for a given patient population and setting. Once identified, these indicators, measurement techniques, and reference standards should be identified in policies and procedures or other documents for use in patient/client records, quality or performance improvement, or in formal research projects.

---

*If a synonym for the term "breastmilk" is helpful or needed, an approved alternative is "human milk."

Breastfeeding (FH-7.1)

Evaluation

Criteria for Evaluation

Comparison to Goal or Reference Standard:

1. Goal (tailored to patient/client's needs)

    OR

2. Reference Standard

Patient/Client Example(s)

Example(s) of one or two of the Nutrition Care Indicators (includes sample initial and reassessment documentation for one of the indicators)

Indicator(s) Selected

Initiation of breastfeeding

Criteria for Evaluation

Comparison to Goal or Reference Standard:

1. Goal: Patient/client currently fears that her breastmilk* supply is not adequate and worries about how she will manage when she returns to work in four weeks. Goal is for mother to breastfeed for six months.

    OR

2. Reference Standard: No validated standard exists.

Sample Nutrition Assessment	Monitoring and Evaluation Documentation
Initial encounter with patient/client	Postpartum patient/client states that she is planning to use a combination of formula and breastfeeding and start solids at 3 months. Will educate and refer to lactation support group.
Reassessment after nutrition intervention	Patient/client reports that she has exclusively breastfed for three months and plans to delay introduction of solids. Will reinforce and educate. Continue to monitor.

*If a synonym for the term "breastmilk" is helpful or needed, an approved alternative is "human milk."

Nutrition-Related Activities of Daily Living and Instrumental Activities of Daily Living (FH-7.2)

Definition

Level of cognitive and physical ability to perform nutrition-related activities of daily living and instrumental activities of daily living by older and/or disabled persons

Nutrition Assessment and Monitoring and Evaluation

Indicators

- Physical ability to complete tasks for meal preparation (plan meals, shop for meals, finances, meal preparation) (yes/no)
- Physical ability to self-feed (yes/no)
- Ability to position self in relation to plate (within 12 to 18 inches (30-45 cm) from mouth to plate) (yes/no)
- Receives assistance with intake (yes/no)
- Ability to use adaptive eating devices (those that have been deemed necessary and that improve self-feeding skills) (yes/no)
- Cognitive ability to complete tasks for meal preparation (planning meals, shopping for meals, finances, meal preparation) (yes/no)
- Remembers to eat (yes/no)
- Recalls eating (yes/no)
- Mini Mental State Examination score (score)
- Nutrition-related activities of daily living (ADL) score (score)
- Nutrition-related instrumental activities of daily living (IADL) score (score)

Note: Sufficient intake of food can be found on the Food Intake reference sheet. Sufficient intake of fluid can be found on the Fluid/Beverage Intake reference sheet. Food security and ability to maintain sanitation can be found on the Safe Food/Meal Availability reference sheet.

Ability to maintain weight can be found on the Body Composition/Growth/Weight History reference sheet.

Examples of the measurement methods or data sources for these indicators: Patient/client report, caregiver report, home visit, targeted questionnaires and monitoring devices, ADL and/or IADL measurement tool, congregate meal site attendance records

Typically used with the following domains of nutrition interventions: Coordination of nutrition care by nutrition professional

Typically used to determine and to monitor and evaluate change in the following nutrition diagnoses: Inability to manage self-care, impaired ability to prepare foods/meals

Note: Clinical judgment must be used to select indicators and determine the appropriate measurement techniques and reference standards for a given patient population and setting. Once identified, these indicators, measurement techniques, and reference standards should be identified in policies and procedures or other documents for use in patient/client records, quality or performance improvement, or in formal research projects.

Nutrition-Related Activities of Daily Living and Instrumental Activities of Daily Living (FH-7.2)

Evaluation

Criteria for Evaluation

Comparison to Goal or Reference Standard:

1. Goal (tailored to patient/client's needs)

   OR

2. Reference Standard

Patient/Client Example(s)

Example(s) of one or two of the Nutrition Care Indicators (includes sample initial and reassessment documentation for one of the indicators)

Indicator(s) Selected

Nutrition-related instrumental activities of daily living (IADL) score

Criteria for Evaluation

Comparison to Goal or Reference Standard:

1. Goal: Patient/client with decreased food intake due to an inability to drive, no close relatives living in the vicinity, and difficulty in performing meal preparation tasks due to weakness.

   OR

2. Reference Standard: No validated standard exists.

Sample Nutrition Assessment	Monitoring and Evaluation Documentation
Initial encounter with patient/client	Patient/client with inadequate food intake due to inability to drive, no close relatives living in the vicinity, subsequent weight loss, and difficulties in performing ADLs and IADLs due to weakness. Patient/client is to use new strategies and community resources to facilitate attendance at senior center congregate meals 5 times per week, use of community-provided transportation offered to grocery store 1 x per week, and attendance in strength training at senior center.
Reassessment after nutrition intervention	Significant progress in nutrition-related activities of daily living. Patient/client able to attend senior center for meals and strength training 3 times this week. Goal is 5 times. Will continue to assess at next encounter. Patient/client going to grocery store 1 x per week.

Physical Activity (FH-7.3)

Definition

Level of physical activity and/or amount of exercise performed

Nutrition Assessment and Monitoring and Evaluation

Indicators

- Physical activity history (eg, activities, preferences, attitudes)
- Consistency (yes/no)
- Frequency (number of times per week)
- Duration (number of minutes per session, number of total minutes per day)
- Intensity (eg, talk test, Borg Rating of Perceived Exertion, % of predetermined max heart rate)
- Type of physical activity (eg, cardiovascular, muscular strength/endurance, flexibility; lifestyle, programmed)
- Strength (eg, handgrip or other muscle strength measure)
  - Handgrip strength (normal, measurably reduced) defined as a proxy measure of upper extremity muscle function
- TV/screen time (minutes per day)
- Other sedentary activity time (eg, commuting; sitting at desk, in meetings, at sporting or arts events) (minutes per day)
- Involuntary physical movement (present/absent)
- Nonexercise activity thermogenesis (NEAT) (present/absent, level)

Examples of the measurement methods or data sources for these indicators: History interview/questionnaire, physical activity log, step counter, accelerometer, attendance at strength training, balance training (for older adults), and/or aerobic classes, caretaker records, medical record, dynamometer

Typically used with the following domains of nutrition interventions: Nutrition education, nutrition counseling

Typically used to determine and to monitor and evaluate change in the following nutrition diagnoses: Physical inactivity, excessive exercise, underweight, overweight/obesity, unintended weight loss or weight gain

Note: Clinical judgment must be used to select indicators and determine the appropriate measurement techniques and reference standards for a given patient population and setting. Once identified, these indicators, measurement techniques, and reference standards should be identified in policies and procedures or other documents for use in patient/client records, quality or performance improvement, or in formal research projects.

Evaluation

Criteria for Evaluation

Comparison to Goal or Reference Standard:

1. Goal (tailored to patient/client's needs)

   OR

2. Reference Standard

Physical Activity (FH-7.3)

Patient/Client Example(s)

Example(s) of one or two of the Nutrition Care Indicators (includes sample initial and reassessment documentation for one of the indicators)

Indicator(s) Selected

Consistency and duration

Criteria for Evaluation

Comparison to Goal or Reference Standard:

1. Goal: Patient/client typically walks approximately 10 minutes twice per week. Patient/client's goal is to walk approximately 15 minutes 5 days per week.

   OR

2. Reference Standard: Patient/client's typical 10-minute walk twice a week is well below the recommended at least 30 minutes of moderate-intensity physical activity (in bouts of 10 minutes or longer) 5 days per week or at least 20 minutes of vigorous intensity physical activity (in bouts of 10 minutes or longer) 3 days per week (ACSM/AHA Physical Activity Guidelines for Public Health for adults and seniors).

Sample Nutrition Assessment	Monitoring and Evaluation Documentation
Initial encounter with patient/client	Based on exercise log, patient/client doing moderate-intensity physical activities 30 minutes per day 2 days per week. Goal is to do at least 30 minutes per day (in bouts of 10 minutes or longer) of moderate-intensity activities 5 or more days per week. Will monitor physical activity level at next appointment.
Reassessment after nutrition intervention	Significant progress toward goal of exercising for 30 minutes per day doing moderate-intensity activities 5 or more days per week. Patient/client reports doing moderate-intensity activities 30 minutes per day 4 days per week.

Factors Affecting Access to Physical Activity (FH-7.4)

Definition

Factors influencing access to physical activity opportunities and physical activity participation

Nutrition Assessment and Monitoring and Evaluation

Indicators

- Neighborhood safety (patient/client's perception of crime and traffic, presence of gangs, witness to physical attacks, presence of community members walking or playing outside, and feeling it is safe to walk outside. Patient/client rates on a scale of 1 to 10 [1 = unsafe, 10 = safe])
- Walkability of neighborhood (patient/client's perception of his or her ability to walk in a neighborhood related to street connectivity, road type, dwelling density, and land use attributes (ie, residential, commercial, institutional, or industrial land use. Patient/client rates on a scale of 1 to 10 [1 = not walkable, 10 = very walkable])
- Proximity to parks/green space (patient/client's perception of the distance from patient/client's home/workplace to the nearest park/green space. Patient/client rates on a scale of 1 to 10 [1 = large distance to nearest park/green space, 10 = small distance to nearest park/green space])
- Access to physical activity facilities/programs (patient/client's perception of the availability of physical activity facilities/programs in the patient/client's environment. Patient/client rates on a scale of 1 to 10 [1 = no availability of facilities/programs, 10 = excellent availability of facilities/programs])

Note: Physical disability, mobility, and socioeconomic factors affecting physical activity can be documented in the Personal Data (CH-1.1) and Social History (CH-3.1) reference sheets.

Examples of the measurement methods or data sources for these indicators: Patient perception, neighborhood crime statistics, neighborhood traffic statistics, geographic information systems data to map a neighborhood, availability of retail establishments within walking distance

Typically used with the following domains of nutrition interventions: Nutrition education, nutrition counseling, and coordination of nutrition care by nutrition professional

Typically used to determine and to monitor and evaluate change in the following nutrition diagnoses: Overweight/obesity, physical inactivity, not ready for diet/lifestyle change

Note: Clinical judgment must be used to select indicators and determine the appropriate measurement techniques and reference standards for a given patient population and setting. Once identified, these indicators, measurement techniques, and reference standards should be identified in policies and procedures or other documents for use in patient/client records, quality or performance improvement, or in formal research projects.

Factors Affecting Access to Physical Activity (FH-7.4)

Evaluation

Criteria for Evaluation

Comparison to Goal or Reference Standard:

1. Goal (tailored to patient/client's needs)

   OR

2. Reference Standard

Patient/Client Example(s)

Example(s) of one or two of the Nutrition Care Indicators (includes sample initial and reassessment documentation for one of the indicators)

Indicator(s) Selected

Neighborhood safety

Criteria for Evaluation

Comparison to Goal or Reference Standard:

1. Goal: Patient rated neighborhood as unsafe when increased physical activity is a goal.

   OR

2. Reference Standard:

Sample Nutrition Assessment	Monitoring and Evaluation Documentation
Initial encounter with patient/client	Patient perceives that the neighborhood is unsafe (self-perception rating of a 2) for an individual to engage in outdoor exercise alone because of environmental factors (eg crime, traffic, gang presence, witness to physical attack) and has limited compliance with increasing physical activity.
Reassessment after nutrition intervention	Patient has joined a neighborhood outdoor exercise group and now rates neighborhood safety as a 7 and has increasing compliance with regular physical activity.

Nutrition Quality of Life* (FH-8.1)

Assessment

Definition

Extent to which the Nutrition Care Process impacts a patient/client's physical, mental, and social well-being related to food and nutrition

Nutrition Assessment and Monitoring and Evaluation

Indicators

- Nutrition quality of life responses

Examples of the measurement methods or data sources for these outcome indicators: Nutrition quality of life measurement tool, other quality of life tools

Typically used with the following domains of nutrition interventions: Food and/or nutrient delivery, supplements, nutrition education, nutrition counseling, coordination of nutrition care by nutrition professional

Typically used to determine and to monitor and evaluate change in the following nutrition diagnoses: Poor nutrition quality of life, inadequate or excessive energy or macronutrient intake, underweight, unintended weight loss, overweight/obesity, unintended weight gain, disordered eating pattern, inability to manage self-care, swallowing difficulty, chewing difficulty, self-feeding difficulty, altered GI function, limited access to food

Note: Clinical judgment must be used to select indicators and determine the appropriate measurement techniques and reference standards for a given patient population and setting. Once identified, these indicators, measurement techniques, and reference standards should be identified in policies and procedures or other documents for use in patient/client records, quality or performance improvement, or in formal research projects.

Evaluation

Criteria for Evaluation

Comparison to Goal or Reference Standard:

1. Goal (tailored to patient/client's needs)

   OR

2. Reference Standard

---

*This nutrition indicator is included to encourage further research.

Nutrition Quality of Life* (FH-8.1)

Patient/Client Example(s)

Example(s) of one or two of the Nutrition Care Indicators (includes sample initial and reassessment documentation for one of the indicators)

Indicator(s) Selected

Nutrition quality of life score

Criteria for Evaluation

Comparison to Goal or Reference Standard:

1. Goal: Patient/client with chronic renal disease currently reports poor nutrition quality of life, especially decreased walking ability (physical) and limited food choices on renal diet (food impact). The goal of medical nutrition therapy is to educate and coach patient/client and his family on options and strategies to significantly enhance his nutrition quality of life.

   OR

2. Reference Standard: No validated standard exists.

Sample Nutrition Assessment	Monitoring and Evaluation Documentation
Initial encounter with patient/client	Patient/client with chronic renal disease reports poor nutrition quality of life, particularly in physical and food impact aspects. Patient/client to receive intensive medical nutrition therapy with a goal to improve patient/client's overall nutrition quality of life over a 6-month period. Will monitor nutrition quality of life in 6 months.
Reassessment after nutrition intervention	Some progress toward goal. Patient/client's nutrition quality of life is increased, but further improvement is desired in the physical dimension. Will continue medical nutrition therapy and reassess in 3 months.

*This nutrition indicator is included to encourage further research.

Body Composition/Growth/ Weight History (AD-1.1)

Assessment (sidebar)

Definition

Measures of the body, including fat, muscle, and bone components and growth

Nutrition Assessment and Monitoring and Evaluation

Indicators

- Height—defined as measures of a body's length, typically from head to foot
  - Measured height (in./cm)—defined as measured standing height
  - Measured length (in./cm)—defined as measured recumbent length
  - Birth length (in./cm)—defined as measured recumbent length at birth
  - Pre-amputation measured height (in./cm)—defined as body height prior to removal of a limb or part of a limb
  - Pre-amputation estimated height (in./cm)—defined as estimated body height prior to removal of a limb or part of a limb
  - Estimated height (in./cm)—defined as estimated body height
  - Stated height (in./cm)—defined as stated body height
  - Measured peak adult height (in./cm)—defined as tallest measured height recorded in adulthood
  - Stated peak adult height (in./cm)—defined as stated body height at age 25
  - Knee height (in./cm)—defined as the measured distance from the posterior surface of the thigh, just proximal to the patella, to the sole of the foot when the knee is bent at a 90° angle (adapted from Chumlea et al. *J Am Diet Assoc.* 1994;94:1385–1391)
  - Tibia length (cm)—defined as the measured distance from the superomedial edge of the tibia to the inferior edge of the medial malleolus (adapted from Stevenson RD. *Arch Pediatr Adolesc Med.* 1995;149:658–662))
  - Arm span (in./cm)—defined as the measured distance of outstretched arms between the tip of the middle finger to the tip of the other middle finger with arms parallel to the ground (adapted from the Nutrition Care Manual 2016)
  - Arm demispan (cm)—defined as the measured distance from the midline at the sternal notch to the web between the middle and ring fingers along outstretched arm (Mini Nutrition Assessment)
  - Arm halfspan (cm)—defined as the measured distance from the midline at the sternal notch to the tip of the middle finger (Mini Nutrition Assessment)
  - Height measurement device—defined as the tool used to measure height or length
- Weight—defined as measures of a body's mass; heaviness or lightness of a body
  - Measured weight (lb, oz, kg, g)—defined as measured body weight
  - Stated weight (lb, oz, kg, g)—defined as reported body weight
  - Stated peak weight (lb, kg)—defined as reported maximum body weight
  - Measured peak weight (lb, kg)—defined as the measured maximum body weight
  - Usual stated body weight (UBW) (lb, oz, kg, g)—defined as the reported body weight that is typical for the individual
  - UBW percentage (%)—defined as the calculation using actual body weight divided by usual weight and then multiplied by 100

Body Composition/Growth/ Weight History (AD-1.1)

- Birth weight (lb, oz, kg, g)—defined as the measured body weight at birth
- Stated pre-pregnancy weight (lb, oz, kg, g)—defined as the reported weight prior to pregnancy
- Dosing weight (lb, oz, kg, g)—defined as the calculated body weight that may be used to determine the appropriate dose for medications, enteral nutrition, parenteral nutrition, and IVs
- Estimated dry weight (lb, oz, kg, g)—defined as the estimated body weight without excess fluid volume (euvolemic)
- Pre-amputation measured weight (lb, oz, kg, g)—defined as the measured body weight prior to removal of a limb or part of a limb
- Pre-amputation estimated weight (lb, oz, kg, g)—defined as the estimated body weight prior to removal of a limb or part of a limb
- Post-amputation measured weight (lb, oz, kg, g)—defined as the measured body weight after removal of a limb or part of a limb
- Post-amputation estimated weight (lb, oz, kg, g)—defined as the estimated body weight after removal of a limb or part of a limb
- Pre-dialysis weight (lb, oz, kg, g)—defined as measured body weight prior to dialysis
- Post-dialysis weight (lb, oz, kg, g)—defined as measured body weight after dialysis
- Frame—defined as estimate of a body frame based upon height and wrist measure
  - Frame size (small/medium/large)—defined as calculation using measured wrist circumference and measured height to estimate frame size
  - Wrist circumference (in./cm)—defined as the measured circumference of the wrist
- Weight change—defined as measures of the difference in body weight typically over time
  - Weight gain (lb, kg, oz, g)—defined as the measured increase in body weight over a specified period of time
  - Weight loss (lb, kg, oz, g)—defined as the measured decrease in body weight over a specified period of time
  - Weight change percentage (%)—defined as the weight change value divided by the original weight and multiplied by 100
  - Measured interdialytic weight gain (lb, oz, kg, g)—defined as the measured increase in body weight between dialysis treatments
  - Measured interdialytic weight loss (lb, oz, kg, g)—defined as the measured decrease in body weight between dialysis treatments
  - Weight change intent (intentional/unintentional)—defined as the purpose of weight gain or weight loss
  - Measured gestational weight gain (lb, oz, kg, g)—defined as measured weight increase during pregnancy
  - Measured gestational weight loss (lb, oz, kg, g)—defined as measured weight decrease during pregnancy
- Body mass—defined as measures of a body's weight relative to height
  - Body mass index (BMI) (kg/m^2)—defined as weight in kilograms divided by the square height in meters
  - BMI prime ratio (ratio)—defined as the ratio of actual BMI to the upper limit BMI of 25
- Growth pattern indices—defined as measures used to monitor growth
  - BMI-for-age percentile (percentile)—defined as weight in kilograms divided by the square of height in meters at the child's age
  - BMI-for-age z score—defined as the standard deviation score for BMI at the child's age
  - Head circumference (in/cm)—defined as the largest occipital-frontal circumference

Body Composition/Growth/ Weight History (AD-1.1)

- ○ Birth head circumference (in./cm)—defined as the largest occipital-frontal circumference at birth.
- ○ Head circumference-for-age percentile (percentile)—defined as attained head circumference at the child's age
- ○ Head circumference-for-age z score (z score)—defined as the standard deviation score for attained head circumference at the child's age
- ○ Length-for-age percentile (percentile)—defined as attained growth in recumbent length at the child's age.
- ○ Length-for-age z score (z score)—defined as the standard deviation score for attained length at the child's age
- ○ Stature-for-age percentile (percentile)—defined as attained growth in standing height at the child's age.
- ○ Stature-for-age z score (z score)—defined as the standard deviation score for attained height at the child's age
- ○ Weight-for-length percentile (percentile)—defined as body weight in proportion to attained growth in recumbent length
- ○ Weight-for-length z score (z score)—defined as the standard deviation score for body weight in proportion to attained growth in recumbent length
- ○ Weight-for-age percentile (percentile)—defined as body weight relative to the child's age
- ○ Weight-for-age z score (z score)—defined as the standard deviation score for attained body weight at the child's age
- ○ Weight-for-stature percentile (percentile)—defined as body weight in proportion to attained growth in standing height
- ○ Weight-for-stature z score (z score)—defined as the standard deviation score for body weight in proportion to attained growth in height
- ○ Mid parental height comparator (in/cm)—defined as the parental heights used to predict a child's expected adult height centile
- Body compartment estimates—defined as measures of fat, muscle, and bone components of a body.)
  - ○ Body fat percentage (%)—defined as the portion of the body attributed to body fat and excludes muscle, fluids, bone, or organs
  - ○ Body fat percentage technique—defined as the tool used to estimate body fat
  - ○ Body surface area (m^2)—defined as the measured surface area of a human body
  - ○ Calculated body surface area (m^2)—defined as the calculated surface area of a human body
  - ○ Bone age (years)—defined as the degree of maturation of a child's skeleton
  - ○ Bone mineral density t score (t score)—defined as the measure of minerals in bone compared with a healthy young adult of the same sex
  - ○ Bone mineral density z score (z score)—defined as the measure of minerals in bone compared with a person of the same age, sex, weight, and ethnic or racial origin
  - ○ Bone mineral density technique—defined as the test to measure bone mineral density
  - ○ Mid arm muscle circumference (in./cm)—defined as the measure of the muscle area of the upper arm
  - ○ Mid arm muscle circumference percentile (percentile)—defined as the rank of the muscle area of the upper arm
  - ○ Triceps skinfold thickness (in./cm)—defined as measure of the fold of skin taken over the tricep muscle
  - ○ Triceps skinfold percentile (percentile)—defined as the percentile rank of the skinfold thickness over the tricep muscle

Body Composition/Growth/ Weight History (AD-1.1)

- Triceps skinfold z score (z score)—defined as the standard deviation score for the skinfold thickness over the tricep muscle
- Waist circumference (in./cm)—defined as the circumference around the waist measured at the umbilicus
- Waist circumference narrowest point (in/ cm). Defined as the circumference around the waist measured at the narrowest point
- Waist circumference iliac crest (in./cm)—defined as the circumference around the waist measured at the midpoint between the lower margin of the least palpable rib and the top of the iliac crest
- Hip circumference (in/cm)—defined as the circumference of the hips measure at the widest portion of the buttocks
- Waist to hip ratio (ratio)—defined as the calculated waist circumference measurement divided by the hip measurement
- Mid upper arm circumference (in./cm)—defined as the circumference of the upper right arm measured between the tip of the shoulder and the tip of the elbow
- Mid upper arm circumference, left arm (in./cm)—defined as the circumference of the upper left arm measured between the tip of the shoulder and the tip of the elbow
- Mid upper arm circumference z score (z score)—defined as the standard deviation score for mid upper arm circumference

Examples of the measurement methods or data sources for these indicators: Referring health care provider or agency, direct measurement, patient/client report, medical record

Typically used with the following domains of nutrition interventions: Food and nutrient delivery, nutrition education, nutrition counseling, coordination of nutrition care by nutrition professional

Typically used to determine and to monitor and evaluate change in the following nutrition diagnoses: Excessive or inadequate intake of energy, fat, protein, carbohydrate, alcohol, and/or mineral intake; underweight; overweight; physical inactivity; excessive exercise

Note: Clinical judgment must be used to select indicators and determine the appropriate measurement techniques and reference standards for a given patient population and setting. Once identified, these indicators, measurement techniques, and reference standards should be identified in policies and procedures or other documents for use in patient/client records, quality or performance improvement, or formal research projects.

Evaluation

Criteria for Evaluation

Comparison to Goal or Reference Standard:

1. Goal (tailored to patient/client's needs)

   OR

2. Reference Standard

Body Composition/Growth/ Weight History (AD-1.1)

Patient/Client Example(s)

Example(s) of one or two of the Nutrition Care Indicators (includes sample initial and reassessment documentation for one of the indicators)

Indicator(s) Selected

Weight change per day

BMI percentile/age

Criteria for Evaluation

Comparison to Goal or Reference Standard:

1. Goal: The infant is only gaining, on average, 10 g/day compared with a goal weight gain of 20 to 30 g/day.

   OR

2. Reference Standard: Child's (>3 years of age) BMI percentile/age per growth curve has crossed 2 percentile channels from 50% to 10% in the last 6 months.

Sample Nutrition Assessment	Monitoring and Evaluation Documentation
Initial nutrition assessment with patient/client	Child's BMI percentile/age per growth curve has crossed 2 percentile channels from 50% to 10% in the last 6 months. Will monitor BMI percentile/age at next encounter.
Reassessment after nutrition intervention	Child's BMI percentile/age per growth curve is unchanged from baseline measure.

Assessment

Acid Base Balance (BD-1.1)

Definition

Balance between acids and bases in the body fluids. The pH (hydrogen ion concentration) of the arterial blood provides an index for the total body acid-base balance.

Nutrition Assessment

Indicators

- pH (number)
- Arterial bicarbonate, HCO3 (mmol/L)
- Partial pressure of carbon dioxide in arterial blood (PaCO2) (mmHg)
- Partial pressure of oxygen in arterial blood (PaO2) (mmHg)
- Venous pH (number)
- Venous bicarbonate (mmol/L)

Note: Sodium and chloride can be found on the Electrolyte and Renal Profile reference sheet.

Examples of the measurement methods or data sources for these indicators: Biochemical measurement, laboratory report

Typically used with the following domains of nutrition interventions: Food and/or nutrient delivery, coordination of nutrition care by nutrition professional

Typically used to determine and to monitor and evaluate change in the following nutrition diagnoses: Altered nutrition-related laboratory values

Note: Clinical judgment must be used to select indicators and determine the appropriate measurement techniques and reference standards for a given patient population and setting. Once identified, these indicators, measurement techniques, and reference standards should be identified in policies and procedures or other documents for use in patient/client records, quality or performance improvement, or in formal research projects.

Evaluation

Criteria for Evaluation

Comparison to Goal or Reference Standard:

1. Goal (tailored to patient/client's needs)
   OR
2. Reference Standard

Acid Base Balance (BD-1.1)

Patient/Client Example

Example(s) of one or two of the Nutrition Care Indicators (includes sample initial and reassessment documentation for one of the indicators)

Indicator(s) Selected

pH, serum (number)

Criteria for Evaluation

Comparison to Goal or Reference Standard:

1. Goal: Not generally used.

   OR

2. Reference Standard: The patient/client's pH is 7.48, which is above (above, below, or within expected range) the reference standard (7.35–7.45).

Sample Nutrition Assessment	Monitoring and Evaluation Documentation
Initial nutrition assessment with patient/client	Patient/client's pH is 7.48, which is above expected range. Will monitor change in pH at next arterial blood gas.
Reassessment after nutrition intervention	Significant progress toward reference standard. Patient/client's pH is 7.40, within expected range.

Assessment

Electrolyte and Renal Profile (BD-1.2)

Definition

Laboratory measures associated with electrolyte balance and kidney function

Nutrition Assessment and Monitoring and Evaluation

Indicators

- BUN (mg/dL or mmol/L)
- Creatinine (mg/dL or μmol/L)
- BUN:creatinine ratio (ratio number)
- Glomerular filtration rate (mL/min/1.73 m^2)
- Sodium (mEq/L or mmol/L)
- Chloride (mEq/L or mmol/L)
- Potassium (mEq/L or mmol/L)
- Magnesium (mEq/L or mmol/L)
- Calcium, serum (mg/dL or mmol/L)
- Calcium, ionized (mg/dL or mmol/L)
- Phosphorus (mg/dL or mmol/L)
- Serum osmolality (mOsm/kg or mmol/kg)
- Parathyroid hormone (pg/mL or ng/L)

Note: Bicarbonate can be found on the Acid Base Balance reference sheet.

Serum albumin can be found on the Protein Profile reference sheet for adjustment of serum calcium.

Examples of the measurement methods or data sources for these indicators: Biochemical measurement, laboratory report

Typically used with the following domains of nutrition interventions: Food and/or nutrient delivery, coordination of nutrition care by nutrition professional

Typically used to determine and to monitor and evaluate change in the following nutrition diagnoses: Excessive or inadequate intake of protein or minerals

Note: Clinical judgment must be used to select indicators and determine the appropriate measurement techniques and reference standards for a given patient population and setting. Once identified, these indicators, measurement techniques, and reference standards should be identified in policies and procedures or other documents for use in patient/client records, quality or performance improvement, or in formal research projects.

Evaluation

Criteria for Evaluation

Comparison to Goal or Reference Standard:

1. Goal (tailored to patient/client's needs)
   OR
2. Reference Standard

Electrolyte and Renal Profile (BD-1.2)

Assessment

Patient/Client Example

Example(s) of one or two of the Nutrition Care Indicators (includes sample initial and reassessment documentation for one of the indicators)

Indicator(s) Selected

Potassium (mEq/L)

Criteria for Evaluation

Comparison to Goal or Reference Standard:

1. Goal: A goal of serum K^+ 3.5 to 5.5 mEq/L in patient/client on medications that block the renin–angiotensin system.

   OR

2. Reference Standard: The patient/client's potassium is 2.9 mEq/L, which is below (above, below, within expected range) the expected range (3.5–5.0 mEq/L).

Sample Nutrition Assessment	Monitoring and Evaluation Documentation
Initial nutrition assessment with patient/client	Patient/client's serum potassium is 2.9 mEq/L, which is below the expected range. Will monitor change in potassium at next encounter.
Reassessment after nutrition intervention	Regression from reference standard. Patient/client's potassium is 2.7 mEq/L, below the expected range.

Essential Fatty Acid Profile (BD-1.3)

Definition

Laboratory measures of essential fatty acids

Nutrition Assessment and Monitoring and Evaluation

Indicators

- Triene:tetraene ratio (ratio number)

Examples of the measurement methods or data sources for these indicators: Biochemical measurement, laboratory report/record

Typically used with the following domains of nutrition interventions: Food and/or nutrient delivery, coordination of nutrition care by nutrition professional

Typically used to determine and to monitor and evaluate change in the following nutrition diagnoses: Inadequate intake of fat, parenteral nutrition; parenteral nutrition composition inconsistent with needs; parenteral nutrition administration inconsistent with needs; altered nutrition-related laboratory values; impaired nutrient utilization

Note: Clinical judgment must be used to select indicators and determine the appropriate measurement techniques and reference standards for a given patient population and setting. Once identified, these indicators, measurement techniques, and reference standards should be identified in policies and procedures or other documents for use in patient/client records, quality or performance improvement, or formal research projects.

Evaluation

Criteria for Evaluation

Comparison to Goal or Reference Standard:

1. Goal (tailored to patient/client's needs)

   OR

2. Reference Standard

Patient/Client Example

Example(s) of one or two of the Nutrition Care Indicators (includes sample initial and reassessment documentation for one of the indicators)

Indicator(s) Selected

Triene:tetraene ratio (ratio number)

Criteria for Evaluation

Comparison to Goal or Reference Standard:

1. Goal: Not generally used.

   OR

2. Reference Standard: The patient/client's triene:tetraene ratio is 0.45, which is (above, below, or within expected range) above expected range (>0.2–0.4 essential fatty acid deficiency).

Essential Fatty Acid Profile (BD-1.3)

Assessment

Sample Nutrition Assessment	Monitoring and Evaluation Documentation
Initial nutrition assessment with patient/client	Patient/client's triene:tetraene ratio is 0.45, above the expected range (essential fatty acid deficiency). Will monitor change in triene:tetraene ratio at next encounter.
Reassessment after nutrition intervention	Significant progress toward the expected range. Patient/client's triene:tetraene ratio is 0.1.

Gastrointestinal Profile (BD-1.4)

Definition

Laboratory measures and medical tests associated with function of the gastrointestinal tract and related organs

Nutrition Assessment and Monitoring and Evaluation

Indicators

- Alkaline phosphatase (U/L)
- Alanine aminotransferase (ALT) (U/L)
- Aspartate aminotransferase (AST) (U/L)
- Gamma glutamyl transferase (GGT) (U/L)
- Gastric residual volume (mL)
- Bilirubin, total (mg/dL or µmol/L)
- Ammonia, serum (µg/dL or µmol/L)
- Toxicology report, including alcohol (by report)
- Prothrombin time (PT) (seconds)
- Partial thromboplastin time (PTT) (seconds)
- INR ratio (ratio number)
- Amylase (U/L)
- Lipase (U/L)
- Fecal fat, 24 hour (g/24 hours)
- Fecal fat, 72 hour (g/24 hours)
- Fecal fat, qualitative (by report)
- Fecal calprotectin (µg/g stool)
- Fecal lactoferrin (ordinal)
- Pancreatic elastase (µg/g stool)
- 5'-nucleotidase (U/L)
- D-xylose (mg/dL)
- Lactulose hydrogen breath test (ppm above baseline/by report)
- Lactose hydrogen breath test (ppm above baseline/by report)
- Fructose hydrogen breath test (ppm above baseline/by report)
- Glucose hydrogen breath test (ppm above baseline/by report)
- Urea hydrogen breath test (ppm above baseline/by report)
- Intestinal biopsy (by report)
- Stool culture (by report)
- Gastric emptying time (minutes)
- Small bowel transit time (minutes, hours)
- Abdominal X-ray (by report)
- Abdominal CT (computed tomography) (by report)
- Abdominal ultrasound (by report)
- Endoscopic ultrasound (EUS) (by report)
- Pelvic CT (computed tomography) scan (by report)
- Modified barium swallow (by report)
- Barium swallow (by report)
- Esophagogastroduodenoscopy (EGD) (by report)
- Endoscopic retrograde cholangiopancreatography (ERCP) (by report)
- Capsule endoscopy (by report)
- Esophageal manometry (by report)
- Esophageal pH test (pH)
- Gastroesophageal reflux monitoring (by report)
- Gastrointestinal sphincter monitoring (by report)
- Urate (mg/dL or µmol/L)

Gastrointestinal Profile (BD-1.4)

Assessment

Examples of the measurement methods or data sources for these indicators: Biochemical measurement, laboratory report

Typically used with the following domains of nutrition interventions: Food and/or nutrient delivery, nutrition education, nutrition counseling

Typically used to determine and to monitor and evaluate change in the following nutrition diagnoses: Altered nutrition-related laboratory values, excess intake of protein or fat

> **Note:** Clinical judgment must be used to select indicators and determine the appropriate measurement techniques and reference standards for a given patient population and setting. Once identified, these indicators, measurement techniques, and reference standards should be identified in policies and procedures or other documents for use in patient/client records, quality or performance improvement, or in formal research projects.

Evaluation

Criteria for Evaluation

Comparison to Goal or Reference Standard:

1. Goal (tailored to patient/client's needs)

    OR

2. Reference Standard

Patient/Client Example

Example(s) of one or two of the Nutrition Care Indicators (includes sample initial and reassessment documentation for one of the indicators)

Indicator(s) Selected

Ammonia, serum (µg/dL)

Criteria for Evaluation

Comparison to Goal or Reference Standard:

1. Goal: The patient/client's serum ammonia is 105 µg/dL, which is above the goal (<75 µg/dL) for this patient/client with end-stage liver disease.

    OR

2. Reference Standard: The patient/client serum ammonia is 85 µg/dL, which is above (above, below, or percent of) the expected range (11–35 µg/dL).

Sample Nutrition Assessment	Monitoring and Evaluation Documentation
Initial nutrition assessment with patient/client	Patient/client's serum ammonia is 85 µg/dL, above the expected range. Will monitor change in serum ammonia at next encounter.
Reassessment after nutrition intervention	Significant progress toward expected range. Patient/client's serum ammonia is 45 µg/dL.

Glucose/Endocrine Profile (BD-1.5)

Definition

Laboratory measures associated with glycemic control and endocrine findings

Nutrition Assessment and Monitoring and Evaluation

Indicators

- Glucose, fasting (mg/dL, mmol/L)
- Glucose, casual (mg/dL, mmol/L)
- Hemoglobin A1c (%, mmol/mol)
- Preprandial capillary plasma glucose (mg/dL, mmol/L)
- Peak postprandial capillary plasma glucose (mg/dL, mmol/L)
- Glucose tolerance test (mg/dL, mmol/L)
- Cortisol level (µg/dL, mmol/L)
- IGF-binding protein (ng/mL, mg/L)
- Thyroid-stimulating hormone (µmol/mL, mmol/L)
- Thyroxine test or T4 (µg/dL, pmol/L)
- Triiodothyronine or T3 (ng/dL, pmol/L)
- Adrenocorticotropic hormone (pg/mL, pmol/L)
- Follicle-stimulating hormone (mU/mL, IU/L)
- Growth hormone (ng/mL, µg/L)
- Luteinizing hormone (mU/mL, IU/L)

Examples of the measurement methods or data sources for these indicators: Biochemical measurement, laboratory report

Typically used with the following domains of nutrition interventions: Food and/or nutrient delivery, nutrition education, nutrition counseling

Typically used to determine and to monitor and evaluate change in the following nutrition diagnoses: Excessive or inadequate intake of carbohydrate or energy; less than optimal intake of types of carbohydrate; inconsistent carbohydrate intake

Note: Clinical judgment must be used to select indicators and determine the appropriate measurement techniques and reference standards for a given patient population and setting. Once identified, these indicators, measurement techniques, and reference standards should be identified in policies and procedures or other documents for use in patient/client records, quality or performance improvement, or in formal research projects.

Evaluation

Criteria for Evaluation

Comparison to Goal or Reference Standard:

1. Goal (tailored to patient/client's needs)
   OR
2. Reference Standard

Glucose/Endocrine Profile (BD-1.5)

Assessment

Patient/Client Example

Example(s) of one or two of the Nutrition Care Indicators (includes sample initial and reassessment documentation for one of the indicators)

Indicator(s) Selected

Hemoglobin A1c (%, mmol/mol)

Criteria for Evaluation

Comparison to Goal or Reference Standard:

1. Goal: The patient/client's HgbA1c is 7.8% (60 mmol/mol), which is above the expected limit but is an acceptable goal in a pediatric patient.

   OR

2. Reference Standard: The patient/client's Hemoglobin A1c is 11% (97 mmol/mol), which is above the expected limit (<6%, 42 mmol/mol).

Sample Nutrition Assessment	Monitoring and Evaluation Documentation
Initial nutrition assessment with patient/client	Patient/client's Hemoglobin A1c is 9% (75 mmol/mol), which is above the expected limit. Will monitor change in HgbA1c at next encounter.
Reassessment after nutrition intervention	Regression from the expected limit. Patient/client's Hemoglobin A1c is 10% (86 mmol/mol).

Inflammatory Profile (BD-1.6)

Definition

Laboratory measures of inflammatory proteins

Nutrition Assessment

Indicators

- C-reactive protein, highly sensitive, or hs-CRP (mg/L) (cardiovascular disease)

Examples of the measurement methods or data sources for these indicators: Direct measurement, medical record

Typically used with the following domains of nutrition interventions: Food and/or nutrient delivery

Typically used to determine the following nutrition diagnoses: Increased nutrient need, less than optimal intake of types of fats inconsistent with needs, excessive physical activity

Note: Clinical judgment must be used to select indicators and determine the appropriate measurement techniques and reference standards for a given patient population and setting. Once identified, these indicators, measurement techniques, and reference standards should be identified in policies and procedures or other documents for use in patient/client records, quality or performance improvement, or in formal research projects.

Evaluation

Criteria for Evaluation

Comparison to Goal or Reference Standard:

1. Goal (tailored to patient/client's needs)

    OR

2. Reference Standard

Inflammatory Profile (BD-1.6)

Assessment

Patient/Client Example

Example(s) of one or two of the Nutrition Care Indicators (includes sample initial and reassessment documentation for one of the indicators)

Indicator(s) Selected

C-reactive protein (mg/L)

Criteria for Evaluation

Comparison to Goal or Reference Standard:

1. Goal: Not generally used.

   OR

2. Reference Standard: A patient/client has a C-reactive protein level of 4.0 mg/L, which is above (above, below, within expected range) the expected range of 1.0 to 3.0 mg/L.

Sample Nutrition Assessment	Monitoring and Evaluation Documentation
Nutrition assessment with patient/client	Patient/client's C-reactive protein level is 4.0 mg/L, which is above (above, below, within expected range) the expected range of 1.0 to 3.0 mg/L.

Lipid Profile (BD-1.7)

Definition

Laboratory measures associated with lipid disorders

Nutrition Assessment and Monitoring and Evaluation

Indicators

- Cholesterol, serum (mg/dL or mmol/L)
- Cholesterol, HDL (mg/dL or mmol/L)
- Cholesterol, LDL (mg/dL or mmol/L)
- Cholesterol, non-HDL (mg/dL or mmol/L)
- Total cholesterol:HDL cholesterol ratio (ratio number)
- LDL:HDL ratio (ratio number)
- Triglycerides, serum (mg/ dL or mmol/L)

Examples of the measurement methods or data sources for these indicators: Biochemical measurement, laboratory report, patient/client report

Typically used with the following domains of nutrition interventions: Nutrition education, nutrition counseling

Typically used to determine and to monitor and evaluate change in the following nutrition diagnoses: Excessive or inadequate intake of fat or energy

Note: Clinical judgment must be used to select indicators and determine the appropriate measurement techniques and reference standards for a given patient population and setting. Once identified, these indicators, measurement techniques, and reference standards should be identified in policies and procedures or other documents for use in patient/client records, quality or performance improvement, or in formal research projects.

Evaluation

Criteria for Evaluation

Comparison to Goal or Reference Standard:

1. Goal (tailored to patient/client's needs)

   OR

2. Reference Standard

Lipid Profile (BD-1.7)

Assessment

Patient/Client Example

Example(s) of one or two of the Nutrition Care Indicators (includes sample initial and reassessment documentation for one of the indicators)

Indicator(s) Selected

LDL cholesterol (mg/dL)

Criteria for Evaluation

Comparison to Goal or Reference Standard:

1. Goal: The patient/client's LDL cholesterol is 200 mg/dL, compared to a goal of <100 mg/dL. (**Note:** While reference standards are generally used for laboratory measures, a goal might be used in a special situation such as this example. The patient/client has a familial hypercholesterolemia where a normal reference standard may not be realistic.)

   OR

2. Reference Standard: The patient/client's LDL cholesterol is 159 mg/dL, which is above the expected limit of the NHLBI recommendation of <100 mg/dL.

Sample Nutrition Assessment	Monitoring and Evaluation Documentation
Initial nutrition assessment with patient/client	The patient/client LDL cholesterol is 159 mg/dL compared to the reference standard (eg, National Heart, Lung, and Blood Institute [NHLBI]) recommended level of <100 mg/dL. Will monitor LDL cholesterol at next encounter.
Reassessment after nutrition intervention	Some progress toward goal/reference standard, as patient/client's LDL cholesterol is 145 mg/dL.

Metabolic Rate Profile (BD-1.8)

Definition

Measures associated with or having implications for assessing metabolic rate

Nutrition Assessment and Monitoring and Evaluation

Indicators

- Resting metabolic rate, measured (calories, kcal or kJ/day)
- Respiratory quotient, measured ($RQ = CO_2$ produced/O_2 consumed)

Note: Use of RQ is considered valid if respiratory factors (hyper- or hypoventilation), equipment failure, measurement protocol violations, or operator errors have not occurred.

Examples of the measurement methods or data sources for these indicators: Direct measurement (indirect calorimetry), medical record

Typically used with the following domains of nutrition interventions: Food and/or nutrient delivery

Typically used to determine the following nutrition diagnoses: Excessive or inadequate intake of parenteral/enteral nutrition, enteral/parenteral nutrition composition or administration inconsistent with needs, excessive energy intake, excessive mineral intake, disordered eating pattern, excessive exercise, increased energy expenditure, increased nutrient needs (energy), inadequate protein-energy intake

Note: Clinical judgment must be used to select indicators and determine the appropriate measurement techniques and reference standards for a given patient population and setting. Once identified, these indicators, measurement techniques, and reference standards should be identified in policies and procedures or other documents for use in patient/client records, quality or performance improvement, or in formal research projects.

Evaluation

Criteria for Evaluation

Comparison to Goal or Reference Standard:

1. Goal (tailored to patient/client's needs)

   OR

2. Reference Standard

Metabolic Rate Profile (BD-1.8)

Patient/Client Example

Example(s) of one or two of the Nutrition Care Indicators (includes sample initial and reassessment documentation for one of the indicators)

Indicator(s) Selected

Respiratory quotient

Criteria for Evaluation

Comparison to Goal or Reference Standard:

1. Goal: Not generally used.

   OR

2. Reference Standard: A patient/client on parenteral nutrition support with an RQ of 1.04, which is above (above, below, within expected range) the expected range (0.7–1.0) with no apparent errors in the measurement.

Sample Nutrition Assessment	Monitoring and Evaluation Documentation
Initial nutrition assessment with patient/client	Patient/client's RQ is 1.04, with energy intake from parenteral nutrition 400 kcal (1,670 kJ) higher than measured metabolic rate. No apparent respiratory factors (hyper- or hypoventilation), equipment failure, measurement protocol violations, or operator errors. Will adjust content of parenteral nutrition and remeasure RQ.
Reassessment after nutrition intervention	RQ has dropped to 0.92 with no apparent measurement error. Metabolic rate and calorie/kcal/kJ intake are matched. Parenteral nutrition has been appropriately adjusted to equal patient/client's energy requirement.

Mineral Profile (BD-1.9)

Definition

Laboratory measures associated with body mineral status

Nutrition Assessment and Monitoring and Evaluation

Indicators

- Copper, serum or plasma (µg/dL or µmol/L)
- Iodine, urinary excretion (µg/24hr)
- Zinc, serum or plasma (µg/dL or µmol/L)
- Boron, serum or plasma (µg/L)
- Chromium, serum (ng/mL or nmol/L), urinary (µg/L)

- Fluoride, plasma (µmol/L)
- Manganese, urinary excretion (µg/L or nmol/L), blood (µg/L or nmol/L), plasma (µg/L or nmol/L)
- Molybdenum, serum (ng/mL)
- Selenium, serum (µmol/L), urinary excretion (µg/L or µg per day)

Note: Other measures of body mineral status, such as urinary manganese excretion, are provided to offer complete information in the reference sheet. These are rarely used in practice, but may be warranted in limited circumstances.

Serum calcium, magnesium, phosphorus, and potassium can be found on the Electrolyte and Renal Profile reference sheet.

Serum iron, serum ferritin, and transferrin saturation can be found on the Nutritional Anemia Profile reference sheet.

Thyroid stimulating hormone (↑ TSH as an indicator of excess iodine supplementation) can be found on the Glucose/Endocrine Profile reference sheet.

Examples of the measurement methods or data sources for these indicators: Biochemical measurement, laboratory record

Typically used with the following domains of nutrition interventions: Food and/or nutrient delivery, nutrition education, nutrition counseling

Typically used to determine and to monitor and evaluate change in the following nutrition diagnoses: Excessive or inadequate intake of minerals, parenteral nutrition

Note: Clinical judgment must be used to select indicators and determine the appropriate measurement techniques and reference standards for a given patient population and setting. Once identified, these indicators, measurement techniques, and reference standards should be identified in policies and procedures or other documents for use in patient/client records, quality or performance improvement, or in formal research projects.

Evaluation

Criteria for Evaluation

Comparison to Goal or Reference Standard:

1. Goal (tailored to patient/client's needs)

   OR

2. Reference Standard

Mineral Profile (BD-1.9)

Patient/Client Example

Example(s) of one or two of the Nutrition Care Indicators (includes sample initial and reassessment documentation for one of the indicators)

Indicator(s) Selected

Zinc, plasma (µg/dL)

Criteria for Evaluation

Comparison to Goal or Reference Standard:

1. Goal: There is no goal generally associated with mineral status.

   OR

2. Reference Standard: The patient/client's plasma zinc is 40 µg/dL, which is below (above, below, within expected range) the expected range (66–110 µg/dL) for adults.

Sample Nutrition Assessment	Monitoring and Evaluation Documentation
Initial nutrition assessment with patient/client	Patient/client's plasma zinc is 40 µg/dL, which is below the expected range for adults. Will monitor change in plasma zinc at next encounter.
Reassessment after nutrition intervention	Goal/reference standard achieved, as patient/client's plasma zinc is 90 µg/dL.

Nutritional Anemia Profile (BD-1.10)

Definition

Laboratory measures associated with nutritional anemias

Nutrition Assessment and Monitoring and Evaluation

Indicators

- Hemoglobin (g/dL, g/L, or mmol/L)
- Hematocrit (% or proportion of one [1])
- Mean corpuscular volume, MCV (fL)
- RBC folate (ng/mL or nmol/L)
- Red cell distribution width, RDW (%)
- Serum B12 (pg/mL or pmol/L)
- Methylmalonic acid, serum (nmol/L)

- Serum folate (ng/mL or nmol/L)
- Serum homocysteine (µmol/L)
- Serum ferritin (ng/mL or pmol/L)
- Serum iron (µg/dL or µmol/L)
- Total iron-binding capacity (µg/dL or µmol/L)
- Transferrin saturation (%)

Examples of the measurement methods or data sources for these indicators: Biochemical measurement, patient/client laboratory record, national/state/local nutrition monitoring and surveillance data

Typically used with the following domains of nutrition interventions: Food and/or nutrient delivery, nutrition education, nutrition counseling, coordination of nutrition care by nutrition professional

Typically used to determine and to monitor and evaluate change in the following nutrition diagnoses: Excessive or inadequate intake of vitamins or minerals (eg, iron, B12, folate); altered nutrition-related laboratory values; impaired nutrient utilization

> **Note:** Clinical judgment must be used to select indicators and determine the appropriate measurement techniques and reference standards for a given patient population and setting. Once identified, these indicators, measurement techniques, and reference standards should be identified in policies and procedures or other documents for use in patient/client records, quality or performance improvement, or in formal research projects.

Evaluation

Criteria for Evaluation

Comparison to Goal or Reference Standard:

1. Goal (tailored to patient/client's needs)
   OR
2. Reference Standard

Nutritional Anemia Profile (BD-1.10)

Patient/Client Example

Example(s) of one or two of the Nutrition Care Indicators (includes sample initial and reassessment documentation for one of the indicators)

Indicator(s) Selected

Hemoglobin (gm/dL)

Serum ferritin (ng/mL)

Criteria for Evaluation

Comparison to Goal or Reference Standard:

1. Goal: The patient/client's hemoglobin and hematocrit are below the expected limits for adult males, but are within the goal range for a patient/client receiving hemodialysis.

   OR

2. Reference Standard: The patient/client's serum ferritin is 8 ng/mL, which is below (above, below, or within expected range) the expected range for adult females.

Sample Nutrition Assessment	Monitoring and Evaluation Documentation
Initial nutrition assessment with patient/client	Patient/client's serum ferritin is 8 ng/mL, which is below the expected range for adult females. Will monitor change in serum ferritin at next encounter.
Reassessment after nutrition intervention	Patient/client's serum ferritin is 10.9 ng/mL, within the expected range.

Protein Profile (BD-1.11)

Definition

Laboratory measures associated with hepatic and circulating proteins and protein metabolism

Nutrition Assessment and Monitoring and Evaluation

Indicators

- Albumin (g/dL or g/L)
- Prealbumin (mg/dL or mg/L)
- Transferrin (mg/dL or g/L)
- Phenylalanine, plasma (mg/dL or µmol/L)
- Tyrosine, plasma (mg/dL or µmol/L)
- Amino acid panel (by report)
- Phenylalanine, dried blood spot (ordinal)
- Tyrosine, dried blood spot (ordinal)
- Phenylalanine:tyrosine ratio (ratio number)
- Hydroxyproline (mg/dL or µmol/L)
- Threonine (mg/dL or µmol/L)
- Serine (mg/dL or µmol/L)
- Asparagine (mg/dL or µmol/L)
- Glutamate (mg/dL or µmol/L)
- Glutamine (mg/dL or µmol/L)
- Proline (mg/dL or µmol/L)
- Glycine (mg/dL or µmol/L)
- Alanine (mg/dL or µmol/L)
- Citrulline (mg/dL or µmol/L)
- Valine (mg/dL or µmol/L)
- Cysteine (mg/dL or µmol/L)
- Methionine (mg/dL or µmol/L)
- Isoleucine (mg/dL or µmol/L)
- Leucine (mg/dL or µmol/L)
- Ornithine (mg/dL or µmol/L)
- Lysine (mg/dL or µmol/L)
- Histidine (mg/dL or µmol/L)
- Arginine (mg/dL or µmol/L)
- Lysine:arginine ratio (ratio number)
- Tryptophan, plasma or serum
- Plasma organic acid panel (by report)
- Organic acids/creatinine (mmol/mol creatinine)
- Lactate (mg/dL or µmol/L)
- Pyruvate (mg/dL or µmol/L)
- Lactate:pyruvate ratio (ratio number)
- 3-hydroxybutyrate (mg/dL or µmol/L)
- 3-hydroxyisovalerate (mg/dL or µmol/L)
- Acetoacetate (mg/dL or µmol/L)
- Ethylmalonate (mg/dL or µmol/L)
- Succinate (mg/dL or µmol/L)
- Fumarate (mg/dL or µmol/L)
- Glutarate (ng/dL or nmol/L)
- 3-methylglutarate (mg/dL or µmol/L)
- Adipate (mg/dL or µmol/L)
- 2-hydroxyglutarate (mg/dL or µmol/L)
- 3-hydroxypheylacetate (mg/dL or µmol/L)
- 2-ketoglutarate (mg/dL or µmol/L)
- Citrate (mg/dL or µmol/L)
- Propionate (mg/dL or µmol/L)
- Methylcitrate (mg/dL or µmol/L)
- 3-hydroxy propionate (mg/dL or µmol/L)
- ß-hydroxy butyrate (mg/dL or µmol/L)
- Creatine kinase (U/L)
- Troponin I cardiac (ng/mL)
- Troponin T cardiac (ng/mL)
- B-type natriuretic peptide (pg/mL)
- Succinylacetone (mg/dL or µmol/L)
- Total serum immunoglobulin A (IgA) (mg/dL or µmol/L)
- Tissue transglutaminase antibodies (IgA) (U/mL)
- Tissue transglutaminase antibodies (IgG) (U/mL)
- Deamidated gliadin peptide antibodies (IgG) (U/mL)
- Endomysial antibodies (ordinal)
- Carbohydrate-deficient transferrin (mg/dL or %)

Protein Profile (BD-1.11)

Assessment

Note: Methylmalonic acid can be found on the Nutritional Anemia Profile reference sheet. In the past, hepatic transport protein measures (eg, albumin and prealbumin) were used as indicators of malnutrition. See the Evidence Analysis Library questions on this topic at https://www.andevidencelibrary.com/topic.cfm?cat=4302.

Examples of the measurement methods or data sources for these indicators: Biochemical measurement, laboratory report

Typically used with the following domains of nutrition interventions: Food and/or nutrient delivery, nutrition education, nutrition counseling, coordination of nutrition care by nutrition professional

Typically used to determine and to monitor and evaluate change in the following nutrition diagnoses: Increased nutrient needs, malnutrition, inadequate enteral/parenteral nutrition infusion

Note: Clinical judgment must be used to select indicators and determine the appropriate measurement techniques and reference standards for a given patient population and setting. Once identified, these indicators, measurement techniques, and reference standards should be identified in policies and procedures or other documents for use in patient/client records, quality or performance improvement, or in formal research projects.

Evaluation

Criteria for Evaluation

Comparison to Goal or Reference Standard:

1. Goal (tailored to patient/client's needs)

   OR

2. Reference Standard

Patient/Client Example

Example(s) of one or two of the Nutrition Care Indicators (includes sample initial and reassessment documentation for one of the indicators)

Indicator(s) Selected

Prealbumin (mg/dL)

Criteria for Evaluation

Comparison to Goal or Reference Standard:

1. Goal: Not generally used.

   OR

2. Reference Standard: The patient/client's prealbumin is 7 mg/dL, which is below (above, below, or within the expected range) the expected range (16–40 mg/dL) for adults.

Protein Profile (BD-1.11)

Sample Nutrition Assessment	Monitoring and Evaluation Documentation
Initial nutrition assessment with patient/client	Patient/client's prealbumin is 7.0 mg/dL, below the expected range (16–40 mg/dL) for adults. Will monitor change in prealbumin at next encounter.
Reassessment after nutrition intervention	Significant progress toward expected range, as patient/client's serum prealbumin is 13.0 mg/dL.

Urine Profile (BD-1.12)

Assessment

Definition

Physical and/or chemical properties of urine

Nutrition Assessment and Monitoring and Evaluation

Indicators

- Urine color (by visualization)
- Urine osmolality (mOsm/kg H2O)
- Urine specific gravity (number)
- Urine volume (mL/24 hours; however, in certain populations, eg, infants, this indicator may be reported in number of wet diapers/day)
- Urine calcium, 24 hour (mg/day or mmol/day)
- Urine d-xylose (mg/dL or mmol/L)
- Urine glucose (ordinal)
- Urine ketones (ordinal)
- Urine sodium (mg/dL or mmol/L)
- Urine microalbumin (mg/dL or mmol/L)
- Urine protein, random (mg/dL or mmol/L)
- Urine protein, 24 hour (mg/day or mmol/day)
- Urine uric acid, random (mg/dL or µmol/L)
- Urine uric acid, 24 hour (mg/day or mmol/day)
- Urine organic acid panel (by report)
- Urine glutarate (ordinal)
- Urine methylmalonate (µg/dL)
- Urine acylglycines/creatinine (mg/g creatinine or mmol/mol creatinine)
- Urine argininosuccinate (mmol/L)
- Urine succinylacetone/creatinine (µmol/mmol creatinine)
- Urine orotate (µmol/L)
- Urine orotate/creatinine (µmol/mmol creatinine)
- Urine 2-hydroxyisovalerate (ordinal)
- Urine 2-oxoisovalerate (ordinal)
- Urine galactitol (ordinal)
- Urine reducing substances (ordinal)
- Urine porphyrins (ordinal)

Examples of the measurement methods or data sources for these indicators: Observation, biochemical measurement, laboratory report, patient/client report

Typically used with the following domains of nutrition interventions: Food and/or nutrient delivery, nutrition education, nutrition counseling, coordination of nutrition care by nutrition professional

Typically used to determine and to monitor and evaluate change in the following nutrition diagnoses: Inadequate or excessive fluid intake, inadequate or excessive enteral/parenteral nutrition infusion

Note: Clinical judgment must be used to select indicators and determine the appropriate measurement techniques and reference standards for a given patient population and setting. Once identified, these indicators, measurement techniques, and reference standards should be identified in policies and procedures or other documents for use in patient/client records, quality or performance improvement, or in formal research projects.

Urine Profile (BD-1.12)

Evaluation

Criteria for Evaluation

Comparison to Goal or Reference Standard:

1. Goal (tailored to patient/client's needs)

   OR

2. Reference Standard

Patient/Client Example

Example(s) of one or two of the Nutrition Care Indicators (includes sample initial and reassessment documentation for one of the indicators)

Indicator(s) Selected

Urine specific gravity

Criteria for Evaluation

Comparison to Goal or Reference Standard:

1. Goal: Not generally used for this indicator.

   OR

2. Reference Standard: The patient/client's urine specific gravity is 1.050, which is above (above, below, within expected range) the expected range (1.003–1.030).

Sample Nutrition Assessment	Monitoring and Evaluation Documentation
Initial nutrition assessment with patient/client	Patient/client's urine specific gravity is 1.050, which is above the expected range. Will monitor change in urine specific gravity at next encounter.
Reassessment after nutrition intervention	Significant progress toward goal; patient/client's urine specific gravity is 1.025 which is within the expected range.

Vitamin Profile (BD-1.13)

Definition

Laboratory measures associated with body vitamin status

Nutrition Assessment and Monitoring and Evaluation

Indicators

- Vitamin A, serum or plasma retinol (µg/dL or µmol/L)
- Vitamin C, plasma or serum (mg/dL or µmol/L)
- Vitamin D, 25-hydroxy (ng/mL or nmol/L)
- Vitamin E, plasma alpha tocopherol (mg/dL or µmol/L)
- Thiamin, activity coefficient for erythrocyte transketolase activity (µg/mL/hr)
- Riboflavin, activity coefficient for erythrocyte glutathione reductase activity (IU/g hemoglobin)
- Niacin, urinary N'methyl-nicotinamide concentration (µmol/day)
- Vitamin B6, plasma or serum pyridoxal 5'phosphate concentration (ng/mL or nmol/L)
- Pantothenic acid, urinary pantothenate excretion (mg/day), plasma (ng/mL or nmol/L)
- Biotin, urinary 3-hydroxyisovaleric acid excretion (mmol/mmol creatinine)
- Biotin, lymphocyte propionyl-CoA carboxylase in pregnancy [pmol/(min × mg)], serum (ng/mL or nmol/L)
- Biotinidase (U/L)
- Protein induced by vitamin K absence or antagonist II (PIVKA-II) (ng/mL or nmol/L)

Note: Other measures of body vitamin status, such as urinary pantothenate excretion, are provided to offer complete information in the reference sheet. These are rarely used in practice but may be warranted in limited circumstances.

Measures for folate and vitamin B12 can be found on the Nutritional Anemia Profile reference sheet.

Measures related to vitamin K (PT, PTT, INR) can be found on the GI Profile reference sheet.

A test for choline is not available. According to the DRIs, it should be evaluated in light of serum alanine amino transferase (ALT) levels, which can be found on the GI Profile (BD-1.4) reference sheet.

Examples of the measurement methods or data sources for these indicators: Biochemical measurement, patient/client record

Typically used with the following domains of nutrition interventions: Food and/or nutrient delivery, coordination of nutrition care by nutrition professional

Typically used to determine and to monitor and evaluate change in the following nutrition diagnoses: Excessive or inadequate intake of vitamins

Note: Clinical judgment must be used to select indicators and determine the appropriate measurement techniques and reference standards for a given patient population and setting. Once identified, these indicators, measurement techniques, and reference standards should be identified in policies and procedures or other documents for use in patient/client records, quality or performance improvement, or in formal research projects.

Vitamin Profile (BD-1.13)

Evaluation

Criteria for Evaluation

Comparison to Goal or Reference Standard:

1. Goal (tailored to patient/client's needs)

   OR

2. Reference Standard

Patient/Client Example

Example(s) of one or two of the Nutrition Care Indicators (includes sample initial and reassessment documentation for one of the indicators)

Indicator(s) Selected

Vitamin A, serum retinol (µg/dL)

Criteria for Evaluation

Comparison to Goal or Reference Standard:

1. Goal: Not generally used for this indicator.

   OR

2. Reference Standard: The patient/client's serum retinol is 95 µg/dL, which is above (above, below, within expected range) the expected range (10–60 µg/dL).

Sample Nutrition Assessment	Monitoring and Evaluation Documentation
Initial nutrition assessment with patient/client	Patient/client's serum retinol is 95 µg/dL, which is above the expected range. Will monitor change in serum retinol at next encounter, along with vitamin A and beta-carotene intake.
Reassessment after nutrition intervention	Significant progress toward expected range. Patient/client's retinol is 70 µg/dL.

Nutrition-Focused Physical Findings (PD-1.1)

Definition

Nutrition-related physical signs or symptoms associated with pathophysiological states derived from a nutrition-focused physical exam, interview, and/or the health record

Nutrition Assessment and Monitoring and Evaluation

Indicators

Note: Presence or absence unless otherwise specified.

- Overall appearance
  - Asthenia (weakness)
  - Buffalo hump
  - Cachexia
  - Cushingoid appearance
  - Ectomorph
  - Endomorph
  - Lethargic
  - Mesomorph
  - Neglect of personal hygiene
  - Obese
  - Short stature for age
  - Tall stature
- Adipose
  - Atrophy of orbital fat
  - Excess subcutaneous fat
  - Loss of subcutaneous fat
  - Central adiposity
  - Loss of subcutaneous triceps fat
  - Loss of subcutaneous biceps fat
  - Loss of subcutaneous fat overlying the ribs
- Bones
  - Bow legs
  - Frontal bossing
  - Harrison's sulcus
  - Rachitic rosary
  - Rickets
  - Scoliosis
  - Acromion abnormal prominence
  - Bone widening at ends
  - Clavicle abnormal prominence
  - Rib abnormal prominence
  - Scapula abnormal prominence
  - Spine abnormal prominence
  - Iliac crest abnormal prominence
  - Patella abnormal prominence
- Cardiovascular–pulmonary system
  - Absent breath sounds
  - Bradycardia
  - Bradypnea (slow respiration)
  - Decreased breath sounds
  - Dyspnea (shortness of breath)
  - Increased breath sounds
  - Normal breath sounds
  - Tachypnea
  - Tachycardia
  - Respiratory crackles (rales)
- Digestive system
  - Abdominal bloating
  - Abdominal cramping
  - Abdominal distension
  - Abdominal pain
  - Absence of bowel sounds
  - Anorexia (loss of appetite)
  - Ascites
  - Bulky stool
  - Constipation
  - Decrease in appetite
  - Diarrhea
  - Early satiety

Nutrition-Focused Physical Findings (PD-1.1)

- ○ Epigastric pain
- ○ Excessive appetite
- ○ Excessive belching
- ○ Excessive flatus
- ○ Fatty stool
- ○ Heartburn
- ○ Hyperactive bowel sounds
- ○ Hypoactive bowel sounds
- ○ Increased appetite
- ○ Liquid stool
- ○ Loose stool
- ○ Nausea
- ○ Normal bowel sounds
- ○ Retching
- ○ Vomiting
- ○ Gastrointestinal drainage volume
- ○ Gastric drainage volume
- ○ Bile duct drainage volume
- ○ Pancreatic drainage volume
- ○ Wound drainage volume
- ○ Intestinal fistula drainage volume
- Edema
  - ○ +1 pitting edema
  - ○ +2 pitting edema
  - ○ +3 pitting edema
  - ○ +4 pitting edema
  - ○ Anasarca
  - ○ Ankle edema
  - ○ Edema of calf
  - ○ Edema of eyelid
  - ○ Edema of foot
  - ○ Edema of the hand
  - ○ Edema of the scrotum
  - ○ Edema of thigh
  - ○ Edema of the vulva
  - ○ Mucosal edema
  - ○ Sacral edema
- Extremities
  - ○ Amputated foot
  - ○ Amputated hand

- ○ Amputated leg
- ○ Athetoid movement
- ○ Decreased range of ankle movement
- ○ Decreased range of cervical spine movement
- ○ Decreased range of elbow movement
- ○ Decreased range of finger movement
- ○ Decreased range of foot movement
- ○ Decreased range of hip movement
- ○ Decreased range of knee movement
- ○ Decreased range of lumbar spine movement
- ○ Decreased range of shoulder movement
- ○ Decreased range of subtalar movement
- ○ Decreased range of thumb movement
- ○ Decreased range of toe movement
- ○ Decreased range of thoracic spine movement
- ○ Decreased range of wrist movement
- ○ Hypertonia
- ○ Hypotonia
- ○ Joint arthralgia (joint pain)
- ○ Lower limb spasticity
- ○ Peripheral cyanosis
- ○ Spasticity
- ○ Tetany
- ○ Upper limb spasticity
- Eyes
  - ○ Abnormal vision
  - ○ Angular blepharitis
  - ○ Bitot's spots
  - ○ Circles under eyes
  - ○ Corneal arcus
  - ○ Conjunctival discoloration
  - ○ Conjunctival hemorrhage
  - ○ Conjunctival keratinization
  - ○ Excessive tear production
  - ○ Keratomalacia
  - ○ Jaundiced sclera
  - ○ Night blindness
  - ○ Ophthalmoplegia
  - ○ Sunken eyes
  - ○ Xerophthalmia

Nutrition-Focused Physical Findings (PD-1.1)

- Xanthelasma
- Pale conjunctiva
- Genitourinary
  - Amenorrhea
  - Anuria
  - Delay in sexual development and/or puberty
  - Menorrhagia
  - Oliguria
  - Polyuria
- Hair
  - Abnormal keratinization of hair follicle
  - Alopecia
  - Brittle hair
  - Corkscrew hairs
  - Dry hair
  - Fine hair
  - Follicular hyperkeratosis
  - Hair changes due to malnutrition
  - Hair lacks luster
  - Hypertrichosis
  - Increased loss of hair
  - Nutritional hair color change
  - White hair
  - Easily pluckable hair
  - Lanugo hair formation
- Head
  - Altered olfactory sense
  - Anosmia (loss of sense of smell)
  - Bulging fontanelle
  - Epistaxis
  - Headache
  - Hyposmia (decreased sense of smell)
  - Macrocephaly
  - Microcephaly
  - Nasal mucosa dry
  - Sunken fontanelle
- Hand and nails
  - Beau's lines
  - Clubbing of nails
  - Flaking of nails

- Koilonychia (spoon shaped nails)
- Leukonychia
- Longitudinal grooving of nails
- Muehrcke's lines
- Nail changes
- Palmar erythema
- Ridged nails
- Splits in nails
- Thin nails
- Trachyonychia (brittle nails)
- Splinter hemorrhages under nail
- White flecks in nails
- Blue nail beds
- Pale nail beds
- Russell's sign
- Mouth
  - Ageusia (loss of taste)
  - Angular stomatitis
  - Aphthous ulcer of mouth
  - Aptyalism (xerostomia)
  - Blue lips
  - Blue line on gingiva
  - Candidiasis of the mouth
  - Cheilosis (dry lips)
  - Cheilitis
  - Cleft palate
  - Cracked lips
  - Drooling
  - Dry mucus membranes
  - Dysgeusia
  - Excessive salivation
  - Excessive thirst
  - Gingival hypertrophy
  - Gingivitis
  - Halitosis (breath smells unpleasant)
  - Hemorrhagic gingivitis (bleeding gums)
  - Hypogeusia
  - Ketotic breath
  - Micrognathia
  - Swollen gums

Nutrition-Focused Physical Findings (PD-1.1)

- o Oral candidiasis
- o Oral lesion
- o Parotid swelling
- o Poor oral hygiene
- o Retains food in mouth
- o Stomatitis
- o Uremic breath
- o Pale gums
- Muscles
  - o Muscle atrophy
  - o Muscle contracture
  - o Muscle cramp
  - o Muscle pain
  - o Muscle weakness
  - o Quadricep muscle atrophy
  - o Deltoid muscle atrophy
  - o Gastrocnemius (calf) muscle atrophy
  - o Gluteal muscle atrophy
  - o Interosseous hand muscle atrophy
  - o Latissiumus dorsi muscle atrophy
  - o Pectoral muscle atrophy
  - o Temporalis muscle atrophy
  - o Trapezius muscle atrophy
- Neck
  - o Goiter (thyroid enlargement)
- Nerves, cognition, and feeling
  - o Abnormal gait
  - o Absent reflex
  - o Asterixis
  - o Ataxia
  - o Clouded consciousness (confusion)
  - o Cranial nerve finding
  - o Decreased vibratory sense
  - o Delirious
  - o Dementia
  - o Depressed mood
  - o Disoriented
  - o Dizziness
  - o Feels cold
  - o Flat affect
  - o Hyperreflexia (exaggeration of deep reflexes)
  - o Hyporeflexia (diminished reflexes)
  - o Inappropriate affect
  - o Many seizures a day
  - o Numbness of foot
  - o Numbness of hand
  - o Peripheral nerve disease
  - o Tremor of outstretched hand
  - o Tingling of foot
  - o Tingling of hand
- Skin
  - o Acanthosis nigricans
  - o Calcinosis
  - o Carotenemia
  - o Cutaneous xanthoma
  - o Decreased skin turgor
  - o Dermatitis
  - o Diaper rash
  - o Dry skin
  - o Ecchymosis
  - o Erythema
  - o Eczema
  - o Flushing
  - o Hirsutism
  - o Hyperpigmentation of skin
  - o Impaired skin integrity
  - o Jaundice
  - o Keratinization of skin
  - o Pale complexion
  - o Peeling skin
  - o Petechiae
  - o Impaired wound healing
  - o Pressure injury of ankles
  - o Pressure injury of back
  - o Pressure injury of breast
  - o Pressure injury of buttock
  - o Pressure injury of dorsum of foot
  - o Pressure injury of elbow
  - o Pressure injury of head
  - o Pressure injury of heel

Nutrition-Focused Physical Findings (PD-1.1)

- o Pressure injury of hip
- o Pressure injury of knee
- o Pressure injury of natal cleft
- o Pressure injury of shoulder
- o Pressure injury stage 1
- o Pressure injury stage 2
- o Pressure injury stage 3
- o Pressure injury stage 4
- o Pruritus of the skin
- o Psoriasis
- o Scaly skin
- o Seborrheic dermatitis
- o Skin rash
- o Stasis ulcer
- o Yellow skin
- o Perifollicular hemorrhages
- o Pressure injury of the coccyx
- o Pressure injury of the sacrum
- o Vesiculobullous rash
- Teeth
  - o Baby bottle tooth decay
  - o Broken denture
  - o Broken teeth
  - o Dental caries
  - o Dental fluorosis
  - o Dental plaque
  - o Denture loose
  - o Denture lost
  - o Denture present
  - o Edentulous
  - o Erosion of teeth
  - o Impaired dentition
  - o Ill fitting denture
  - o Mottling of enamel
  - o Partially edentulous mandible
  - o Partially edentulous maxilla
  - o Rampant dental caries
- Throat and swallowing
  - o Choking during swallowing

- o Cough
- o Dysphagia
- o Esophageal lesion
- o Food sticks on swallowing
- o Gagging
- o Hoarse voice
- o Hypoactive gag reflex
- o Odynophagia (painful swallowing)
- o Swallow impairment
- o Suck, swallow, breath incoordination (infants)
- o Wet voice
- Tongue
  - o Atrophy of tongue papillae
  - o Beefy red tongue
  - o Difficulty moving tongue
  - o Dry tongue
  - o Glossitis
  - o Glossodynia (painful tongue)
  - o Hypertrophy of tongue papillae
  - o Lesion of the tongue
  - o Macroglossia
  - o Strawberry tongue
  - o Short frenulum of tongue
  - o Split frenulum of tongue
  - o Blue tongue
  - o Cracked tongue
  - o Magenta tongue
  - o Pale tongue
- Vital signs
  - o Blood pressure
  - o Heart rate
  - o Jugular venous pressure
  - o Mean arterial pressure
  - o Pulse rate
  - o Respiratory rate
  - o Temperature

Nutrition-Focused Physical Findings (PD-1.1)

Examples of the measurement methods or data sources for these indicators: Direct observation, patient/client report, health record

Typically used with the following domains of nutrition interventions: Food and nutrient delivery, nutrition education, nutrition counseling, coordination of nutrition care by nutrition professional

Typically used to determine and to monitor and evaluate change in the following nutrition diagnoses: Excessive or inadequate intake of vitamins/minerals, or fluid, parenteral/enteral nutrition; overweight/obesity; underweight; unintended weight loss; malnutrition (undernutrition)

> **Note:** Clinical judgment must be used to select indicators and determine the appropriate measurement techniques and reference standards for a given patient population and setting. Once identified, these indicators, measurement techniques, and reference standards should be identified in policies and procedures or other documents for use in patient/client records, quality or performance improvement, or in formal research projects.

Evaluation

Criteria for Evaluation

Comparison to Goal or Reference Standard:

1. Goal (tailored to patient/client's needs)

   OR

2. Reference Standard

Patient/Client Example

Example(s) of one or two of the Nutrition Care Indicators (includes sample initial and reassessment documentation for one of the indicators)

Indicator(s) Selected

Muscle atrophy

Loss of subcutaneous fat

Criteria for Evaluation

Comparison to Goal or Reference Standard:

1. Goal: The patient/client maintains or gains muscle and subcutaneous fat (as appropriate) as determined by a nutrition focused physical exam.

   OR

2. Reference Standard: The patient/client's muscle atrophy and subcutaneous fat loss are mild undernutrition in the context of acute illness or injury, which is consistent with the nutrition diagnosis of non-severe (moderate) malnutrition. Normal reference standard is no muscle atrophy and fat pads slightly bulged.

Nutrition-Focused Physical Findings (PD-1.1)

Assessment

Sample Nutrition Assessment	Monitoring and Evaluation Documentation
Initial nutrition assessment with patient/client	Patient/client's muscle atrophy and subcutaneous fat loss is mild, which is abnormal for a well-nourished individual and consistent with non-severe (moderate) malnutrition. Will monitor for adequate protein-calorie intake and changes in muscle and subcutaneous fat status at next encounter.
Reassessment after nutrition intervention	Progress toward maintaining or gaining of muscle mass and (as appropriate) subcutaneous fat. Patient/client's muscle and subcutaneous fat status is improved upon re-assessment by nutrition focused physical exam.

Personal Data (CH-1.1)

Definition

General patient/client information such as age, gender, sex, race, ethnicity, occupation, tobacco use, and physical disability

Nutrition Assessment and Monitoring and Evaluation

Indicators

Age***
- Age in days (neonates)***
- Age in months (up to 36 months)***
- Age in years***
- Other (eg, age adjusted)***

Gender*** (as the behavioral, cultural, or psychological traits typically associated with one sex)
- Female***
- Male***

Sex*** (as female or male based upon reproductive organs and structures)
- Female***
- Male***

Race*** (a group of people connected by common descent or origin)
- American Indian or Alaska Native***
- Asian***
- Black or African American***
- Native Hawaiian or Other Pacific Islander***
- White***
- Other***

Ethnicity*** (pertaining to or having common racial, cultural, religious, or linguistic characteristics)
- Hispanic or Latino***
- Not Hispanic or Latino***
- Other***

Language***
- English***
- Spanish***
- Other (specify)***

Literacy factors***
- Language barrier***
- Low literacy***

Education***
- Years of education***

Role in family***
- Specify* (patient/client's reported role, eg, mother, cousin, in the description of his/her family)

Tobacco use***
- Yes***
  - Average number of cigarettes smoked per day (number per day)***
  - Total number of other tobacco products used per day (number per day)***
  - Number years tobacco products used on a regular basis (years)***
- No***

Physical disability***
- Eyesight impaired***
- Hearing impaired***
- Other (specify)***

Mobility***
- House bound***
- Bed or chair bound***
- Tremors (Parkinson's)***

Other (specify)***

***Indicator is used for nutrition assessment only. Other indicators are used for both nutrition assessment and nutrition monitoring and evaluation.

Personal Data (CH-1.1)

Assessment

Examples of the measurement methods or data sources for these outcome indicators: Patient/client report, medical record, referring health care provider or agency, surveys, administrative data sets

Typically used with the following domains of nutrition interventions: Food and/or nutrient delivery, nutrition education, nutrition counseling, coordination of nutrition care by nutrition professional

Typically used to determine and to monitor and evaluate change in the following nutrition diagnoses: N/A

> **Note:** Clinical judgment must be used to select indicators and determine the appropriate measurement techniques and reference standards for a given patient population and setting. Once identified, these indicators, measurement techniques, and reference standards should be identified in policies and procedures or other documents for use in patient/client records, quality or performance improvement, or in formal research projects.

Evaluation

Criteria for Evaluation

Comparison to Goal or Reference Standard:

1. Goal (tailored to patient/client's needs)

   OR

2. Reference Standard

Patient/Client Example(s)

Example(s) of one or two of the Nutrition Care Indicators (includes sample initial assessment documentation for one of the indicators)

Indicator(s) Selected

Age, sex, and education level

Criteria for Evaluation

Comparison to Goal or Reference Standard:

1. Goal: Not typically used

   OR

2. Reference Standard: No standard exists

Sample Nutrition Assessment	Monitoring and Evaluation Documentation
Initial nutrition assessment with patient/client	Patient/client is a 40-year-old male with new onset type 2 diabetes and a 7th-grade education level.

Patient/Client or Family Nutrition-Oriented Medical/Health History (CH-2.1)

Definition

Patient/client or family member disease states, conditions, and illnesses that may impact nutritional status

Nutrition Assessment

Indicators

- Patient/client chief nutrition complaint (specify)***
- Cardiovascular***
  - Cardiovascular disease***
  - Congestive heart failure***
  - Hyperlipidemia***
  - Hypertension***
  - Stroke***
  - Other***
- Endocrine/metabolism***
  - Cystic fibrosis***
  - Diabetes mellitus***
  - Diabetes, gestational***
  - Inborn errors***
  - Malnutrition/failure to thrive***
  - Metabolic syndrome***
  - Obesity***
  - Overweight (specify duration)***
  - Other (specify)***
- Excretory***
  - Dehydration***
  - Renal failure, acute***
  - Renal failure, chronic***
  - Other (specify)***
- Gastrointestinal***
  - Crohn's disease***
  - Diverticulitis/osis***
  - Dyspepsia***
  - Inflammatory bowel disease***
  - Lactase deficiency***
  - Liver disease***

- Pancreatic disease (specify)***
- Other (specify)***
- Gynecological***
  - Amenorrhea***
  - Lactating***
  - Mastitis***
  - Perimenopausal/postmenopausal***
  - Pregnant***
    - Gestational age (weeks)***
    - Single fetus***
    - Multiple fetuses (specify)***
  - Other (specify)***
- Hematology/oncology***
  - Anemia (specify)***
  - Cancer (specify)***
  - Other (specify)***
- Immune***
  - AIDS/HIV***
  - Food allergies***
  - Sepsis/severe infection***
  - Other (specify)***
- Integumentary***
  - Burns***
  - Other (specify)***
- Musculoskeletal***
  - Multiple traumas/fractures***
  - Osteoporosis***
  - Other (specify)***
- Neurological***
  - Developmental delay***

***Indicator is used for nutrition assessment only. Other indicators are used for both nutrition assessment and nutrition monitoring and evaluation.

Patient/Client or Family Nutrition-Oriented Medical/Health History (CH-2.1)

- o Other (specify)***
- Psychological***
  - o Alcoholism***
  - o Cognitive impairment***
  - o Dementia/Alzheimer's***
  - o Depression***
  - o Eating disorder (specify)***

- o Psychosis***
- o Other (specify)***
- Respiratory***
  - o Chronic obstructive pulmonary disease***
  - o Other (specify)***
- Other***

Examples of the measurement methods or data sources for these outcome indicators: Medical record, referring health care provider or agency

Typically used with the following domains of nutrition interventions: Nutrition education, nutrition counseling

Typically used to determine and to monitor and evaluate change in the following nutrition diagnoses: All

> **Note:** Clinical judgment must be used to select indicators and determine the appropriate measurement techniques and reference standards for a given patient population and setting. Once identified, these indicators, measurement techniques, and reference standards should be identified in policies and procedures or other documents for use in patient/client records, quality or performance improvement, or in formal research projects.

Evaluation

Criteria for Evaluation

Comparison to Goal or Reference Standard:

1. Goal (tailored to patient/client's needs)

   OR

2. Reference Standard

Patient Example(s)

Example(s) of one or two of the Nutrition Care Indicators (includes sample initial assessment documentation for one of the indicators)

Indicator(s) Selected

Cardiovascular disease (CVD)

Criteria for Evaluation

Comparison to Goal or Reference Standard:

1. Goal: Not typically used

   OR

2. Reference Standard: No reference standard exists.

***Indicator is used for nutrition assessment only. Other indicators are used for both nutrition assessment and nutrition monitoring and evaluation.

Patient/Client or Family Nutrition-Oriented Medical/Health History (CH-2.1)

Sample Nutrition Assessment	Monitoring and Evaluation Documentation
Initial nutrition assessment with patient/client	Patient/client with history of CVD. Recommend the Therapeutic Lifestyle Changes (TLC) diet in accordance with the reference standard (eg, NHLBI Adult Treatment Panel III guidelines).

Treatments/Therapy (CH-2.2)

Definition

Documented medical or surgical treatments that may impact nutritional status of the patient/client

Nutrition Assessment

Indicators

- Medical treatment/therapy***
  - Chemotherapy***
  - Dialysis***
  - Mechanical ventilation/oxygen therapy***
  - Ostomy (specify)***
  - Radiation therapy***
  - Other (specify, eg, speech, OT, PT)***
- Surgical treatment***
  - Coronary artery bypass (CABG)***
  - Gastric bypass (specify type)***
  - Intestinal resection***
  - Joint/orthopedic surgery/replacement***
  - Limb amputation***
  - Organ transplant (specify)***
  - Total gastrectomy***
  - Other (specify)***
- Palliative/end-of-life care (care of patient/client with terminal or life-threatening condition)***

Examples of the measurement methods or data sources for these indicators: Patient/client interview, medical record, referring health care provider or agency

Typically used with the following domains of nutrition interventions: Food and/or nutrient delivery, nutrition education, nutrition counseling, coordination of nutrition care by nutrition professional

Typically used to determine and to monitor and evaluate change in the following nutrition diagnoses: Impaired nutrient utilization, increased nutrient needs, altered gastrointestinal function, biting/chewing (masticatory) difficulty, unintended weight loss.

Note: Clinical judgment must be used to select indicators and determine the appropriate measurement techniques and reference standards for a given patient population and setting. Once identified, these indicators, measurement techniques, and reference standards should be identified in policies and procedures or other documents for use in patient/client records, quality or performance improvement, or in formal research projects.

***Indicator is used for nutrition assessment only. Other indicators are used for both nutrition assessment and nutrition monitoring and evaluation.

Assessment

Treatments/Therapy (CH-2.2)

Evaluation

Criteria for Evaluation

Comparison to Goal or Reference Standard:

1. Goal (tailored to patient/client's needs)

   OR

2. Reference Standard

Patient/Client Example(s)

Example(s) of one or two of the Nutrition Care Indicators (includes sample initial assessment documentation for one of the indicators)

Indicator(s) Selected

Radiation therapy

Criteria for Evaluation

Comparison to Goal or Reference Standard:

1. Goal: Patient/client receiving radiation therapy for lung cancer and experiencing decreased appetite and pain with eating. Goal is to optimize nutrition during radiation therapy.

   OR

2. Reference Standard: No standards exist.

Sample Nutrition Assessment	Monitoring and Evaluation Documentation
Initial nutrition assessment with patient/client	Patient/client receiving radiation therapy for lung cancer and experiencing decreased appetite due to fatigue and pain with eating.

Social History (CH-3.1)

Assessment

Definition

Patient/client socioeconomic status, housing situation, medical support, and involvement in social groups

Nutrition Assessment

Indicators

- Socioeconomic factors***
  - Economic constraints (major/minor)***
  - Access to medical care (full/limited/none)***
  - Diverts food money to other needs***
  - Other (specify)***
- Living/housing situation***
  - Lives alone***
  - Lives with family member/caregiver***
  - Homeless***
- Domestic issues***
  - Specify***
- Social and medical support***
  - Family members***
  - Caregivers***
  - Community group/senior center/church***
  - Support group attendance (eg, weight control, substance abuse, etc)***
  - Other (specify)***
- Geographic location of home***
  - Urban***
  - Rural***
- Limited exposure to sunlight (vitamin D)***
- Other (specify)***
- Occupation***
  - Stay-at-home mother***
  - Student***
  - Retired***
  - Specify***
- Religion***
  - Catholic***
  - Jewish***
  - Protestant***
- Specify***
  - Islam***
  - Specify***
- History of recent crisis***
  - Job loss***
  - Family member death***
  - Trauma, surgery***
  - Other (specify)***
- Daily stress level (high, moderate, low bodily or mental tension)***

Examples of the measurement methods or data sources for these outcome indicators: Patient/client report, medical record, referring health care provider or agency

Typically used with the following domains of nutrition interventions: Food and/or nutrient delivery, nutrition education, nutrition counseling, coordination of nutrition care by nutrition professional

Typically used to determine and to monitor and evaluate change in the following nutrition diagnoses: All

Note: Clinical judgment must be used to select indicators and determine the appropriate measurement techniques and reference standards for a given patient population and setting. Once identified, these indicators, measurement techniques, and reference standards should be identified in policies and procedures or other documents for use in patient/client records, quality or performance improvement, or in formal research projects.

***Indicator is used for nutrition assessment only. Other indicators are used for both nutrition assessment and nutrition monitoring and evaluation.

Social History (CH-3.1)

Evaluation

Criteria for Evaluation

Comparison to Goal or Reference Standard:

1. Goal (tailored to patient/client's needs)

   OR

2. Reference Standard

Patient/Client Example(s)

Example(s) of one or two of the Nutrition Care Indicators (includes sample initial assessment documentation for one of the indicators)

Indicator

Living/housing situation and geographic location of home

Criteria for Evaluation

Comparison to Goal or Reference Standard:

1. Goal: Not typically used

   OR

2. Reference Standard: No reference standard exists.

Sample Nutrition Assessment	Monitoring and Evaluation Documentation
Initial nutrition assessment with patient/client	Patient/client is house bound, lives in a rural area, and receives one meal/day from Meals on Wheels.

Estimated Energy Needs (CS-1.1)

Definition

Estimated quantity of total energy needed for nutritional adequacy

Purpose

Identify appropriate reference standard of energy intake needs for individual patients/clients. Utilized as a basis of comparison to assess adequacy or excessiveness of patient/client's estimated total energy intake as compared to estimated needs and for development of the nutrition prescription

Indicators

- Total energy estimated needs in 24 hours (specify, eg, calories, kcal, or kJ/day)—defined as the estimated quantity of total energy needed for nutritional adequacy in one day
- Total energy estimated needs per kg body weight: (specify, eg, calories, kcal, or kJ/kg/day)

	EAR	RDA	AI	UL	Other
Energy*					Formula

EAR	—	Estimated Average Requirement
RDA	—	Recommended Dietary Allowance
AI	—	Adequate Intake
UL	—	Tolerable Upper Intake Level

*See DRI interpretation table.

- Method for estimating total energy needs: (specify, eg, patient/client goal or nutrition prescription, equation/method of adjustments—for example, for activity, stress, pregnancy, breastfeeding, fever)—defined as the approach for estimating total energy needs for one day

Note: Comparison to the Dietary Reference Intakes is assumed, but other reference intake standards may be used.

Estimated Fat Needs (CS-2.1)

Definition

Estimated quantity of total and/or type of fat intake needed for nutritional adequacy

Purpose

Identify appropriate reference standard of fat intake needs for individual patients/clients. Utilized as a basis of comparison to assess adequacy or excessiveness of patient/client's estimated total fat intake as compared to needs and for development of the nutrition prescription

Indicators

- Total fat estimated needs in 24 hours (specify, eg, g/day)—defined as the total fat needed for nutritional adequacy in one day

Macronutrients*	EAR	RDA	AI	UL	Other
Fat			X Infants only		Acceptable Macronutrient Distribution Range (AMDR) (children and adults)
n-6 polyunsaturated fatty acids (alpha linolenic acid)			X (All ages)		Acceptable Macronutrient Distribution Range (AMDR) (children and adults)
n-3 polyunsaturated fatty acids (alpha linolenic acid)			X (All ages)		Acceptable Macronutrient Distribution Range (AMDR) (children and adults)
Dietary cholesterol Trans fatty acids Saturated fatty acids					As low as possible while consuming a nutritionally adequate diet

EAR — Estimated Average Requirement

RDA — Recommended Dietary Allowance

AI — Adequate Intake

UL — Tolerable Upper Intake Level

*See DRI interpretation table.

- Total fat estimated need per kilogram of body weight (specify, eg, calories, kcal, or kJ/kg/day)—defined as the estimated quantity of total fat needed for nutrition adequacy for each kg of body weight in one day
- Method for estimating total fat needs (specify, eg, patient/client goal or nutrition prescription, disease/condition-based reference standard, Dietary Reference Intake)—defined as the approach for estimating total fat needs for one day
- Proportion of energy needs from fat in 24 hours (specify, eg, percent)—defined as the portion of total estimated energy needs to be derived from fat

Note: Comparison to the Dietary Reference Intakes is assumed, but other reference intake standards may be used.

Estimated Protein Needs (CS-2.2)

Definition

Estimated quantity and/or type of protein needed for nutritional adequacy

Purpose

Identify appropriate reference standard of protein intake needs for individual patients/clients. Utilized as a basis of comparison to assess adequacy or excessiveness of patient/client's estimated total protein intake as compared to estimated needs and for development of the nutrition prescription

Indicators

- Total protein estimated needs in 24 hours (specify, eg, grams/day)—defined as the estimated quantity of total protein needed for nutritional adequacy in one day

Macronutrient*	EAR	RDA	AI	UL	Other
Protein	X All except infants 0 to 6 months	X All except infants 0 to 6 months	X Infants 0 to 6 months		Acceptable Macronutrient Distribution Range (children and adults)

EAR — Estimated Average Requirement

RDA — Recommended Dietary Allowance

AI — Adequate Intake

UL — Tolerable Upper Intake Level

*See DRI interpretation table.

- Total protein estimated needs per kilogram of body weight (specify, eg, g/kg/day)—defined as the estimated quantity of total protein needed for nutritional adequacy for each kg of body weight in one day
- Method for estimating total protein needs (specify, eg, patient/client goal or nutrition prescription, disease/condition-based reference standard, Dietary Reference Intake)—defined as the approach for estimating total protein needs for one day
- Proportion of energy needs from protein in 24 hours (specify, percent)—defined as the portion of total estimated energy needs to be derived from protein

Note: Comparison to the Dietary Reference Intakes is assumed, but other reference intake standards may be used.

Estimated Carbohydrate Needs (CS-2.3)

Definition

Estimated quantity of total and/or type of carbohydrates needed for nutritional adequacy.

Purpose

Identify appropriate reference standard of carbohydrate intake needs for individual patients/clients. Utilized for assessing the adequacy or excessiveness of patient/client's estimated total carbohydrate intake as compared to estimated needs and for development of the nutrition prescription.

Indicators

- Total carbohydrate estimated needs in 24 hours (specify, eg, g/day)—defined as the estimated quantity of total carbohydrate needed for nutritional adequacy in one day

Macronutrients*	EAR	RDA	AI	UL	Other
Carbohydrates		X	X infants		Acceptable Macronutrient Distribution Range (children and adults) Added sugars—limit to no more than 25% of total energy (all ages)

EAR	—	Estimated Average Requirement
RDA	—	Recommended Dietary Allowance
AI	—	Adequate Intake
UL	—	Tolerable Upper Intake Level

*See DRI interpretation table.

- Total carbohydrate estimated needs per kilogram of body weight (specify, eg, g/kg/day)—defined as the estimated quantity of carbohydrate needed for nutritional adequacy for each kg of body weight in one day
- Method for estimating total carbohydrate needs (specify, eg, patient/client goal or nutrition prescription, disease-/condition-based reference standard, Dietary Reference Intake)—defined as the approach for estimating total carbohydrate needs for one day
- Proportion of energy needs from carbohydrate in 24 hours (specify, percent)—defined as the portion of estimated energy needs to be derived from carbohydrate

Note: Comparison to the Dietary Reference Intakes is assumed, but other reference intake standards may be used.

Estimated Fiber Needs (CS-2.4)

Definition

Estimated quantity of total and/or type of fiber needed for nutritional adequacy

Purpose

Identify appropriate reference standard of fiber intake needs for individual patients/clients. Utilized as a basis of comparison to assess adequacy or excessiveness of patient/client's estimated total fiber intake as compared to estimated needs and for development of the nutrition prescription

Indicators

- Total fiber estimated needs in 24 hours (specify, eg, g/day)—defined as the estimated quantity of total fiber needed for nutritional adequacy in one day

Macronutrients*	EAR	RDA	AI	UL	Other
Fiber			X		
			Children and adults		

EAR — Estimated Average Requirement

RDA — Recommended Dietary Allowance

AI — Adequate Intake

UL — Tolerable Upper Intake Level

*See DRI interpretation table.

- Method for estimating total fiber needs (specify, eg, patient/client goal or nutrition prescription, disease/condition-based reference standard, Dietary Reference Intake)—defined as the approach for estimating total fiber needs for one day

Note: Comparison to the Dietary Reference Intakes is assumed, but other reference intake standards may be used.

Estimated Fluid Needs (CS-3.1)

Definition

Estimated quantity of fluid needed for nutritional adequacy

Purpose

Identify appropriate reference standard of fluid intake needs for individual patients/clients. Utilized as a basis of comparison to assess adequacy or excessiveness of patient/client's estimated total fluid intake as compared to estimated need and for development of the nutrition prescription

Indicators

- Total estimated fluid needs, assumed to be consistent with the Dietary Reference Intakes unless otherwise specified (specify, eg, mL or L/day, mL/kg/day, mL/calories or kcal expended, mL/m^2/day, mL output)

Macronutrients*	EAR	RDA	AI	UL	Other
Total water			X		

EAR	—	Estimated Average Requirement
RDA	—	Recommended Dietary Allowance
AI	—	Adequate Intake
UL	—	Tolerable Upper Intake Level

*See DRI interpretation table.

- Method for estimating fluid needs (specify, eg, patient/client goal or nutrition prescription, disease/condition-based reference standard, Dietary Reference Intake, and adjustments, if needed, eg, patient/client goal or nutrition prescription, increased due to fever, sweating, hyperventilation, hyperthyroid, extraordinary gastric/renal losses, or decreased due to, for example, renal or liver disease)

Note: Comparison to the Dietary Reference Intakes is assumed, but other reference intake standards may be used.

Estimated Vitamin Needs (CS-4.1)

Assessment

Definition

Estimated quantity of one or more vitamins needed for nutritional adequacy and avoidance of toxicity

Purpose

Identify appropriate reference standard of vitamin intake needs for individual patients/clients. Utilized as a basis of comparison to assess adequacy or excessiveness of patient/client's estimated total vitamin intake as compared to estimated needs and for development of the nutrition prescription

Indicators

- Total estimated vitamin needs, assumed to be consistent with the Dietary Reference Intakes unless otherwise specified

Micronutrients—Vitamins*	EAR	RDA	AI	UL
Vitamin A (µg/day)	X	X	X Infants	X
Vitamin C (mg/day)	X	X	X Infants	X Children and adults
Vitamin D (µg/day)	X	X	X Infants	X
Vitamin E (mg/day)	X	X	X Infants	X Children and adults
Vitamin K (µg/day)			X	
Thiamin (mg/day)	X	X	X Infants	
Riboflavin (mg/day)	X	X	X Infants	
Niacin (mg/day)	X	X	X Infants	X Children and adults
Vitamin B6 (mg/day)	X	X	X Infants	X Children and adults
Folate (µg/day)	X	X	X Infants	X Children and adults
Vitamin B12 (µg/day)	X	X	X Infants	
Pantothenic acid (mg/day)			X	
Biotin (µg/day)			X	
Choline (mg/day)			X	X Children and adults

Estimated Vitamin Needs (CS-4.1)

EAR — Estimated Average Requirement

RDA — Recommended Dietary Allowance

AI — Adequate Intake

UL — Tolerable Upper Intake Level

*See DRI interpretation table.

- Method for estimating vitamin needs (specify, eg, patient/client goal or nutrition prescription, disease/condition-based reference standard, any adjustments for special conditions or situations, Dietary Reference Intake)

Note: Comparison to the Dietary Reference Intakes is assumed, but other reference intake standards may be used.

Estimated Mineral Needs (CS-4.2)

Definition

Estimated quantity of one or more minerals needed for nutritional adequacy and avoidance of toxicity

Purpose

Identify appropriate reference standard of mineral intake needs for individual patients/clients. Utilized as a basis of comparison to assess adequacy or excessiveness of patient/client's estimated mineral intake as compared to estimated needs and for development of the nutrition prescription

Indicators

- Total estimated mineral needs, assumed to be consistent with the Dietary Reference Intakes unless otherwise specified

Micronutrients— Minerals/elements*	EAR	RDA	AI	UL	Other
Boron (mg/day)				X Children and adults	
Calcium (mg/day)	X	X	X Infants	X Children and adults	
Chloride (g/day)			X	X Children and adults	
Chromium (µg/day)			X		
Cobalt (µg/day)					Not addressed in the DRIs
Copper (µg/day)	X	X	X Infants	X Children and adults	
Fluoride (mg/day)			X	X	
Iodine (µg/day)	X	X	X Infants	X Children and adults	
Iron (mg/day)	X	X	X Infants 0-6 mos.	X	
Magnesium (mg/day)	X	X	X Infants	X Children and adults	
Manganese (mg/day)			X	X Children and adults	
Molybdenum (mg/day)	X Children and adults	X Children and adults	X Infants	X Children and adults	
Phosphorus (mg/day)	X	X	X Infants	X Children and adults	
Potassium (g/day)			X		

Estimated Mineral Needs (CS-4.2)

Micronutrients—Minerals/elements* (cont.)	EAR	RDA	AI	UL	Other
Selenium (µg/day)	X	X	X	X	
			Infants		
Sodium (g/day)			X	X	
				Children and adults	
Sulfate (g/day)	X	X	X	X	
			Infants		
Zinc (mg/day)	X	X	X	X	
			Infants 0 to 6 mos.		

EAR — Estimated Average Requirement

RDA — Recommended Dietary Allowance

AI — Adequate Intake

UL — Tolerable Upper Intake Level

*See DRI interpretation table.

- Method for estimating mineral needs (specify, eg, patient/client goal or nutrition prescription, disease/condition-based reference standard, any adjustments for special conditions or situations, Dietary Reference Intake)

Note: Comparison to the Dietary Reference Intakes is assumed, but other reference intake standards may be used.

Recommended Body Weight/ Body Mass Index/Growth (CS-5.1)

Definition

Estimated reference ideal body weight (known as desirable body weight), body mass index, and/or growth parameter used to evaluate nutritional status

Purpose

Identify appropriate reference standard for body weight for individual patients/clients. Utilized as a basis of comparison to assess patient/client's body weight as compared to recommendations and for development of the nutrition prescription

Indicators (Measures)

- Ideal/reference body weight
  - Method for determining ideal body weight (IBW)/desirable body weight (specify, eg, Hamwi equation, growth chart)
  - IBW adjustment
  - % IBW
  - Adjusted body weight/metabolically active weight for overweight/obesity (specify, eg, equation)
- Recommended body mass index (BMI)[*] (kg/m^2)—defined as advised weight in kilograms divided by square height in meters
- Goal weight (pounds, ounces, kilograms, or grams)—defined as stated desired weight
- Goal weight gain/day (g/day)—defined as desired weight gain per day
- Goal weight-for-length z score (z score)—defined as desired standard deviation score for body weight in proportion to attained growth in length
- Goal mid upper arm circumference z score (z score)—defined as desired standard deviation score for mid upper arm circumference
- Goal BMI-for-age z score (z score)—defined as desired standard deviation score for BMI at the child's age
- Percent median BMI (%)—defined as comparison of the child's BMI to the median BMI-for-age expressed as a percent

Note: Please refer to the Academy Evidence Analysis Library at www.andevidencelibrary.com for recommendations related to using actual weight versus IBW or ABW for estimating energy expenditure.

---

[*]BMI is a measure of the weight of an individual scaled according to height. It is a common method for assessing body fat in the clinical setting and is compared to a population reference standard (eg, US National Institutes of Health guidelines or World Health Organization guidelines). BMI was designed for use within a physically inactive population.

SNAPSHOT   NCP Step 2: Nutrition Diagnosis

Purpose: The purpose of a nutrition diagnosis is to identify and describe a specific nutrition problem that can be resolved or improved through treatment/nutrition intervention by a nutrition and dietetics practitioner. A nutrition diagnosis (eg, inconsistent carbohydrate intake) is different from a medical diagnosis (eg, diabetes).

Determining a nutrition diagnosis: Nutrition and dietetics practitioners use nutrition assessment data to identify and label the patient/client's* nutrition diagnosis using standard nutrition diagnostic terminology. The eNCPT provides a reference sheet for each nutrition diagnosis that includes its definition, possible etiology/causes, and common signs or symptoms identified in the nutrition assessment step.

Terminology for nutrition diagnosis is organized in 3 domains (categories):

Intake	Clinical	Behavioral–Environmental
Too much or too little of a food or nutrient compared to actual or estimated needs	Nutrition problems that relate to medical or physical conditions	Knowledge, attitudes, beliefs, physical environment, access to food, or food safety

Documenting a nutrition diagnosis: Nutrition and dietetics practitioners write a PES (Problem, Etiology, Signs and Symptoms) statement to describe the problem, its root cause, and the assessment data that provide evidence for the nutrition diagnosis.

The format for the PES statement is "[Nutrition diagnosis term (Problem)] related to [Etiology] as evidenced by [Signs/Symptoms]."

(P) Problem or Nutrition Diagnosis Term	(E) Etiology	(S) Signs/Symptoms
Describes alterations in the patient/client's nutritional status.	Cause/Contributing Risk Factors Linked to the nutrition diagnosis term by the words "related to."	Data or indicators used to determine the patient/client's nutrition diagnosis. Linked to the etiology by the words "as evidenced by."

No nutrition diagnosis at this time (NO-1.1) may be documented if the assessment indicates that no nutrition problem exists to justify a nutrition intervention or if further nutrition assessment data are needed to identify a nutrition diagnosis.

Guidelines for selecting the nutrition diagnosis and writing a clear PES statement: Select the most important and urgent problem to be addressed. When writing the PES statement, nutrition and dietetics practitioners can ask a series of questions (identified in the critical thinking skills section below) that help clarify the nutrition diagnosis.

Critical Thinking Skills

P – Can the nutrition and dietetics practitioner resolve or improve the nutrition diagnosis of the patient/client? When all things are equal and there is a choice between stating the PES statement using two nutrition diagnoses from different domains, consider the Intake nutrition diagnosis as the one more specific to the role of the RDN.

E – Evaluate whether the etiology is the specific "root cause" that can be addressed with a nutrition intervention. If addressing the etiology cannot resolve the problem, can the RDN intervention at least lessen the signs and symptoms?

S – Will measuring the signs and symptoms indicate if the problem is resolved or improved? Are the signs and symptoms specific enough that the RDN can monitor (measure/evaluate changes) and document resolution or improvement of the nutrition diagnosis?

PES Overall – Do the nutrition assessment data support the nutrition diagnosis, etiology, and signs and symptoms?

For more information, sign in as a subscriber at https://ncpt.webauthor.com.

*Patient/client refers to individuals, groups, populations, family members, and/or caregivers.

Each term is designated with an alphanumeric NCPT hierarchical code, followed by a five-digit (e.g., 99999) Academy SNOMED CT/LOINC unique identifier (ANDUID). Neither should be used in nutrition documentation. The ANDUID is for data tracking purposes in electronic health records.

	NCPT Code	ANDUID

INTAKE (NI)

Actual problems related to intake of energy, nutrients, fluids, bioactive substances through oral diet or nutrition support

Energy Balance (1)

Actual or estimated changes in energy (calorie/kcal/kJ) balance

	NCPT Code	ANDUID
❑ Increased energy expenditure	NI-1.1	10633
❑ Inadequate energy intake	NI-1.2	10634
❑ Excessive energy intake	NI-1.3	10635

Oral or Nutrition Support Intake (2)

Actual or estimated food and beverage intake from oral diet or nutrition support compared with patient/client goal

	NCPT Code	ANDUID
❑ Inadequate oral intake	NI-2.1	10639
❑ Excessive oral intake	NI-2.2	10640
❑ Inadequate enteral nutrition infusion	NI-2.3	10641
❑ Excessive enteral nutrition infusion	NI-2.4	10642
❑ Enteral nutrition composition inconsistent with needs	NI-2.5	11142
❑ Enteral nutrition administration inconsistent with needs	NI-2.6	11143
❑ Inadequate parenteral nutrition infusion	NI-2.7	10644
❑ Excessive parenteral nutrition infusion	NI-2.8	10645
❑ Parenteral nutrition composition inconsistent with needs	NI-2.9	11144
❑ Parenteral nutrition administration inconsistent with needs	NI-2.10	11145
❑ Limited food acceptance	NI-2.11	10647

Fluid Intake (3)

Actual or estimated fluid intake compared with patient/client goal

	NCPT Code	ANDUID
❑ Inadequate fluid intake	NI-3.1	10649
❑ Excessive fluid intake	NI-3.2	10650

Bioactive Substances (4)

Actual or estimated intake of bioactive substances, including single or multiple functional food components, ingredients, dietary supplements, alcohol

	NCPT Code	ANDUID
❑ Inadequate bioactive substance intake	NI-4.1	10859
❑ Inadequate psyllium intake	NI-4.1.4	11079
❑ Inadequate β-glucan intake	NI-4.1.5	11076
❑ Excessive bioactive substance intake	NI-4.2	10653
❑ Excessive psyllium intake	NI-4.2.4	11086

Bioactive Substances (4) (continued)

	NCPT Code	ANDUID
❑ Excessive β-glucan intake	NI-4.2.5	11081
❑ Excessive caffeine intake	NI-4.2.7	11082
❑ Excessive alcohol intake	NI-4.3	10654

Nutrient (5)

Actual or estimated intake of specific nutrient groups or single nutrients as compared with desired levels

	NCPT Code	ANDUID
❑ Increased nutrient needs (specify) _____	NI-5.1	10656
❑ Inadequate protein-energy intake	NI-5.2	10658
❑ Decreased nutrient needs (specify) _____	NI-5.3	10659
❑ Imbalance of nutrients	NI-5.4	10660

Fat and Cholesterol (5.5)

	NCPT Code	ANDUID
❑ Inadequate fat intake	NI-5.5.1	10662
❑ Excessive fat intake	NI-5.5.2	10663
❑ Intake of types of fats inconsistent with needs (specify) _____	NI-5.5.3	10854

Protein (5.6)

	NCPT Code	ANDUID
❑ Inadequate protein intake	NI-5.6.1	10666
❑ Excessive protein intake	NI-5.6.2	10667
❑ Intake of types of proteins inconsistent with needs (specify) _____	NI-5.6.3	10855

Amino Acid (5.7)

	NCPT Code	ANDUID
❑ Intake of types of amino acids inconsistent with needs (specify) _____	NI-5.7.1	12007

Carbohydrate and Fiber (5.8)

	NCPT Code	ANDUID
❑ Inadequate carbohydrate intake	NI-5.8.1	10670
❑ Excessive carbohydrate intake	NI-5.8.2	10671
❑ Intake of types of carbohydrate inconsistent with needs (specify) _____	NI-5.8.3	10856
❑ Inconsistent carbohydrate intake	NI-5.8.4	10673
❑ Inadequate fiber intake	NI-5.8.5	10675
❑ Excessive fiber intake	NI-5.8.6	10676

Diagnosis

Diagnosis

	NCPT Code	ANDUID
Vitamin (5.9)		
❑ Inadequate vitamin intake (specify)	NI-5.9.1	10678
❑ A (1)		10679
❑ C (2)		10680
❑ D (3)		10681
❑ Folate (9)		10687
❑ B6 (10)		10688
❑ B12 (11)		10689
❑ Excessive vitamin intake (specify)	NI-5.9.2	10693
❑ A (1)		10694
❑ C (2)		10695
❑ D (3)		10696
❑ Folate (9)		10702
❑ B6 (10)		10703
❑ B12 (11)		10704
Mineral (5.10)		
❑ Inadequate mineral intake (specify)	NI-5.10.1	10709
❑ Calcium (1)		10710
❑ Iron (3)		10712
❑ Potassium (5)		10714
❑ Phosphorus (6)		10715
❑ Sodium (7)		10716
❑ Zinc (8)		10717
❑ Excessive mineral intake (specify)	NI-5.10.2	10729
❑ Calcium (1)		10730
❑ Iron (3)		10732
❑ Potassium (5)		10734
❑ Phosphorus (6)		10735
❑ Sodium (7)		10736
❑ Zinc (8)		10737

	NCPT Code	ANDUID
CLINICAL (NC)		

Nutritional findings/problems identified that relate to medical or physical conditions

Functional (1)

Change in physical or mechanical functioning that interferes with or prevents desired nutritional consequences

	NCPT Code	ANDUID
❑ Swallowing difficulty	NC-1.1	10754
❑ Biting/chewing (masticatory) difficulty	NC-1.2	10755
❑ Breastfeeding difficulty	NC-1.3	10756
❑ Altered GI function	NC-1.4	10757

Biochemical (2)

Change in capacity to metabolize nutrients as a result of medications, surgery, or as indicated by altered laboratory values

	NCPT Code	ANDUID
❑ Impaired nutrient utilization	NC-2.1	10759
❑ Altered nutrition-related laboratory values	NC-2.2	10760
(specify) _____		
❑ Food–medication interaction	NC-2.3	10761
(specify) _____		

Weight (3)

Chronic weight or changed weight status when compared with usual or desired body weight

	NCPT Code	ANDUID
❑ Underweight	NC-3.1	10764
❑ Unintended weight loss	NC-3.2	10765
❑ Overweight/obesity	NC-3.3	10766
❑ Overweight, adult or pediatric	NC-3.3.1	10767
❑ Obese, pediatric	NC-3.3.2	10768
❑ Obese, Class I	NC-3.3.3	10769
❑ Obese, Class II	NC-3.3.4	10818
❑ Obese, Class III	NC-3.3.5	10819
❑ Unintended weight gain	NC-3.4	10770
❑ Growth rate below expected	NC-3.5	10802

Malnutrition Disorders (4)

Health consequences resulting from insufficient or excessive energy and/or nutrient intake compared to physiologic needs and/or utilization.

	NCPT Code	ANDUID
❑ Malnutrition (undernutrition)	NC-4.1	10657
❑ Starvation related malnutrition	NC-4.1.1	12069
❑ Chronic disease or condition related malnutrition	NC-4.1.2	11131
❑ Acute disease or injury related malnutrition	NC-4.1.3	11132
❑ Non illness related pediatric malnutrition	NC-4.1.4	12072
❑ Illness related pediatric malnutrition	NC-4.1.5	12073

Diagnosis

	NCPT Code	ANDUID

Behavioral–Environmental (NB)

Nutritional findings/problems identified that relate to knowledge, attitudes/beliefs, physical environment, access to food, or food safety

Knowledge and Beliefs (1)

Actual knowledge and beliefs as related, observed, or documented

	NCPT Code	ANDUID
❑ Food- and nutrition-related knowledge deficit	NB-1.1	10773
❑ Not ready for diet/lifestyle change	NB-1.3	10775
❑ Disordered eating pattern	NB-1.5	10777
❑ Limited adherence to nutrition-related recommendations	NB-1.6	10778
❑ Undesirable food choices	NB-1.7	10779

Physical Activity and Function (2)

Actual physical activity, self-care, and quality-of-life problems as reported, observed, or documented

	NCPT Code	ANDUID
❑ Physical inactivity	NB-2.1	10782
❑ Excessive physical activity	NB-2.2	10783
❑ Inability to manage self-care	NB-2.3	10780

Food Safety and Access (3)

Actual problems with food safety or access to food, water, or nutrition-related supplies

	NCPT Code	ANDUID
❑ Intake of unsafe food	NB-3.1	10789
❑ Limited access to food	NB-3.2	12009

Other (NO)

Nutrition findings that are not classified as intake, clinical or Behavioral–Environmental problems.

Other (1)

	NCPT Code	ANDUID
❑ No nutrition diagnosis at this time	NO-1.1	10795

Increased Energy Expenditure (NI-1.1)

Diagnosis

Definition

Resting metabolic rate (RMR) more than predicted requirements due to body composition; medications; or endocrine, neurologic, or genetic changes

> **Note:** RMR is the sum of metabolic processes of active cell mass related to the maintenance of normal body functions and regulatory balance during rest.

Etiology (Cause/Contributing Risk Factors)

Factors gathered during the nutrition assessment process that contribute to the existence or the maintenance of pathophysiological, psychosocial, situational, developmental, cultural, and/or environmental problems:

- Physiological causes increasing nutrient needs due to anabolism, growth, maintenance of body temperature
- Voluntary or involuntary physical activity/movement

Signs/Symptoms (Defining Characteristics)

A typical cluster of subjective and objective signs and symptoms gathered during the nutrition assessment process that provide evidence that a problem exists; quantify the problem and describe its severity.

Nutrition Assessment Category	Potential Indicators of This Nutrition Diagnosis (one or more must be present)
Biochemical Data, Medical Tests, and Procedures	
Anthropometric Measurements	Unintentional weight loss of ≥10% in 6 months, ≥5% in 1 month (adults and pediatrics), and >2% in 1 week (pediatrics)
	Evidence of need for accelerated or catch-up growth or weight gain in children; absence of normal growth
	Increased proportion of lean body mass
Nutrition-Focused Physical Findings	Fever
	Measured RMR > estimated or expected RMR
Food/Nutrition-Related History	Increased physical activity, eg, endurance athlete
	Medications that increase energy expenditure
Client History	Conditions associated with a diagnosis or treatment, eg, Parkinson's disease, cerebral palsy, Alzheimer's disease, cystic fibrosis, chronic obstructive pulmonary disease (COPD)

Inadequate* Energy Intake (NI-1.2)

Definition

Energy intake that is less than energy expenditure, established reference standards, or recommendations based on physiological needs.

Note: May not be an appropriate nutrition diagnosis when the goal is weight loss, during end-of-life care, upon initiation of EN/PN, or acute stressed state (eg, surgery, organ failure).

Whenever possible, nutrient intake data should be considered in combination with clinical, biochemical, anthropometric information, medical diagnosis, clinical status, and/or other factors as well as diet to provide a valid assessment of nutritional status based on a totality of the evidence. (Institute of Medicine. Dietary Reference Intakes: Applications in Dietary Assessment.Washington, DC: National Academies Press; 2000.)

Etiology (Cause/Contributing Risk Factors)

Factors gathered during the nutrition assessment process that contribute to the existence or the maintenance of pathophysiological, psychosocial, situational, developmental, cultural, and/or environmental problems:

- Pathological or physiological causes that result in increased energy requirements, eg, increased nutrient needs due to prolonged catabolic illness
- Decreased ability to consume sufficient energy
- Lack of access to food or artificial nutrition, eg, economic constraints, restricting food given to older adults and/or children
- Cultural practices that affect ability to access food
- Food- and nutrition-related knowledge deficit concerning energy intake
- Psychological causes such as depression and disordered eating

*If a synonym for the term "inadequate" is helpful or needed, an approved alternative is the word "suboptimal."

Diagnosis

Inadequate* Energy Intake (NI-1.2)

Signs/Symptoms (Defining Characteristics)

A typical cluster of subjective and objective signs and symptoms gathered during the nutrition assessment process that provide evidence that a problem exists; quantify the problem and describe its severity.

Diagnosis

Nutrition Assessment Category	Potential Indicators of This Nutrition Diagnosis (one or more must be present)
Biochemical Data, Medical Tests, and Procedures	
Anthropometric Measurements	Failure to gain or maintain appropriate weight
Nutrition-Focused Physical Findings	Poor dentition
Food/Nutrition-Related History	Reports or observations of: • Estimated energy intake from diet less than needs based on estimated or measured resting metabolic rate • Restriction or omission of energy-dense foods from diet • Food avoidance and/or lack of interest in food • Inability to independently consume foods/fluids (diminished joint mobility of wrist, hand, or digits) • Estimated parenteral or enteral nutrition intake insufficient to meet needs based on estimated or measured resting metabolic rate • Excessive consumption of alcohol or other drugs that reduce hunger • Medications that affect appetite
Client History	Conditions associated with diagnosis or treatment, eg, mental illness, eating disorders, dementia, alcoholism, substance abuse, and acute or chronic pain management

---

*If a synonym for the term "inadequate" is helpful or needed, an approved alternative is the word "suboptimal."

Excessive Energy Intake (NI-1.3)

Definition

Energy intake that exceeds energy expenditure, established reference standards, or recommendations based on physiological needs

Note: May not be an appropriate nutrition diagnosis when weight gain is desired.

Etiology (Cause/Contributing Risk Factors)

Factors gathered during the nutrition assessment process that contribute to the existence or the maintenance of pathophysiological, psychosocial, situational, developmental, cultural, and/or environmental problems:

- Unsupported beliefs/attitudes about food, nutrition, and nutrition-related topics
- Food- and nutrition-related knowledge deficit concerning energy intake
- Lack of or limited access to healthful food choices, eg, healthful food choices not provided as an option by caregiver or parent; homeless
- Lack of value for behavior change, competing values
- Medications that increase appetite, eg, steroids, antidepressants
- Overfeeding of parenteral/enteral nutrition (PN/EN)
- Calories/kcal/kJ unaccounted for from IV infusion and/or medications
- Unwilling or disinterested in reducing energy intake
- Failure to adjust for lifestyle changes and decreased metabolism (eg, aging)
- Failure to adjust for restricted mobility due to recovery from injury, surgical procedure, other
- Resolution of prior hypermetabolism without reduction in intake

Excessive Energy Intake (NI-1.3)

Signs/Symptoms (Defining Characteristics)

A typical cluster of subjective and objective signs and symptoms gathered during the nutrition assessment process that provide evidence that a problem exists; quantify the problem and describe its severity.

Nutrition Assessment Category	Potential Indicators of This Nutrition Diagnosis (one or more must be present)
Biochemical Data, Medical Tests, and Procedures	Abnormal liver function tests after prolonged exposure (3 to 6 weeks) to parenteral nutrition ↑ Respiratory quotient >1.0
Anthropometric Measurements	Body fat percentage >25% for men and >32% for women BMI >25 (adults); BMI >95th percentile (pediatrics) Weight gain
Nutrition-Focused Physical Findings	Increased body adiposity Increased respiratory rate
Food/Nutrition-Related History	Reports or observations of: • Intake of energy in excess of estimated or measured energy needs • Intake of high caloric density or large portions of foods/beverages • EN/PN more than estimated or measured (eg, indirect calorimetry) energy expenditure
Client History	

Arrows used with laboratory values: ↑ represents above reference standard and ↓ represents below reference standard.

Inadequate* Oral Intake (NI-2.1)

Definition

Oral food/beverage intake that is less than established reference standards or recommendations based on physiological needs

> **Note:** This nutrition diagnosis does not include intake via oroenteric tube.
>
> May not be an appropriate nutrition diagnosis when the goal is weight loss, during end-of-life care, upon initiation of feeding, or during combined oral/EN/PN therapy.
>
> Whenever possible, nutrient intake data should be considered in combination with clinical, biochemical, anthropometric information, medical diagnosis, clinical status, and/or other factors as well as diet to provide a valid assessment of nutritional status based on a totality of the evidence (Institute of Medicine. Dietary Reference Intakes: Applications in Dietary Assessment. Washington, DC: National Academies Press; 2000).

Etiology (Cause/Contributing Risk Factors)

Factors gathered during the nutrition assessment process that contribute to the existence or the maintenance of pathophysiological, psychosocial, situational, developmental, cultural, and/or environmental problems:

- Physiological causes increasing nutrient needs, eg, due to prolonged catabolic illness
- Decreased ability to consume sufficient energy, eg, increased nutrient needs due to prolonged catabolic illness
- Lack of or limited access to food, eg, economic constraints, restricting food given to older adults and/or children
- Limited food acceptance due to physiological or behavioral issues, aversion, or unsupported beliefs/attitudes
- Cultural practices that affect ability to access food
- Food- and nutrition-related knowledge deficit concerning appropriate oral food/beverage intake
- Psychological causes such as depression and disordered eating

*If a synonym for the term "inadequate" is helpful or needed, an approved alternative is "suboptimal."

Inadequate* Oral Intake (NI-2.1)

Signs/Symptoms (Defining Characteristics)

A typical cluster of subjective and objective signs and symptoms gathered during the nutrition assessment process that provide evidence that a problem exists; quantify the problem and describe its severity.

Nutrition Assessment Category	Potential Indicators of This Nutrition Diagnosis (one or more must be present)
Biochemical Data, Medical Tests, and Procedures	
Anthropometric Measurements	Weight loss, insufficient growth velocity
Nutrition-Focused Physical Findings	Dry skin, mucous membranes, poor skin turgor Anorexia, nausea, or vomiting Change in appetite or taste Clinical evidence of vitamin/mineral deficiency
Food/Nutrition-Related History	Reports or observations of: • Estimates of insufficient intake of energy or high-quality protein from diet when compared to requirements • Economic constraints that limit food availability • Excessive consumption of alcohol or other drugs that reduce hunger • Medications that cause anorexia • Limited food/beverage intake inconsistent with nutrition reference standards for type, variety, diet quality • Less than optimal reliance on foods, food groups, supplements, or nutrition support
Client History	Conditions associated with a diagnosis or treatment of catabolic illness such as AIDS, tuberculosis, anorexia nervosa, sepsis or infection from recent surgery, depression, acute or chronic pain Protein and/or nutrient malabsorption

Diagnosis

---

* If a synonym for the term "inadequate" is helpful or needed, an approved alternative is "suboptimal."

Excessive Oral Intake (NI-2.2)

Definition

Oral food/beverage intake that exceeds estimated energy needs, established reference standards, or recommendations based on physiological needs

> **Note:** This nutrition diagnosis does not include intake via oroenteric tube.
>
> May not be an appropriate nutrition diagnosis when weight gain is desired.

Etiology (Cause/Contributing Risk Factors)

Factors gathered during the nutrition assessment process that contribute to the existence or the maintenance of pathophysiological, psychosocial, situational, developmental, cultural, and/or environmental problems:

- Unsupported beliefs/attitudes about food, nutrition, and nutrition-related topics
- Food- and nutrition-related knowledge deficit concerning appropriate oral food/beverage intake
- Lack of or limited access to healthful food choices, eg, healthful food choices not provided as an option by caregiver or parent; homeless
- Lack of value for behavior change, competing values
- Inability to limit or refuse offered foods
- Lack of food planning, purchasing, and preparation skills
- Loss of appetite awareness
- Medications that increase appetite, eg, steroids, antidepressants
- Psychological causes such as depression and disordered eating
- Unwilling or disinterested in reducing intake

Excessive Oral Intake (NI-2.2)

Signs/Symptoms (Defining Characteristics)

A typical cluster of subjective and objective signs and symptoms gathered during the nutrition assessment process that provide evidence that a problem exists; quantify the problem and describe its severity.

Nutrition Assessment Category	Potential Indicators of This Nutrition Diagnosis (one or more must be present)
Biochemical Data, Medical Tests, and Procedures	
Anthropometric Measurements	Weight gain not attributed to fluid retention or normal growth
Nutrition-Focused Physical Findings	
Food/Nutrition-Related History	Reports or observations of: • Intake of high caloric-density foods/beverages (juice, soda, or alcohol) at meals and/or snacks • Intake of large portions of foods/beverages, food groups, or specific food items • Estimated intake that exceeds estimated or measured energy needs • Highly variable estimated daily energy intake • Binge eating patterns • Frequent, excessive fast food or restaurant intake
Client History	Conditions associated with a diagnosis or treatment, eg, obesity, overweight, or metabolic syndrome, depression, anxiety disorder

Diagnosis

Inadequate* Enteral Nutrition Infusion (NI-2.3)

Definition

Enteral infusion that provides fewer calories/kcal/kJ or nutrients compared to established reference standards or recommendations based on physiological needs

Note: May not be an appropriate nutrition diagnosis when recommendation is for weight loss, during end-of-life care, upon initiation of feeding, or during acute stressed states (eg, surgery, organ failure).

Whenever possible, nutrient intake data should be considered in combination with clinical, biochemical, anthropometric information, medical diagnosis, clinical status, and/or other factors as well as diet to provide a valid assessment of nutritional status based on a totality of the evidence (Institute of Medicine. Dietary Reference Intakes: Applications in Dietary Assessment. Washington, DC: National Academies Press; 2000).

Etiology (Cause/Contributing Risk Factors)

Factors gathered during the nutrition assessment process that contribute to the existence or the maintenance of pathophysiological, psychosocial, situational, developmental, cultural, and/or environmental problems:

- Altered absorption or metabolism of nutrients, eg, medications
- Food- and nutrition-related knowledge deficit concerning appropriate formula/formulation given for EN
- Lack of, compromised, or incorrect access for delivering EN
- Physiological causes increasing nutrient needs, eg, due to accelerated growth, wound healing, chronic infection, multiple fractures
- Intolerance of EN
- Infusion volume not reached or schedule for infusion interrupted

Signs/Symptoms (Defining Characteristics)

A typical cluster of subjective and objective signs and symptoms gathered during the nutrition assessment process that provide evidence that a problem exists; quantify the problem and describe its severity.

Nutrition Assessment Category	Potential Indicators of This Nutrition Diagnosis (one or more must be present)
Biochemical Data, Medical Tests, and Procedures	↓ Metabolic cart/indirect calorimetry measurement, eg, respiratory quotient <0.7
	Vitamin/mineral abnormalities:
	• ↓ Calcium <9.2 mg/dL (2.3 mmol/L)
	• Vitamin K—abnormal international normalized ratio (INR)
	• ↓ Copper <70 µg/dL (11 µmol/L)
	• ↓ Zinc <78 µg/dL (12 µmol/L)
	• ↓ Iron <50 µg/dL (8.9 nmol/L); iron-binding capacity <250 µg/dL (44.8 µmol/L)

Continued on next page

*If a synonym for the term "inadequate" is helpful or needed, an approved alternative is "suboptimal."

Inadequate* Enteral Nutrition Infusion (NI-2.3)

Continued from previous page

Nutrition Assessment Category	Potential Indicators of This Nutrition Diagnosis (one or more must be present)
Anthropometric Measurements	Growth failure based on reference growth standards, eg, National Center for Health Statistics (NCHS) and fetal growth failure
	Insufficient maternal weight gain
	Lack of planned weight gain
	Unintentional weight loss of ≥5% in 1 month or ≥10% in 6 months (not attributed to fluid) in adults
	Any weight loss in infants or children
	Underweight (BMI <18.5)
Nutrition-Focused Physical Findings	Clinical evidence of vitamin/mineral deficiency (eg, hair loss, bleeding gums, pale nail beds, neurologic changes)
	Evidence of dehydration, eg, dry mucous membranes, poor skin turgor
	Loss of skin integrity, delayed wound healing, or pressure ulcers
	Loss of muscle mass and/or subcutaneous fat
	Nausea, vomiting, diarrhea
Food/Nutrition-Related History	Reports or observations of: • Inadequate EN volume compared to estimated or measured (indirect calorimetry) requirements • Feeding tube in wrong position or removed • Altered capacity for desired levels of physical activity or exercise, easy fatigue with increased activity • Suboptimal feeding position
Client History	Conditions associated with a diagnosis or treatment, eg, intestinal resection, Crohn's disease, HIV/AIDS, burns, preterm birth, malnutrition

Arrows used with laboratory values: ↑ represents above reference standard and ↓ represents below reference standard.

---

*If a synonym for the term "inadequate" is helpful or needed, an approved alternative is "suboptimal."

Diagnosis

Excessive Enteral Nutrition Infusion (NI-2.4)

Definition

Enteral infusion that provides more calories/kcal/kJ or nutrients compared to established reference standards or recommendations based on physiological needs

Etiology (Cause/Contributing Risk Factors)

Factors gathered during the nutrition assessment process that contribute to the existence or the maintenance of pathophysiological, psychosocial, situational, developmental, cultural, and/or environmental problems:

- Physiological causes, eg, decreased needs related to low activity levels with critical illness or organ failure
- Food- and nutrition-related knowledge deficit concerning appropriate amount of enteral nutrition

Signs/Symptoms (Defining Characteristics)

A typical cluster of subjective and objective signs and symptoms gathered during the nutrition assessment process that provide evidence that a problem exists; quantify the problem and describe its severity.

Nutrition Assessment Category	Potential Indicators of This Nutrition Diagnosis (one or more must be present)
Biochemical Data, Medical Tests, and Procedures	↑ BUN:creatinine ratio (protein)
	Hyperglycemia (carbohydrate)
	Hypercapnia
Anthropometric Measurements	Weight gain in excess of lean tissue accretion
Nutrition-Focused Physical Findings	Edema with excess fluid administration
Food/Nutrition-Related History	Reports or observations of: • Estimated intake from enteral nutrients that is consistently more than recommended intake for carbohydrate, protein, and fat • Use of drugs that reduce requirements or impair metabolism of energy, protein, fat, or fluid • Unrealistic expectations of weight gain or ideal weight
Client History	

Arrows used with laboratory values: ↑ represents above reference standard and ↓ represents below reference standard.

Diagnosis

Enteral Nutrition Composition Inconsistent With Needs (NI-2.5)

Definition

Enteral nutrition formula that varies from established reference standards or recommendations based on physiological needs

Etiology (Cause/Contributing Risk Factors)

Factors gathered during the nutrition assessment process that contribute to the existence or the maintenance of pathophysiological, psychosocial, situational, developmental, cultural, and/or environmental problems:

- Physiological causes, eg, improvement in patient/client status allowing return to total or partial oral diet; changes in the course of disease resulting in changes in feeding and/or nutrient requirements

- Food and nutrition-related knowledge deficit concerning EN product

- End-of-life care if patient/client or family does not desire nutrition support

Enteral Nutrition Composition Inconsistent With Needs (NI-2.5)

Signs/Symptoms (Defining Characteristics)

A typical cluster of subjective and objective signs and symptoms gathered during the nutrition assessment process that provide evidence that a problem exists; quantify the problem and describe its severity.

Nutrition Assessment Category	Potential Indicators of This Nutrition Diagnosis (one or more must be present)
Biochemical Data, Medical Tests, and Procedures	Abnormal levels of markers specific for various nutrients, eg, hyperphosphatemia in patient/client receiving feedings with a high phosphorus content, hypokalemia in patient/client receiving feedings with low potassium content
Anthropometric Measurements	Weight gain in excess of lean tissue accretion Weight loss
Nutrition-Focused Physical Findings	Edema with excess fluid administration Loss of subcutaneous fat and muscle stores Diarrhea, constipation
Food/Nutrition-Related History	Reports or observations of: • Estimated intake from enteral nutrients that is consistently more or less than recommended intake for carbohydrate, proteins or amino acids, fat or fatty acids, and/or micronutrients • Formula composition that is inconsistent with ability to digest and absorb nutrients • Formula composition or concentration that is inconsistent with evidence-based practice • Verbalizations or written responses that are inaccurate or incomplete for enteral nutrition formula prescribed
Client History	Improved or diminished GI function Conditions associated with a diagnosis or treatment, eg, major elective surgery, trauma, burns, head and neck cancer, and critically ill patients, acute lung injury, acute respiratory distress syndrome, treatments/therapy requiring interruption of infusion, transfer of nutrition care to a new setting or level of care, end-of-life care

Diagnosis

Enteral Nutrition Administration Inconsistent With Needs (NI-2.6)

Definition

Enteral nutrition provision that varies from established reference standards or recommendations based on physiological needs

Etiology (Cause/Contributing Risk Factors)

Factors gathered during the nutrition assessment process that contribute to the existence or the maintenance of pathophysiological, psychosocial, situational, developmental, cultural, and/or environmental problems:

- Physiological causes, eg, improvement in patient/client status allowing return to total or partial oral diet; changes in the course of disease resulting in changes in feeding
- Food and nutrition-related knowledge deficit concerning EN product provision
- End-of-life care if patient/client or family does not desire nutrition support

Diagnosis

Enteral Nutrition Administration Inconsistent With Needs (NI-2.6)

Signs/Symptoms (Defining Characteristics)

A typical cluster of subjective and objective signs and symptoms gathered during the nutrition assessment process that provide evidence that a problem exists; quantify the problem and describe its severity.

Nutrition Assessment Category	Potential Indicators of This Nutrition Diagnosis (one or more must be present)
Biochemical Data, Medical Tests, and Procedures	↑ or ↓ serum glucose
Anthropometric Measurements	
Nutrition-Focused Physical Findings	Nausea, vomiting, diarrhea, high gastric residual volume Satiety
Food/Nutrition-Related History	Reports or observations of: • Access route that may warrant modification • Access type that may warrant modification • Administration that may conflict with oral intake • Administration that may conflict with therapies (including medications) or procedures • Enteral nutrition that may contribute to poor nutrition quality of life • Intolerance of bolus feeding • Intolerance of rate of delivery • Verbalizations or written responses that are inaccurate or incomplete regarding enteral nutrition administration • History of enteral nutrition intolerance
Client History	Improved/diminished GI function Conditions associated with a diagnosis or treatment, eg, major elective surgery, trauma, burns, head and neck cancer, and critical illness, acute lung injury, acute respiratory distress syndrome, treatments/therapy requiring interruption of infusion, transfer of nutrition care to a new setting or level of care, end-of-life care

Diagnosis

Inadequate* Parenteral Nutrition Infusion (NI-2.7)

Definition

Parenteral infusion that provides fewer calories/kcal/kJ or nutrients compared to established reference standards or recommendations based on physiological needs

Note: May not be an appropriate nutrition diagnosis when recommendation is for weight loss, during end-of-life care, upon initiation of feeding, or during acute stressed states (eg, surgery, organ failure).

Whenever possible, nutrient intake data should be considered in combination with clinical, biochemical, anthropometric information, medical diagnosis, clinical status, and/or other factors as well as diet to provide a valid assessment of nutritional status based on a totality of the evidence (Institute of Medicine. Dietary Reference Intakes: Applications in Dietary Assessment. Washington, DC: National Academies Press; 2000).

Etiology (Cause/Contributing Risk Factors)

Factors gathered during the nutrition assessment process that contribute to the existence or the maintenance of pathophysiological, psychosocial, situational, developmental, cultural, and/or environmental problems:

- Altered absorption or metabolism of nutrients, eg, medications
- Food- and nutrition-related knowledge deficit concerning appropriate formula/formulation given for PN
- Lack of, compromised, or incorrect access for delivering PN
- Physiological causes increasing nutrient needs, eg, due to accelerated growth, wound healing, chronic infection, multiple fractures
- Intolerance of PN
- Infusion volume not reached or schedule for infusion interrupted

Signs/Symptoms (Defining Characteristics)

A typical cluster of subjective and objective signs and symptoms gathered during the nutrition assessment process that provide evidence that a problem exists; quantify the problem and describe its severity.

Nutrition Assessment Category	Potential Indicators of This Nutrition Diagnosis (one or more must be present)
Biochemical Data, Medical Tests, and Procedures	↓ Metabolic cart/indirect calorimetry measurement, eg, respiratory quotient <0.7 Vitamin/mineral abnormalities: • ↓ Calcium <9.2 mg/dL (2.3 mmol/L) • Vitamin K—abnormal international normalized ratio (INR) • ↓ Copper <70 µg/dL (11 µmol/L) • ↓ Zinc <78 µg/dL (12 µmol/L) • ↓ Iron <50 µg/dL (nmol/L); iron-binding capacity <250 µg/dL (44.8 µmol/L)

Continued on next page

*If a synonym for the term "inadequate" is helpful or needed, an approved alternative is "suboptimal."

Inadequate* Parenteral Nutrition Infusion (NI-2.7)

Continued from previous page

Nutrition Assessment Category	Potential Indicators of This Nutrition Diagnosis (one or more must be present)
Anthropometric Measurements	Growth failure based on reference growth standards, eg, National Center for Health Statistics (NCHS) and fetal growth failure
	Insufficient maternal weight gain
	Lack of planned weight gain
	Unintentional weight loss of >5% in 1 month or >10% in 6 months (not attributed to fluid) in adults
	Any weight loss in infants or children
	Underweight (BMI <18.5)
Nutrition-Focused Physical Findings	Clinical evidence of vitamin/mineral deficiency (eg, hair loss, bleeding gums, pale nail beds, neurologic changes)
	Evidence of dehydration, eg, dry mucous membranes, poor skin turgor
	Loss of skin integrity, delayed wound healing, or pressure ulcers
	Loss of muscle mass and/or subcutaneous fat
	Nausea, vomiting, diarrhea
Food/Nutrition-Related History	Reports or observations of: • Inadequate PN volume compared to estimated or measured (indirect calorimetry) requirements • Feeding tube or venous access in wrong position or removed • Altered capacity for desired levels of physical activity or exercise, easy fatigue with increased activity
Client History	Conditions associated with a diagnosis or treatment, eg, intestinal resection, Crohn's disease, HIV/AIDS, burns, preterm birth, malnutrition

Arrows used with laboratory values: ↑ represents above reference standard and ↓ represents below reference standard.

*If a synonym for the term "inadequate" is helpful or needed, an approved alternative is "suboptimal."

Excessive Parenteral Nutrition Infusion (NI-2.8)

Definition

Parenteral infusion that provides more calories/kcal/kJ or nutrients compared to established reference standards or recommendations based on physiological needs

Etiology (Cause/Contributing Risk Factors)

Factors gathered during the nutrition assessment process that contribute to the existence or the maintenance of pathophysiological, psychosocial, situational, developmental, cultural, and/or environmental problems:

- Physiological causes, eg, decreased needs related to low activity levels with critical illness or organ failure
- Food- and nutrition-related knowledge deficit concerning appropriate amount of PN

Signs/Symptoms (Defining Characteristics)

A typical cluster of subjective and objective signs and symptoms gathered during the nutrition assessment process that provide evidence that a problem exists; quantify the problem and describe its severity.

Nutrition Assessment Category	Potential Indicators of This Nutrition Diagnosis (one or more must be present)
Biochemical Data, Medical Tests, and Procedures	↑ BUN:creatinine ratio (protein) Hyperglycemia (carbohydrate) Hypercapnia ↑ Liver enzymes
Anthropometric Measurements	Weight gain in excess of lean tissue accretion
Nutrition-Focused Physical Findings	Edema with excess fluid administration
Food/Nutrition-Related History	Reports or observations of: • Estimated intake from parenteral nutrients that is consistently more than recommended intake for carbohydrate, protein, and fat • Use of drugs that reduce requirements or impair metabolism of energy, protein, fat, or fluid • Unrealistic expectations of weight gain or ideal weight
Client History	

Arrows used with laboratory values: ↑ represents above reference standard and ↓ represents below reference standard.

Parenteral Nutrition Composition Inconsistent With Needs (NI-2.9)

Definition

Parenteral nutrition solution that varies from established reference standards or recommendations based on physiological needs

Etiology (Cause/Contributing Risk Factors)

Factors gathered during the nutrition assessment process that contribute to the existence or the maintenance of pathophysiological, psychosocial, situational, developmental, cultural, and/or environmental problems:

- Physiological causes, eg, improvement in patient/client status allowing return to total or partial oral diet or enteral nutrition; changes in the course of disease resulting in changes in feeding and/or nutrient requirements

- Food and nutrition-related knowledge deficit concerning PN composition

- End-of-life care if patient/client or family does not desire nutrition support

Parenteral Nutrition Composition Inconsistent With Needs (NI-2.9)

Signs/Symptoms (Defining Characteristics)

A typical cluster of subjective and objective signs and symptoms gathered during the nutrition assessment process that provide evidence that a problem exists; quantify the problem and describe its severity.

Diagnosis (side tab)

Nutrition Assessment Category	Potential Indicators of This Nutrition Diagnosis (one or more must be present)
Biochemical Data, Medical Tests, and Procedures	↑ Liver function tests in patient/client on long-term (more than 3 to 6 weeks) nutrition support Abnormal levels of markers specific for various nutrients, eg, hyperphosphatemia in patient/client receiving feedings with a high phosphorus content, hypokalemia in patient/client receiving feedings with low potassium content
Anthropometric Measurements	Weight gain in excess of lean tissue accretion Weight loss
Nutrition-Focused Physical Findings	Edema with excess fluid administration Loss of subcutaneous fat and muscle stores Nausea
Food/Nutrition-Related History	Reports or observations of: • Estimated intake from parenteral nutrients that is consistently more or less than recommended intake for carbohydrate, protein or amino acids, fat or fatty acids, vitamins, and/or minerals • Estimated intake of other nutrients that is consistently more or less than recommended • Formula composition or type that is inconsistent with evidence-based practice • Verbalizations or written responses that are inaccurate or incomplete regarding PN solution • History of parenteral nutrition intolerance
Client History	Complications such as fatty liver in the absence of other causes Resolving or improved GI function Conditions associated with a diagnosis or treatment, eg, major elective surgery, trauma, burns, head and neck cancer, and critical illness, acute lung injury, acute respiratory distress syndrome, treatments/therapy requiring interruption of infusion, transfer of nutrition care to a new setting or level of care, end-of-life care

Arrows used with laboratory values: ↑ represents above reference standard and ↓ represents below reference standard.

Parenteral Nutrition Administration Inconsistent With Needs (NI-2.10)

Definition

Parenteral nutrition provision that varies from established reference standards or recommendations based on physiological needs

Etiology (Cause/Contributing Risk Factors)

Factors gathered during the nutrition assessment process that contribute to the existence or the maintenance of pathophysiological, psychosocial, situational, developmental, cultural, and/or environmental problems:

- Physiological causes, eg, improvement in patient/client status allowing return to total or partial oral diet or enteral nutrition; changes in the course of disease resulting in changes in feeding provision
- Food and nutrition-related knowledge deficit concerning PN provision
- End-of-life care if patient/client or family does not desire nutrition support

Parenteral Nutrition Administration Inconsistent With Needs (NI-2.10)

Signs/Symptoms (Defining Characteristics)

A typical cluster of subjective and objective signs and symptoms gathered during the nutrition assessment process that provide evidence that a problem exists; quantify the problem and describe its severity.

Nutrition Assessment Category	Potential Indicators of This Nutrition Diagnosis (one or more must be present)
Biochemical Data, Medical Tests, and Procedures	↑ Liver function tests in patient/client on long-term (more than 3 to 6 weeks) nutrition support
Anthropometric Measurements	
Nutrition-Focused Physical Findings	Infusion site compromise Nausea
Food/Nutrition-Related History	Reports or observations of: • Access route that may warrant modification • Access type that may warrant modification • Parenteral nutrition that may conflict with oral or enteral nutrition intake • Parenteral nutrition that may conflict with therapies or procedures • Parenteral nutrition that may contribute to poor nutrition quality of life • Intolerance of rate of delivery • Verbalizations or written responses that are inaccurate or incomplete regarding parenteral nutrition administration • History of parenteral nutrition intolerance
Client History	Complications such as fatty liver in the absence of other causes Resolving or improved GI function Conditions associated with a diagnosis or treatment, eg, major elective surgery, trauma, burns, head and neck cancer, and critical illness, acute lung injury, acute respiratory distress syndrome, treatments/therapy requiring interruption of infusion, transfer of nutrition care to a new setting or level of care, end-of-life care

Arrows used with laboratory values: ↑ represents above reference standard and ↓ represents below reference standard.

Diagnosis

Limited Food Acceptance (NI-2.11)

Definition

Oral food/beverage intake that is inconsistent with reference standard intake for type, variety, or quality

Note: May not be an appropriate nutrition diagnosis for individuals with anorexia nervosa, bulimia nervosa, binge eating disorder, or eating disorder not otherwise specified (EDNOS). Please consider using Disordered Eating Pattern (NB-1.5).

Signs/Symptoms (Defining Characteristics)

Factors gathered during the nutrition assessment process that contribute to the existence or the maintenance of pathophysiological, psychosocial, situational, developmental, cultural, and/or environmental problems:

- Physiological causes, eg, pain, discomfort, or functional issues in the GI tract; developmental delay; neurological disorders
- Aversion to food/beverages in mouth, throat, or hands
- Self-limitation of foods/food groups due to food preference
- Behavioral issues, including caregiver issues and eating behavior that serves a purpose other than nourishment
- Unsupported beliefs and attitudes

Diagnosi

Limited Food Acceptance (NI-2.11)

Signs/Symptoms (Defining Characteristics)

A typical cluster of subjective and objective signs and symptoms gathered during the nutrition assessment process that provide evidence that a problem exists; quantify the problem and describe its severity.

Nutrition Assessment Category	Potential Indicators of This Nutrition Diagnosis (one or more must be present)
Biochemical Data, Medical Tests, and Procedures	
Anthropometric Measurements	Weight loss, insufficient growth velocity, weight gain due to reliance on low-variety or less than optimal intake
Nutrition-Focused Physical Findings	Clinical evidence of vitamin/mineral deficiency Erratic appetite
Food/Nutrition-Related History	Reports or observations of: • Limited food/beverage intake inconsistent with nutrition reference standards for type, variety, or diet quality • Less than optimal reliance on foods, food groups, supplements, or nutrition support
Client History	Conditions associated with a diagnosis or treatment, eg, developmental disabilities, sensory processing issues, autism, dental caries, long-term nutrition support, prematurity, neurological disorders, altered mental state, affected brain studies (MRI)

Inadequate* Fluid Intake (NI-3.1)

Definition

Lower intake of fluid-containing foods or substances compared to established reference standards or recommendations based on physiological needs

> **Note:** Whenever possible, nutrient intake data should be considered in combination with clinical, biochemical, anthropometric information, medical diagnosis, clinical status, and/or other factors as well as diet to provide a valid assessment of nutritional status based on a totality of the evidence (Institute of Medicine. Dietary Reference Intakes: Applications in Dietary Assessment. Washington, DC: National Academies Press; 2000).

Signs/Symptoms (Defining Characteristics)

Factors gathered during the nutrition assessment process that contribute to the existence or the maintenance of pathophysiological, psychosocial, situational, developmental, cultural, and/or environmental problems:

- Physiological causes increasing fluid needs due to climate/temperature change, increased exercise or conditions leading to increased fluid losses, fever causing increased insensible losses, decreased thirst sensation, or use of drugs that reduce thirst
- Lack of or limited access to fluid, eg, economic constraints, unable to access fluid independently such as older adults or children
- Cultural practices that affect the ability to access fluid
- Food- and nutrition-related knowledge deficit concerning appropriate fluid intake
- Psychological causes, eg, depression or disordered eating
- Impaired cognitive ability, including learning disabilities, neurological or sensory impairment, and/or dementia

Diagnosis

---

*If a synonym for the term "inadequate" is helpful or needed, an approved alternative is "suboptimal."

Inadequate* Fluid Intake (NI-3.1)

Signs/Symptoms (Defining Characteristics)

A typical cluster of subjective and objective signs and symptoms gathered during the nutrition assessment process that provide evidence that a problem exists; quantify the problem and describe its severity.

Nutrition Assessment Category	Potential Indicators of This Nutrition Diagnosis (one or more must be present)
Biochemical Data, Medical Tests, and Procedures	Plasma or serum osmolality greater than 290 mOsm/kg Abnormal BUN, Na ↓ Urine volume ↑ Urine specific gravity Hyperglycemia in diabetic patient/client
Anthropometric Measurements	Acute weight loss
Nutrition-Focused Physical Findings	Dry skin and mucous membranes, poor skin turgor, tachycardia and normal or hypotensive blood pressure, fever, increased respirations, flattened neck veins Thirst Difficulty swallowing Increased insensible loss
Food/Nutrition-Related History	Reports or observations of: • Estimated intake of fluid less than requirements (eg, per body surface area for pediatrics) • Use of drugs that reduce thirst
Client History	Conditions associated with a diagnosis or treatment, eg, dementia resulting in decreased recognition of thirst, dehydration, diabetes mellitus, alterations in renal function, diarrhea, vomiting, ileostomy, colostomy, infection

Arrows used with laboratory values: ↑ represents above reference standard and ↓ represents below reference standard.

*If a synonym for the term "inadequate" is helpful or needed, an approved alternative is "suboptimal."

Excessive Fluid Intake (NI-3.2)

Definition

Higher intake of fluid compared to established reference standards or recommendations based on physiological needs

Signs/Symptoms (Defining Characteristics)

Factors gathered during the nutrition assessment process that contribute to the existence or the maintenance of pathophysiological, psychosocial, situational, developmental, cultural, and/or environmental problems:

- Physiological causes, eg, kidney, liver, cardiac, endocrine, neurological, and/or pulmonary dysfunction; diminished water and sodium losses due to changes in exercise or climate; syndrome of inappropriate antidiuretic hormone (SIADH)
- Food- and nutrition-related knowledge deficit concerning appropriate fluid intake
- Psychological causes such as depression and disordered eating

Excessive Fluid Intake (NI-3.2)

Signs/Symptoms (Defining Characteristics)

A typical cluster of subjective and objective signs and symptoms gathered during the nutrition assessment process that provide evidence that a problem exists; quantify the problem and describe its severity.

Nutrition Assessment Category	Potential Indicators of This Nutrition Diagnosis (one or more must be present)
Biochemical Data, Medical Tests, and Procedures	↓ Plasma osmolality (270–280 mOsm/kg), only if positive fluid balance is in excess of positive sodium balance ↓ Serum sodium in SIADH ↓ Urine specific gravity
Anthropometric Measurements	Weight gain
Nutrition-Focused Physical Findings	Edema in the skin of the legs, sacral area, or diffusely; weeping of fluids from lower legs Ascites Pulmonary edema as evidenced by shortness of breath, orthopnea, crackles or rales Nausea, vomiting, anorexia, headache, muscle spasms, convulsions Shortness of breath or dyspnea with exertion or at rest Providing medications in large amounts of fluid Use of drugs that impair fluid excretion
Food/Nutrition-Related History	Reports or observations of: • Estimated intake of fluid more than requirements (eg, per body surface area for pediatrics) • Estimated salt intake in excess of recommendations
Client History	Conditions associated with a diagnosis or treatment, eg, end-stage renal disease, nephrotic syndrome, heart failure, or liver disease Coma (SIADH)

Arrows used with laboratory values: ↑ represents above reference standard and ↓ represents below reference standard.

Diagnosis

INTAKE DOMAIN—BIOACTIVE SUBSTANCES

Inadequate* Bioactive Substance Intake (Specify) (NI-4.1)

Definition

Lower intake of bioactive substances compared to established reference standards or recommendations based on physiological needs

> **Note:** Bioactive substances are not part of the Dietary Reference Intakes, and therefore there are no established minimum requirements or Tolerable Upper Intake Levels. However, nutrition and dietetics practitioners can assess whether estimated intakes are adequate or excessive using the patient/client goal or nutrition prescription for comparison.
>
> Working definition of bioactive substances—physiologically active components of foods that may have an effect on health. There is no scientific consensus about a definition for bioactive substances/components.

Signs/Symptoms (Defining Characteristics)

Factors gathered during the nutrition assessment process that contribute to the existence or the maintenance of pathophysiological, psychosocial, situational, developmental, cultural, and/or environmental problems:

- Food- and nutrition-related knowledge deficit concerning recommended bioactive substance intake
- Lack of or limited access to food that contains a bioactive substance
- Alteration in gastrointestinal tract structure and/or function

---

*If a synonym for the term "inadequate" is helpful or needed, an approved alternative is "suboptimal."

Inadequate* Bioactive Substance Intake (Specify) (NI-4.1)

Signs/Symptoms (Defining Characteristics)

A typical cluster of subjective and objective signs and symptoms gathered during the nutrition assessment process that provide evidence that a problem exists; quantify the problem and describe its severity.

Nutrition Assessment Category	Potential Indicators of This Nutrition Diagnosis (one or more must be present)
Biochemical Data, Medical Tests, and Procedures	
Anthropometric Measurements	
Nutrition-Focused Physical Findings	

Food/Nutrition-Related History	Reports or observations of:
	
	• Estimated intake of plant foods containing the following lower than recommended:
	   ○ Soluble fiber, eg, psyllium (↓ total and LDL cholesterol)
	   ○ Soy protein (↓ total and LDL cholesterol)
	   ○ ß-glucan, eg, whole oat products (↓ total and LDL cholesterol)
	   ○ Plant sterol and stanol esters, eg, fortified margarines (↓ total and LDL cholesterol)
	   ○ Other substances (for which scientific evidence exists and a recommended intake level has been established)
	• Verbalizes inaccurate or incomplete knowledge about bioactive substances

Client History	Conditions associated with a diagnosis or treatment, eg, cardiovascular disease, elevated cholesterol

Arrows used with laboratory values: ↑ represents above reference standard and ↓ represents below reference standard.

*If a synonym for the term "inadequate" is helpful or needed, an approved alternative is "suboptimal."

Excessive Bioactive Substance Intake (Specify) (NI-4.2)

Definition

Higher intake of bioactive substances compared to established reference standards or recommendations based on physiological needs

> **Note:** Bioactive substances are not part of the Dietary Reference Intakes, and therefore there are no established minimum requirements or Tolerable Upper Intake Levels. However, nutrition and dietetics practitioners can assess whether estimated intakes are adequate or excessive using the patient/client goal or nutrition prescription for comparison.
>
> Working definition of bioactive substances—physiologically active components of foods that may have an effect on health. There is no scientific consensus about a definition for bioactive substances/components.

Signs/Symptoms (Defining Characteristics)

Factors gathered during the nutrition assessment process that contribute to the existence or the maintenance of pathophysiological, psychosocial, situational, developmental, cultural, and/or environmental problems:

- Food- and nutrition-related knowledge deficit concerning recommended bioactive substance intake, including food additives
- Contamination, misname, mislabel or lack of labeling, misuse, recent brand change, recent dose increase, recent formulation change of substance consumed
- Frequent intake of foods containing bioactive substances
- Alteration in gastrointestinal tract structure and/or function
- Lack of or limited access to appropriate foods, eg, inadequate markets with labeled food

Signs/Symptoms (Defining Characteristics)

A typical cluster of subjective and objective signs and symptoms gathered during the nutrition assessment process that provide evidence that a problem exists; quantify the problem and describe its severity.

Nutrition Assessment Category	Potential Indicators of This Nutrition Diagnosis (one or more must be present)
Biochemical Data, Medical Tests, and Procedures	Lab values indicating excessive intake of the specific substance, such as rapid ↓ in cholesterol from intake of stanol or sterol esters and a statin drug and related dietary changes or medications ↑ Hepatic enzyme reflecting hepatocellular damage
Anthropometric Measurements	Weight loss as a result of malabsorption or maldigestion

Continued on next page

Excessive Bioactive Substance Intake (Specify) (NI-4.2)

Continued from previous page

Diagnosis

Nutrition Assessment Category	Potential Indicators of This Nutrition Diagnosis (one or more must be present)
Nutrition-Focused Physical Findings	Constipation, diarrhea, nausea, stomach pain, gas, cramps or bloating, vomiting, heartburn
	Neurologic changes, eg, anxiety, mental status changes
	Cardiovascular changes, eg, heart rate, blood pressure
	Discomfort or pain associated with intake of foods rich in bioactive substances, eg, soluble fiber, ß-glucan, soy protein
	Headache/migraine
	Hives, flushing
	Irritability or nervousness

Food/Nutrition-Related History	Reports or observations of:
	 • High intake of plant foods containing:
	   ○ Soy protein ($\downarrow$ total and LDL cholesterol)
	   ○ ß-glucan, eg, whole oat products ($\downarrow$ total and LDL cholesterol)
	   ○ Plant sterol and stanol esters, eg, fortified margarines ($\downarrow$ total and LDL cholesterol) or other foods based on dietary substance, concentrate, metabolite, constituent, extract, or combination
	   ○ Substances that interfere with digestion or absorption of foodstuffs
	   ○ Ready access to available foods/products with bioactive substance, eg, as from dietary supplement vendors
	   ○ Attempts to use supplements or bioactive substances for weight loss, to treat constipation, or to prevent or cure chronic or acute disease
	   ○ Other substances (for which scientific evidence exists and a recommended intake level has been established)
	   ○ Intake of food additives for which patient/client is intolerant, eg, yellow 5, yellow 6, safrole, FD&C Red #4, carmine, MSG, sulfites
	 • Verbalizes inaccurate or incomplete knowledge about bioactive substances

Client History	Conditions associated with a diagnosis or treatment, eg, cardiovascular disease, elevated cholesterol, hypertension, asthma
	Cardiovascular changes, eg, EKG changes

Arrows used with laboratory values: $\uparrow$ represents above reference standard and $\downarrow$ represents below reference standard.

Excessive Alcohol Intake (NI-4.3)

Definition

Intake more than the suggested limits for alcohol

Signs/Symptoms (Defining Characteristics)

Factors gathered during the nutrition assessment process that contribute to the existence or the maintenance of pathophysiological, psychosocial, situational, developmental, cultural, and/or environmental problems:

- Unsupported beliefs/attitudes about food, nutrition, and nutrition-related topics
- Food- and nutrition-related knowledge deficit concerning appropriate alcohol intake
- Lack of value for behavior change, competing values
- Alcohol addiction

Signs/Symptoms (Defining Characteristics)

A typical cluster of subjective and objective signs and symptoms gathered during the nutrition assessment process that provide evidence that a problem exists; quantify the problem and describe its severity.

Nutrition Assessment Category	Potential Indicators of This Nutrition Diagnosis (one or more must be present)
Biochemical Data, Medical Tests, and Procedures	↑ Aspartate aminotransferase (AST), gamma-glutamyl transferase (GGT), carbohydrate-deficient transferrin, mean corpuscular volume, blood alcohol levels
Anthropometric Measurements	
Nutrition-Focused Physical Findings	
Food/Nutrition-Related History	Reports or observations of: • Intake of >2 drinks/day (men) • Intake of >1 drink/day (women) • Binge drinking • Consumption of any alcohol when contraindicated, eg, during pregnancy
Client History	Conditions associated with a diagnosis or treatment, eg, severe hypertriglyceridemia, elevated blood pressure, depression, liver disease, pancreatitis New medical diagnosis or change in existing diagnosis or condition History of estimated alcohol intake in excess of recommended Giving birth to an infant with fetal alcohol syndrome

Arrows used with laboratory values: ↑ represents above reference standard and ↓ represents below reference standard.

Note: 1 drink = 5 oz (150 mL) wine, 12 oz (350 mL) beer, 1.5 oz (45 mL) distilled alcohol.

Increased Nutrient Needs (Specify) (NI-5.1)

Definition

Increased need for a specific nutrient compared to established reference standards or recommendations based on physiological needs

Signs/Symptoms (Defining Characteristics)

Factors gathered during the nutrition assessment process that contribute to the existence or the maintenance of pathophysiological, psychosocial, situational, developmental, cultural, and/or environmental problems:

- Altered absorption or metabolism of nutrient, eg, from medications
- Compromise of organs related to GI function, eg, pancreas, liver
- Decreased functional length of intestine, eg, short-bowel syndrome
- Decreased or compromised function of intestine, eg, celiac disease, Crohn's disease
- Increased demand for nutrient, eg, accelerated growth, wound healing, chronic infection

Diagnosis

Increased Nutrient Needs (Specify) (NI-5.1)

Signs/Symptoms (Defining Characteristics)

A typical cluster of subjective and objective signs and symptoms gathered during the nutrition assessment process that provide evidence that a problem exists; quantify the problem and describe its severity.

Nutrition Assessment Category	Potential Indicators of This Nutrition Diagnosis (one or more must be present)
Biochemical Data, Medical Tests, and Procedures	↓ Total cholesterol <160 mg/dL, albumin, prealbumin, C-reactive protein, indicating increased stress and increased metabolic needs
	Electrolyte/mineral (eg, potassium, magnesium, phosphorus) abnormalities
	Urinary or fecal losses of specific or related nutrient (eg, fecal fat, d-xylose test)
	Vitamin and/or mineral deficiency
Anthropometric Measurements	Growth failure based on reference growth standards, eg, National Center for Health Statistics (NCHS) and fetal growth failure
	Unintentional weight loss of ≥5% in 1 month or ≥10% in 6 months
	Underweight (BMI <18.5)
	Low percent body fat and muscle mass
Nutrition-Focused Physical Findings	Clinical evidence of vitamin/mineral deficiency (eg, hair loss, bleeding gums, pale nail beds)
	Loss of skin integrity, delayed wound healing, or pressure ulcers
	Loss of muscle mass, subcutaneous fat
Food/Nutrition-Related History	Reports or observations of: • Estimated intake of foods/supplements containing needed nutrient less than estimated requirements • Intake of foods that do not contain sufficient quantities of available nutrient (eg, overprocessed, overcooked, or stored improperly) • Food- and nutrition-related knowledge deficit (eg, lack of information, incorrect information, or noncompliance with intake of needed nutrient) • Medications affecting absorption or metabolism of needed nutrient • Athletes or active individuals engaged in intense physical activity
Client History	Conditions associated with a diagnosis or treatment, eg, intestinal resection, Crohn's disease, HIV/AIDS, burns, preterm birth, malnutrition

Arrows used with laboratory values: ↑ represents above reference standard and ↓ represents below reference standard.

Diagnosis

Inadequate* Protein–Energy Intake (NI-5.2)

Definition

Inadequate intake of protein and/or energy compared to established reference standards or recommendations based on physiological needs of short or recent duration

> **Note:** Whenever possible, nutrient intake data should be considered in combination with clinical, biochemical, anthropometric information, medical diagnosis, clinical status, and/or other factors as well as diet to provide a valid assessment of nutritional status based on a totality of the evidence (Institute of Medicine. Dietary Reference Intakes: Applications in Dietary Assessment. Washington, DC: National Academies Press; 2000).

Etiology (Cause/Contributing Risk Factors)

Factors gathered during the nutrition assessment process that contribute to the existence or the maintenance of pathophysiological, psychosocial, situational, developmental, cultural, and/or environmental problems:

- Physiological causes increasing nutrient needs due to catabolic illness, malabsorption
- Decreased ability to consume sufficient protein and/or energy
- Lack of or limited access to food, eg, economic constraints, restricting food given or food selected
- Cultural or religious practices that affect ability to access food
- Food- and nutrition-related knowledge deficit concerning appropriate amount and type of dietary fat and/or protein
- Psychological causes such as depression and disordered eating

*If a synonym for the term "inadequate" is helpful or needed, an approved alternative is "suboptimal."

Inadequate* Protein–Energy Intake (NI-5.2)

Signs/Symptoms (Defining Characteristics)

A typical cluster of subjective and objective signs and symptoms gathered during the nutrition assessment process that provide evidence that a problem exists; quantify the problem and describe its severity.

Nutrition Assessment Category	Potential Indicators of This Nutrition Diagnosis (one or more must be present)
Biochemical Data, Medical Tests, and Procedures	Normal albumin (in the setting of normal liver function despite decreased protein-energy intake)
Anthropometric Measurements	Inadequate maternal weight gain (mild but not severe)
	Weight loss of 7% in 3 months, >5% in 1 month, or 1% to 2% in 1 week in adults; any weight loss or failure to gain weight in children
	Growth failure in children
Nutrition-Focused Physical Findings	Slow wound healing in pressure ulcer or surgical patient/client
Food/Nutrition-Related History	Reports or observations of: • Estimated energy intake from diet less than estimated or measured RMR or recommended levels • Restriction or omission of food groups such as dairy or meat group foods (protein); bread or milk group foods (energy) • Recent food avoidance and/or lack of interest in food • Lack of ability to prepare meals • Excessive consumption of alcohol or other drugs that reduce hunger • Hunger in the face of inadequate access to food supply
Client History	Conditions associated with a diagnosis or treatment of mild protein-energy malnutrition, recent illness (eg, pulmonary or cardiac failure, flu, infection, surgery)
	Nutrient malabsorption (eg, bariatric surgery, diarrhea, steatorrhea)
	Lack of funds for purchase of appropriate foods

*If a synonym for the term "inadequate" is helpful or needed, an approved alternative is "suboptimal."

Diagnosis

Decreased Nutrient Needs (Specify) (NI-5.3)

Definition

Decreased need for a specific nutrient compared to established reference standards or recommendations based on physiological needs

Etiology (Cause/Contributing Risk Factors)

Factors gathered during the nutrition assessment process that contribute to the existence or maintenance of pathophysiological, psychosocial, situational, developmental, cultural, and/or environmental problems:

- Renal dysfunction
- Liver dysfunction
- Altered cholesterol metabolism/regulation
- Heart failure
- Food intolerances, eg, irritable bowel syndrome

Decreased Nutrient Needs (Specify) (NI-5.3)

Signs/Symptoms (Defining Characteristics)

A typical cluster of subjective and objective signs and symptoms gathered during the nutrition assessment process that provide evidence that a problem exists; quantify the problem and describe its severity.

Nutrition Assessment Category	Potential Indicators of This Nutrition Diagnosis (one or more must be present)
Biochemical Data, Medical Tests, and Procedures	↑ Total cholesterol >200 mg/dL (5.2 mmol/L), ↑ LDL cholesterol >100 mg/dL (2.59 mmol/L), ↓ HDL cholesterol <40 mg/dL (1.036 mmol/L), ↑ triglycerides >150 mg/dL (1.695 mmol/L)
	↑ Phosphorus >5.5 mg/dL (1.78 mmol/L)
	↓ Glomerular filtration rate (GFR) <90 mL/min/1.73 m^2
	↑ BUN, creatinine, potassium
	↑ Liver function tests indicating severe liver disease
Anthropometric Measurements	Interdialytic weight gain greater than expected
Nutrition-Focused Physical Findings	Edema/fluid retention
Food/Nutrition-Related History	Reports or observations of: • Estimated intake higher than recommended for fat, phosphorus, sodium, protein, fiber
Client History	Conditions associated with a diagnosis or treatment that require a specific type and/or amount of nutrient, eg, cardiovascular disease (fat), early renal disease (protein, phosphorus), ESRD (phosphorus, sodium, potassium, fluid), advanced liver disease (protein), heart failure (sodium, fluid), irritable bowel disease/Crohn's flare-up (fiber)
	Diagnosis of hypertension, confusion related to liver disease

Arrows used with laboratory values: ↑ represents above reference standard and ↓ represents below reference standard.

Diagnosis

Diagnosis

Imbalance of Nutrients (NI-5.4)

Definition

An undesirable combination of nutrients, such that the amount of one nutrient interferes with or alters absorption and/or utilization of another nutrient

Etiology (Cause/Contributing Risk Factors)

Factors gathered during the nutrition assessment process that contribute to the existence or the maintenance of pathophysiological, psychosocial, situational, developmental, cultural, and/or environmental problems:

- Consumption of high-dose nutrient supplements
- Food- and nutrition-related knowledge deficit concerning nutrient interactions
- Unsupported beliefs/attitudes about food, nutrition, and nutrition-related information
- Food faddism
- Insufficient electrolyte replacement when initiating feeding (PN/EN, including oral)

Signs/Symptoms (Defining Characteristics)

A typical cluster of subjective and objective signs and symptoms gathered during the nutrition assessment process that provide evidence that a problem exists; quantify the problem and describe its severity.

Nutrition Assessment Category	Potential Indicators of This Nutrition Diagnosis (one or more must be present)
Biochemical Data, Medical Tests, and Procedures	Severe hypophosphatemia (in the presence of increased carbohydrate) Severe hypokalemia (in the presence of increased protein) Severe hypomagnesemia (in the presence of increased carbohydrate)
Anthropometric Measurements	
Nutrition-Focused Physical Findings	Diarrhea or constipation (iron supplements) Epigastric pain, nausea, vomiting, diarrhea (zinc supplements)
Food/Nutrition-Related History	Reports or observations of: • Estimated intake of iron supplements (decreased zinc absorption) higher than recommended • Estimated intake of zinc supplements (decreased copper status) higher than recommended • Estimated intake of manganese (decreased iron status) higher than recommended
Client History	Refeeding syndrome

Inadequate* Fat Intake (NI-5.5.1)

Definition

Lower fat intake compared to established reference standards or recommendations based on physiological needs

> **Note:** May not be an appropriate nutrition diagnosis when the goal is weight loss or during end-of-life care.
>
> Whenever possible, nutrient intake data should be considered in combination with clinical, biochemical, anthropo-metric information, medical diagnosis, clinical status, and/or other factors as well as diet to provide a valid assessment of nutritional status based on a totality of the evidence (Institute of Medicine. Dietary Reference Intakes: Applications in Dietary Assessment. Washington, DC: National Academies Press; 2000).

Etiology (Cause/Contributing Risk Factors)

Factors gathered during the nutrition assessment process that contribute to the existence or maintenance of patho-physiological, psychosocial, situational, developmental, cultural, and/or environmental problems:

- Alteration in gastrointestinal tract structure and/or function
- Less than optimal food choices, eg, economic constraints, restricting food given to older adults and/or children, specific food choices
- Cultural practices that affect ability to make appropriate food choices
- Food- and nutrition-related knowledge deficit concerning appropriate amount of dietary fat
- Psychological causes such as depression and disordered eating

*If a synonym for the term "inadequate" is helpful or needed, an approved alternative is "suboptimal."

Diagnosis

Inadequate* Fat Intake (NI-5.5.1)

Signs/Symptoms (Defining Characteristics)

A typical cluster of subjective and objective signs and symptoms gathered during the nutrition assessment process that provide evidence that a problem exists; quantify the problem and describe its severity

Nutrition Assessment Category	Potential Indicators of This Nutrition Diagnosis (one or more must be present)
Biochemical Data, Medical Tests, and Procedures	↑ Triene:tetraene ratio >0.2
Anthropometric Measurements	Impaired growth Weight loss if insufficient calories/kcal/kJ consumed
Nutrition-Focused Physical Findings	Scaly skin and dermatitis consistent with essential fatty acid deficiency
Food/Nutrition-Related History	Reports or observations of: • Estimated intake of essential fatty acids less than 10% of energy (primarily associated with parenteral nutrition) • Verbalizes inaccurate or incomplete knowledge • Cultural or religious practices that affect intake
Client History	Conditions associated with a diagnosis or treatment, eg, prolonged catabolic illness (eg, AIDS, tuberculosis, anorexia nervosa, sepsis or severe infection from recent surgery) Severe fat malabsorption with bowel resection, pancreatic insufficiency, or hepatic disease accompanied by steatorrhea

Arrows used with laboratory values: ↑ represents above reference standard and ↓ represents below reference standard.

*If a synonym for the term "inadequate" is helpful or needed, an approved alternative is "suboptimal."

Diagnosis

Excessive Fat Intake (NI-5.5.2)

Definition

Higher fat intake compared to established reference standards or recommendations based on physiological needs

Etiology (Cause/Contributing Risk Factors)

Factors gathered during the nutrition assessment process that contribute to the existence or the maintenance of pathophysiological, psychosocial, situational, developmental, cultural, and/or environmental problems:

- Food- and nutrition-related knowledge deficit concerning appropriate amount of dietary fat
- Unsupported beliefs/attitudes about food, nutrition, and nutrition-related topics
- Lack of or limited access to healthful food choices, eg, healthful food choices not provided as an option by caregiver or parent; homeless
- Changes in taste and appetite or preference
- Lack of value for behavior change, competing values
- Physiological causes decreasing total fat needs or recommendations

Excessive Fat Intake (NI-5.5.2)

Signs/Symptoms (Defining Characteristics)

A typical cluster of subjective and objective signs and symptoms gathered during the nutrition assessment process that provide evidence that a problem exists; quantify the problem and describe its severity.

Nutrition Assessment Category	Potential Indicators of This Nutrition Diagnosis (one or more must be present)
Biochemical Data, Medical Tests, and Procedures	↑ Cholesterol >200 mg/dL (5.2 mmol/L), ↑ LDL cholesterol >100 mg/dL (2.59 mmol/L), ↓ HDL cholesterol <40 mg/dL (1.036 mmol/L), ↑ triglycerides >150 mg/dL (1.695 mmol/L) ↑ Serum amylase and/or lipase ↑ LFTs, Total bilirubin ↑ Fecal fat >7g/24 hours
Anthropometric Measurements	
Nutrition-Focused Physical Findings	Evidence of xanthomas Diarrhea, cramping, steatorrhea, epigastric pain
Food/Nutrition-Related History	Reports or observations of: • Frequent or large portions of high-fat foods • Frequent food preparation with added fat • Frequent consumption of high-risk lipids (ie, saturated fat, trans fat, cholesterol) • Report of foods containing fat more than diet prescription • Medication, eg, pancreatic enzymes, cholesterol- or other lipid-lowering medications • Verbalizes inaccurate or incomplete knowledge • Verbalizes unsupported beliefs or attitudes
Client History	Conditions associated with a diagnosis or treatment, eg, hyperlipidemia; cystic fibrosis; angina; artherosclerosis; pancreatic, liver, and biliary diseases; post-transplantation chyle fluid leak Family history of hyperlipidemia, atherosclerosis, or pancreatitis

Arrows used with laboratory values: ↑ represents above reference standard and ↓ represents below reference standard.

Intake of Types of Fats Inconsistent With Needs (Specify) (NI-5.5.3)

Definition

Intake of wrong type or quality of fats compared to established reference standards or recommendations based on physiological needs

Etiology (Cause/Contributing Risk Factors)

Factors gathered during the nutrition assessment process that contribute to the existence or the maintenance of pathophysiological, psychosocial, situational, developmental, cultural, and/or environmental problems:

- Food- and nutrition-related knowledge deficit concerning type of fat (eg, fats added to food, formula/breastmilk)
- Unsupported beliefs/attitudes about food, nutrition, and nutrition-related topics
- Lack of or limited access to healthful food choices, eg, healthful food choices not provided as an option by caregiver or parent; homeless
- Changes in taste and appetite or preference
- Lack of value for behavior change, competing values
- Physiological causes altering fatty acid needs or recommendations

Diagnosis

Intake of Types of Fats Inconsistent With Needs (Specify) (NI-5.5.3)

Signs/Symptoms (Defining Characteristics)

A typical cluster of subjective and objective signs and symptoms gathered during the nutrition assessment process that provide evidence that a problem exists; quantify the problem and describe its severity.

Nutrition Assessment Category	Potential Indicators of This Nutrition Diagnosis (one or more must be present)
Biochemical Data, Medical Tests, and Procedures	↑ Cholesterol >200 mg/dL (5.2 mmol/L), ↑ LDL cholesterol >100 mg/dL (2.59 mmol/L), ↓ HDL cholesterol <40 mg/dL (1.036 mmol/L) men, ↓ HDL cholesterol <50 mg/dL (1.3 mmol/L) women, ↑ triglycerides >150 mg/dL (1.695 mmol/L)
	↑ Serum amylase and/or lipase
	↑ LFTs, Total bilirubin, C-reactive protein
	Altered acylcarnitine, carnitine, and other measures of fatty acid metabolism
	Elevated triene:tetraene ratio (>0.2)
	Altered fatty acid panel mitochondrial C8–C18, serum or plasma (µmol/L)
	Altered fatty acid panel mitochondrial C2–C22, serum or plasma (µmol/L)
	Altered fatty acid panel mitochondrial C22–C26, serum or plasma (µmol/L)
Anthropometric Measurements	
Nutrition-Focused Physical Findings	Evidence of dermatitis
	Diarrhea, cramping, steatorrhea, epigastric pain
Food/Nutrition-Related History	Reports or observations of:
	• Frequent food preparation with added fat that is not of desired type for condition
	• Frequent consumption of fats that are undesirable for condition (eg, saturated fat, trans fat, cholesterol, n-6 fatty acids, fatty acid chain length)
	• Estimated intake of monounsaturated, polyunsaturated, n-3 fatty acids, or DHA/ARA fatty acid chain length less than recommended or in sub-optimal ratio
	• Verbalization of inaccurate or incomplete knowledge
	• Verbalization of unsupported beliefs and attitudes
Client History	Conditions associated with a diagnosis or treatment, eg, diabetes, cardiac diseases, obesity, liver or biliary disorders, chyle fluid leak, inborn errors of metabolism
	Family history of diabetes-related heart disease, hyperlipidemia, atherosclerosis, or pancreatitis

Arrows used with laboratory values: ↑ represents above reference standard and ↓ represents below reference standard.

Inadequate* Protein Intake (NI-5.6.1)

Definition

Lower intake of protein compared to established reference standards or recommendations based on physiological needs

Note: Whenever possible, nutrient intake data should be considered in combination with clinical, biochemical, anthropometric information, medical diagnosis, clinical status, and/or other factors as well as diet to provide a valid assessment of nutritional status based on a totality of the evidence (Institute of Medicine. Dietary Reference Intakes: Applications in Dietary Assessment. Washington, DC: National Academies Press; 2000).

Etiology (Cause/Contributing Risk Factors)

Factors gathered during the nutrition assessment process that contribute to the existence or the maintenance of pathophysiological, psychosocial, situational, developmental, cultural, and/or environmental problems:

- Physiological causes increasing nutrient needs due to prolonged catabolic illness, malabsorption, age, or condition
- Decreased ability to consume sufficient protein
- Lack of or limited access to food, eg, economic constraints, restricting food given to older adults and/or children
- Cultural practices that affect the ability to access food
- Food- and nutrition-related knowledge deficit concerning amount of protein
- Psychological causes such as depression and disordered eating

*If a synonym for the term "inadequate" is helpful or needed, an approved alternative is "suboptimal."

Inadequate* Protein Intake (NI-5.6.1)

Signs/Symptoms (Defining Characteristics)

A typical cluster of subjective and objective signs and symptoms gathered during the nutrition assessment process that provide evidence that a problem exists; quantify the problem and describe its severity.

Nutrition Assessment Category	Potential Indicators of This Nutrition Diagnosis (one or more must be present)
Biochemical Data, Medical Tests, and Procedures	
Anthropometric Measurements	
Nutrition-Focused Physical Findings	Edema Failure to thrive (infants/children) Poor musculature Dull skin Thin and fragile hair
Food/Nutrition-Related History	Reports or observations of: • Estimated intake of protein insufficient to meet requirements • Cultural or religious practices that limit protein intake • Economic constraints that limit food availability • Prolonged adherence to a very low-protein weight loss diet • Verbalizes inaccurate or incomplete knowledge
Client History	Conditions associated with a diagnosis or treatment, eg, severe protein malabsorption such as bowel resection

*If a synonym for the term "inadequate" is helpful or needed, an approved alternative is "suboptimal."

Excessive Protein Intake (NI-5.6.2)

Definition

Intake more than the recommended level of protein compared to established reference standards or recommendations based on physiological needs

Etiology (Cause/Contributing Risk Factors)

Factors gathered during the nutrition assessment process that contribute to the existence or the maintenance of pathophysiological, psychosocial, situational, developmental, cultural, and/or environmental problems:

- Liver dysfunction
- Renal dysfunction
- Unsupported beliefs/attitudes about food, nutrition, and nutrition-related topics
- Food and nutrition-related knowledge deficit
- Lack of or limited access to specialized protein products
- Metabolic abnormality
- Food faddism

Signs/Symptoms (Defining Characteristics)

A typical cluster of subjective and objective signs and symptoms gathered during the nutrition assessment process that provide evidence that a problem exists; quantify the problem and describe its severity.

Nutrition Assessment Category	Potential Indicators of This Nutrition Diagnosis (one or more must be present)
Biochemical Data, Medical Tests, and Procedures	Altered laboratory values, eg, ↑ BUN, ↓ glomerular filtration rate (altered renal status)
Anthropometric Measurements	Growth stunting or failure based on National Center for Health Statistics growth charts (metabolic disorders)
Nutrition-Focused Physical Findings	
Food/Nutrition-Related History	Reports or observations of: • Estimated total protein intake higher than recommended, eg, early renal disease, advanced liver disease with confusion • Less than optimal supplementation • Verbalizes inaccurate or incomplete knowledge • Verbalizes unsupported beliefs and attitudes
Client History	Conditions associated with a diagnosis or treatment, eg, early renal disease or advanced liver disease with confusion

Arrows used with laboratory values: ↑ represents above reference standard and ↓ represents below reference standard.

Diagnosis

Intake of Types of Proteins Inconsistent With Needs (Specify) (NI-5.6.3)

Definition

Intake of an amount of a specific type of protein compared to established reference standards or recommendations based on physiological needs

Etiology (Cause/Contributing Risk Factors)

Factors gathered during the nutrition assessment process that contribute to the existence or the maintenance of pathophysiological, psychosocial, situational, developmental, cultural, and/or environmental problems:

- Liver dysfunction
- Renal dysfunction
- Unsupported beliefs/attitudes about food, nutrition, and nutrition-related topics
- Misused specialized protein products
- Metabolic abnormality
- Food faddism
- Inborn errors of metabolism
- Celiac disease, dermatitis herpetiformis, or other GI disease
- Cultural or religious practices that affect the ability to regulate types of protein or amino acids consumed
- Food- and nutrition-related knowledge deficit concerning an appropriate amount of a specific types of proteins or amino acids
- Food and nutrition compliance limitations, eg, lack of willingness or failure to modify protein or amino acid intake in response to recommendations from a dietitian, physician, or caregiver
- Insufficient access to appropriate protein sources

Intake of Types of Proteins Inconsistent With Needs (Specify) (NI-5.6.3)

Signs/Symptoms (Defining Characteristics)

A typical cluster of subjective and objective signs and symptoms gathered during the nutrition assessment process that provide evidence that a problem exists; quantify the problem and describe its severity.

Nutrition Assessment Category	Potential Indicators of This Nutrition Diagnosis (one or more must be present)
Biochemical Data, Medical Tests, and Procedures	Altered laboratory values, eg, ↑ BUN, ↓ glomerular filtration rate (altered renal status) ↑ Specific amino acids (inborn errors of metabolism) ↑ Homocysteine or ammonia Positive autoantibody levels (Anti-tTG antibodies, EmA IgA tissue transglutaminase [tTG], and IgA endomysial antibodies [EMA]) Positive small bowel biopsy for celiac or other GI disease
Anthropometric Measurements	Weight loss, Inability to gain weight Delayed growth
Nutrition-Focused Physical Findings	Physical or neurological changes (inborn errors of metabolism) Diarrhea in response to certain types of carbohydrates Abdominal pain, distention, constipation, reflux, GERD, vomiting
Food/Nutrition-Related History	Reports or observations of: • Estimated protein intake from all sources higher or lower than recommended • Estimated energy intake from all sources lower than recommended • Less than optimal supplementation of specific types of protein • Limited knowledge of protein composition or of protein metabolism • Chronic use of medications containing proteins not recommended
Client History	Conditions associated with a diagnosis or treatment of illness that requires EN/PN therapy, celiac disease, dermatitis herpetiformis, allergies, inborn errors of metabolism Uremia, azotemia (renal patients)

Arrows used with laboratory values: ↑ represents above reference standard and ↓ represents below reference standard.

Intake of Types of Amino Acids Inconsistent With Needs (Specify) (NI-5.7.1)

Definition

Intake of an amount of a specific type of amino acid compared to established reference standards or recommendations based on physiological needs

Etiology (Cause/Contributing Risk Factors)

Factors gathered during the nutrition assessment process that contribute to the existence or the maintenance of pathophysiological, psychosocial, situational, developmental, cultural, and/or environmental problems:

- Liver dysfunction
- Renal dysfunction
- Unsupported beliefs/attitudes about food, nutrition, and nutrition-related topics
- Misused specialized amino acid products
- Metabolic demand or abnormality
- Medication with an amino acid interaction
- Inborn errors of metabolism
- Food- and nutrition-related knowledge deficit concerning an appropriate amount of specific amino acids
- Food and nutrition compliance limitations, eg, lack of willingness or failure to modify amino acid intake in response to recommendations from a dietitian, physician, or caregiver
- Insufficient access to appropriate amino acid sources

Intake of Types of Amino Acids Inconsistent With Needs (Specify) (NI-5.7.1)

Signs/Symptoms (Defining Characteristics)

A typical cluster of subjective and objective signs and symptoms gathered during the nutrition assessment process that provide evidence that a problem exists; quantify the problem and describe its severity.

Nutrition Assessment Category	Potential Indicators of This Nutrition Diagnosis (one or more must be present)
Biochemical Data, Medical Tests, and Procedures	↑ or ↓ specific amino acids (serum, plasma, or urine) ↑ ammonia, serum
Anthropometric Measurements	Weight loss Inability to gain weight Delayed growth
Nutrition-Focused Physical Findings	Physical or neurological changes Vomiting Diarrhea Fever
Food/Nutrition-Related History	Reports or observations of: • Estimated amino acid intake higher or lower than recommended via all routes • Less than optimal amino acid supplementation • Incomplete knowledge of amino acid composition or of amino acid metabolism • Estimated energy intake from all sources lower than recommended
Client History	Conditions associated with a diagnosis or treatment of illness that requires EN/PN therapy, food allergy or intolerance, inborn errors of metabolism, liver disease, kidney disease

Arrows used with laboratory values: ↑ represents above reference standard and ↓ represents below reference standard.

Diagnosis

Inadequate* Carbohydrate Intake (NI-5.8.1)

Diagnosis

Definition

Lower intake of carbohydrate compared to established reference standards or recommendations based on physiological needs

> **Note:** Whenever possible, nutrient intake data should be considered in combination with clinical, biochemical, anthropometric information, medical diagnosis, clinical status, and/or other factors as well as diet to provide a valid assessment of nutritional status based on a totality of the evidence (Institute of Medicine. Dietary Reference Intakes: Applications in Dietary Assessment. Washington, DC: National Academies Press; 2000).

Etiology (Cause/Contributing Risk Factors)

Factors gathered during the nutrition assessment process that contribute to the existence or the maintenance of pathophysiological, psychosocial, situational, developmental, cultural, and/or environmental problems:

- Physiological causes, eg, increased energy needs due to increased activity level or metabolic change, malabsorption
- Lack of or limited access to food, eg, economic constraints, restricting food given to older adults and/or children
- Cultural practices that affect the ability to access food
- Food- and nutrition-related knowledge deficit concerning appropriate amount of dietary carbohydrate
- Psychological causes such as depression and disordered eating

---

*If a synonym for the term "inadequate" is helpful or needed, an approved alternative is "suboptimal."

Inadequate* Carbohydrate Intake (NI-5.8.1)

Signs/Symptoms (Defining Characteristics)

A typical cluster of subjective and objective signs and symptoms gathered during the nutrition assessment process that provide evidence that a problem exists; quantify the problem and describe its severity.

Nutrition Assessment Category	Potential Indicators of This Nutrition Diagnosis (one or more must be present)
Biochemical Data, Medical Tests, and Procedures	
Anthropometric Measurements	
Nutrition-Focused Physical Findings	Ketone smell on breath
Food/Nutrition-Related History	Reports or observations of: • Estimated carbohydrate intake less than recommended amounts • Inability to independently consume foods/fluids, eg, diminished mobility in hand, wrist, or digits • Verbalizes inaccurate or incomplete knowledge
Client History	Conditions associated with a diagnosis or treatment, eg, pancreatic insufficiency, hepatic disease, celiac disease, seizure disorder, or carbohydrate malabsorption

Diagnosis

*If a synonym for the term "inadequate" is helpful or needed, an approved alternative is "suboptimal."

Excessive Carbohydrate Intake (NI-5.8.2)

Diagnosis

Definition

Intake more than the recommended level and type of carbohydrate compared to established reference standards or recommendations based on physiological needs

Etiology (Cause/Contributing Risk Factors)

Factors gathered during the nutrition assessment process that contribute to the existence or the maintenance of pathophysiological, psychosocial, situational, developmental, cultural, and/or environmental problems:

- Physiological causes requiring modified carbohydrate intake, eg, diabetes mellitus, lactase deficiency, sucrase-isomaltase deficiency, aldolase B deficiency
- Cultural practices that affect the ability to reduce carbohydrate intake
- Food- and nutrition-related knowledge deficit concerning appropriate amount of carbohydrate intake
- Food and nutrition compliance limitations, eg, lack of willingness or failure to modify carbohydrate intake in response to recommendations from a dietitian or physician
- Psychological causes such as depression and disordered eating

Excessive Carbohydrate Intake (NI-5.8.2)

Signs/Symptoms (Defining Characteristics)

A typical cluster of subjective and objective signs and symptoms gathered during the nutrition assessment process that provide evidence that a problem exists; quantify the problem and describe its severity.

Nutrition Assessment Category	Potential Indicators of This Nutrition Diagnosis (one or more must be present)
Biochemical Data, Medical Tests, and Procedures	Hyperglycemia (↑ fasting blood glucose >126 mg/dL) ↑ Hemoglobin A1C >6% ↑ Oral glucose tolerance test (2-hour postload glucose >200 mg/dL)
Anthropometric Measurements	
Nutrition-Focused Physical Findings	Dental caries Diarrhea
Food/Nutrition-Related History	Reports or observations of: • Cultural or religious practices that do not support modification of dietary carbohydrate intake • Estimated carbohydrate intake that is consistently more than recommended amounts • Chronic use of medications that cause hyperglycemia, eg, steroids • Verbalizes inaccurate or incomplete knowledge
Client History	Conditions associated with a diagnosis or treatment, eg, diabetes mellitus, inborn errors of carbohydrate metabolism, lactase deficiency, severe infection, sepsis or obesity Pancreatic insufficiency resulting in reduced insulin production Economic constraints that limit availability of appropriate foods

Arrows used with laboratory values: ↑ represents above reference standard and ↓ represents below reference standard.

Diagnosis

Intake of Types of Carbohydrate Inconsistent With Needs (Specify) (NI-5.8.3)

Definition

Intake of an amount of a specific type of carbohydrate compared to the established reference standards or recommendations based on physiological needs

> **Note:** Intolerance to the protein component of grains (eg, gluten) should be documented using the Intake of Types of Proteins Inconsistent With Needs (NI-5.6.3) reference sheet.

Etiology (Cause/Contributing Risk Factors)

Factors gathered during the nutrition assessment process that contribute to the existence or the maintenance of pathophysiological, psychosocial, situational, developmental, cultural, and/or environmental problems:

- Physiological causes altering carbohydrate digestion or metabolism, eg, intolerance, inborn errors of carbohydrate metabolism

  > **Note:** Although research does not support restriction of individual types of carbohydrate for glycemic control, nutrition and dietetics practitioners may determine that restriction is warranted in unique patient/client situations for glycemic control and/or for other reasons, such as promotion of healthful eating.

- Cultural or religious practices that affect the ability to regulate types of carbohydrate consumed
- Food- and nutrition-related knowledge deficit concerning an appropriate amount of a specific type of carbohydrate
- Food and nutrition compliance limitations, eg, lack of willingness or failure to modify carbohydrate intake in response to recommendations from a dietitian, physician, or caregiver
- Psychological causes such as depression and disordered eating

Intake of Types of Carbohydrate Inconsistent With Needs (Specify) (NI-5.8.3)

Signs/Symptoms (Defining Characteristics)

A typical cluster of subjective and objective signs and symptoms gathered during the nutrition assessment process that provide evidence that a problem exists; quantify the problem and describe its severity.

Nutrition Assessment Category	Potential Indicators of This Nutrition Diagnosis (one or more must be present)
Biochemical Data, Medical Tests, and Procedures	Hypoglycemia or hyperglycemia ↓ galactose-1-phosphate in red blood cells, ↓ galactose-1-phosphate uridyl transferase, ↓ fructose
Anthropometric Measurements	Weight loss Inability to gain weight Delayed growth Weight gain
Nutrition-Focused Physical Findings	Diarrhea in response to certain types of carbohydrate Abdominal pain, distention, constipation, reflux, GERD
Food/Nutrition-Related History	Reports or observations of: • Carbohydrate intake that is a different type or exceeds amount recommended for that specific type of carbohydrate • Limited knowledge of carbohydrate composition of foods or of carbohydrate metabolism • Chronic use of medications that cause altered glucose levels, eg, steroids, diabetes medication, antidepressants, antipsychotics, or that contain a type of carbohydrate not recommended • Cultural or religious practices that affect intake
Client History	Conditions associated with a diagnosis or treatment, eg, intolerance, inborn errors of metabolism Allergic reactions or intolerance to certain carbohydrate foods or food groups Economic constraints that limit availability of appropriate foods

Arrows used with laboratory values: ↑ represents above reference standard and ↓ represents below reference standard.

Diagnosis

Inconsistent Carbohydrate Intake (NI-5.8.4)

Definition

Inconsistent timing of carbohydrate intake throughout the day, day to day, or a pattern of carbohydrate intake that is not consistent with recommended pattern based on physiological or medication needs

Etiology (Cause/Contributing Risk Factors)

Factors gathered during the nutrition assessment process that contribute to the existence or the maintenance of pathophysiological, psychosocial, situational, developmental, cultural, and/or environmental problems:

- Physiological causes requiring careful timing and consistency in the amount of carbohydrate, eg, diabetes mellitus, hypoglycemia, PN/EN delivery
- Cultural practices that affect the ability to regulate timing of carbohydrate consumption
- Food- and nutrition-related knowledge deficit concerning appropriate timing of carbohydrate intake
- Food and nutrition compliance limitations, eg, lack of willingness or failure to modify carbohydrate timing in response to recommendations from a dietitian, physician, or caregiver
- Psychological causes such as depression and disordered eating

Inconsistent Carbohydrate Intake (NI-5.8.4)

Signs/Symptoms (Defining Characteristics)

A typical cluster of subjective and objective signs and symptoms gathered during the nutrition assessment process that provide evidence that a problem exists; quantify the problem and describe its severity.

Nutrition Assessment Category	Potential Indicators of This Nutrition Diagnosis (one or more must be present)
Biochemical Data, Medical Tests, and Procedures	Hypoglycemia or hyperglycemia documented on a regular basis associated with inconsistent carbohydrate intake Wide variations in blood glucose levels
Anthropometric Measurements	
Nutrition-Focused Physical Findings	
Food/Nutrition-Related History	Reports or observations of: • Estimated carbohydrate intake that is different from recommended types or ingested on an irregular basis • Use of insulin or insulin secretagogues • Chronic use of medications that cause altered glucose levels, eg, steroids, antidepressants, antipsychotics • Verbalizes inaccurate or incomplete knowledge • Cultural or religious practices that affect intake
Client History	Conditions associated with a diagnosis or treatment, eg, diabetes mellitus, obesity, metabolic syndrome, hypoglycemia Economic constraints that limit availability of appropriate foods

Diagnosis

Inadequate* Fiber Intake (NI-5.8.5)

Definition

Lower intake of fiber compared to established reference standards or recommendations based on physiological needs.

> **Note:** Whenever possible, nutrient intake data should be considered in combination with clinical, biochemical, anthropometric information, medical diagnosis, clinical status, and/or other factors as well as diet to provide a valid assessment of nutritional status based on a totality of the evidence (Institute of Medicine. Dietary Reference Intakes: Applications in Dietary Assessment. Washington, DC: National Academies Press; 2000).

Etiology (Cause/Contributing Risk Factors)

Factors gathered during the nutrition assessment process that contribute to the existence or the maintenance of pathophysiological, psychosocial, situational, developmental, cultural, and/or environmental problems:

- Lack of or limited access to fiber-containing foods/fluids
- Food- and nutrition-related knowledge deficit concerning desirable quantities of fiber
- Psychological causes such as depression and disordered eating
- Prolonged adherence to a low-fiber or low-residue diet
- Difficulty chewing or swallowing high-fiber foods
- Economic constraints that limit availability of appropriate foods
- Inability or unwillingness to purchase or consume fiber-containing foods
- Less than optimal food-preparation practices, eg, reliance on overprocessed, overcooked foods

*If a synonym for the term "inadequate" is helpful or needed, an approved alternative is "suboptimal."

Inadequate* Fiber Intake (NI-5.8.5)

Signs/Symptoms (Defining Characteristics)

A typical cluster of subjective and objective signs and symptoms gathered during the nutrition assessment process that provide evidence that a problem exists; quantify the problem and describe its severity.

Nutrition Assessment Category	Potential Indicators of This Nutrition Diagnosis (one or more must be present)
Biochemical Data, Medical Tests, and Procedures	
Anthropometric Measurements	
Nutrition-Focused Physical Findings	Inadequate fecal bulk
Food/Nutrition-Related History	Reports or observations of: • Estimated intake of fiber that is insufficient when compared to recommended amounts (38 g/day for men and 25 g/day for women) • Verbalizes inaccurate or incomplete knowledge
Client History	Conditions associated with a diagnosis or treatment, eg, ulcer disease, inflammatory bowel disease, short-bowel syndrome treated with a low-fiber diet

Diagnosis

*If a synonym for the term "inadequate" is helpful or needed, an approved alternative is "suboptimal."

Excessive Fiber Intake (NI-5.8.6)

Definition

Higher intake of fiber compared to recommendations based on patient/client condition

Etiology (Cause/Contributing Risk Factors)

Factors gathered during the nutrition assessment process that contribute to the existence or the maintenance of pathophysiological, psychosocial, situational, developmental, cultural, and/or environmental problems:

- Food- and nutrition-related knowledge deficit concerning desirable quantities of fiber
- Unsupported beliefs or attitudes about food- or nutrition-related topics, eg, obsession with bowel frequency and habits
- Lack of knowledge about appropriate fiber intake for condition
- Food preparation or eating patterns that involve only high-fiber foods to the exclusion of other nutrient-dense foods

Signs/Symptoms (Defining Characteristics)

A typical cluster of subjective and objective signs and symptoms gathered during the nutrition assessment process that provide evidence that a problem exists; quantify the problem and describe its severity.

Nutrition Assessment Category	Potential Indicators of This Nutrition Diagnosis (one or more must be present)
Biochemical Data, Medical Tests, and Procedures	
Anthropometric Measurements	
Nutrition-Focused Physical Findings	Nausea, vomiting, excessive flatulence, diarrhea, abdominal cramping, high stool volume or frequency that causes discomfort to the individual
Food/Nutrition-Related History	Reports or observations of: • Estimated fiber intake higher than tolerated or generally recommended for current medical condition • Verbalizes inaccurate or incomplete knowledge • Verbalizes unsupported beliefs and attitudes
Client History	Conditions associated with a diagnosis or treatment, eg, ulcer disease, irritable bowel syndrome, inflammatory bowel disease, short-bowel syndrome, diverticulitis, obstructive constipation, prolapsing hemorrhoids, gastrointestinal stricture, eating disorders, or mental illness with obsessive–compulsive tendencies Obstruction, phytobezoar

Inadequate* Vitamin Intake (Specify) (NI-5.9.1)

Definition

Lower intake of one or more vitamins compared to established reference standards or recommendations based on physiological needs

Note: Whenever possible, nutrient intake data should be considered in combination with clinical, biochemical, anthropometric information, medical diagnosis, clinical status, and/or other factors as well as diet to provide a valid assessment of nutritional status based on a totality of the evidence. (Institute of Medicine. Dietary Reference Intakes: Applications in Dietary Assessment. Washington, DC: National Academies Press; 2000.)

Etiology (Cause/Contributing Risk Factors)

Factors gathered during the nutrition assessment process that contribute to the existence or the maintenance of pathophysiological, psychosocial, situational, developmental, cultural, and/or environmental problems:

- Physiological causes increasing nutrient needs, eg, due to prolonged catabolic illness, disease state, malabsorption, or medications
- Decreased ability to consume sufficient amount of a vitamin(s)
- Lack of or limited access to food, eg, economic constraints, restricting food given to older adults and/or children
- Cultural practices that affect ability to access food
- Food- and nutrition-related knowledge deficit concerning food and supplemental sources of vitamins
- Psychological causes, eg, depression or eating disorders
- Access causes, including season, geography, limited access to sunlight

Signs/Symptoms (Defining Characteristics)

A typical cluster of subjective and objective signs and symptoms gathered during the nutrition assessment process that provide evidence that a problem exists; quantify the problem and describe its severity.

*If a synonym for the term "inadequate" is helpful or needed, an approved alternative is "suboptimal."

Inadequate* Vitamin Intake (Specify) (NI-5.9.1)

Nutrition Assessment Category	Potential Indicators of This Nutrition Diagnosis (one or more must be present)
Biochemical Data, Medical Tests, and Procedures	Vitamin A: ↓ serum retinol <10 µg/dL (0.35 µmol/L)
	Vitamin C: ↓ plasma concentrations <0.2 mg/dL (11.4 µmol/L)
	Vitamin D: ↓ 25(OH)D <50 nmol/L, ↓ ionized calcium <3.9 mg/dL (0.98 mmol/L) with ↑ parathyroid hormone, normal serum calcium, and ↓ serum phosphorus <2.6 mg/dL (0.84 mmol/L)
	Vitamin E: ↓ plasma alpha tocopherol <18 µmol/g (41.8 µmol/L)
	Vitamin K: ↑ prothrombin time; altered INR (without anticoagulation therapy)
	Thiamin: ↑ erythrocyte transketolase activity >1.20 µg/mL/h
	Riboflavin: ↑ erythrocyte glutathione reductase >1.2 IU/g hemoglobin
	Niacin: ↓ N'methyl-nicotinamide excretion <5.8 µmol/day
	Vitamin B-6: ↓ plasma pyridoxal 5'phosphate <5 ng/mL (20 nmol/L)
	Vitamin B-12: ↓ serum concentration <24.4 ng/dL (180 pmol/L); ↑ homocysteine
	Folic acid: ↓ serum concentration <0.3 µg/dL (7 nmol/L); ↓ red cell folate <315 nmol/L
	Pantothenic acid: ↓ plasma
	Biotin: ↓ serum
Anthropometric Measurements	
Nutrition-Focused Physical Findings	Vitamin A: night blindness, Bitot's spots, xerophthalmia, follicular hyperkeratosis
	Vitamin C: follicular hyperkeratosis, petichiae, ecchymosis, coiled hairs, inflamed and bleeding gums, perifolicular hemorrhages, joint effusions, arthralgia, and impaired wound healing
	Vitamin D: widening at ends of long bones
	Riboflavin: sore throat; hyperemia; edema of pharyngeal and oral mucous membranes; cheilosis; angular stomatitis; glossitis; magenta tongue; seborrheic dermatitis; normochromic, normocytic anemia with pure erythrocyte cytoplasia of the bone marrow
	Niacin: symmetrical, pigmented rash on areas exposed to sunlight; bright red tongue
	Vitamin B-6: seborrheic dermatitis, stomatitis, cheilosis, glossitis, confusion, depression
	Vitamin B-12: tingling and numbness in extremities; diminished vibratory and position sense; motor disturbances, including gait disturbances
	Pantothenic acid: irritability and restlessness, fatigue, apathy, malaise, sleep disturbances, nausea, vomiting, abdominal cramps, numbness, muscle cramps, hypoglycemia, sensitivity to insulin
	Biotin: dermatitis, conjunctivitis, alopecia, depression, lethargy, hallucinations and paresthesia, hypotonia, developmental delays

Continued on next page

---

*If a synonym for the term "inadequate" is helpful or needed, an approved alternative is "suboptimal."

Inadequate* Vitamin Intake (Specify) (NI-5.9.1)

Continued from previous page

Nutrition Assessment Category	Potential Indicators of This Nutrition Diagnosis (one or more must be present)
Food/Nutrition-Related History	Reports or observations of: • Estimated intake of foods containing specific vitamins less than requirements or recommended level • Intake of foods that do not contain available vitamins, eg, overprocessed, overcooked, or improperly stored foods • Prolonged use of substances known to increase vitamin requirements or reduce vitamin absorption • Lack of interest in foods
Client History	Conditions associated with a diagnosis or treatment, eg, malabsorption as a result of celiac disease, short-bowel syndrome, inflammatory bowel Certain environmental conditions, eg, infants exclusively fed breastmilk with limited exposure to sunlight (vitamin D) History of chronic kidney disease (decreased conversion of 25(OH)D) Premature infant, extremely low-birth-weight infant (vitamin D) Rachitic rosary in children, rickets, osteomalacia Pellegra Vitamin/mineral deficiency

Diagnosis

Arrows used with laboratory values: ↑ represents above reference standard and ↓ represents below reference standard.

*If a synonym for the term "inadequate" is helpful or needed, an approved alternative is "suboptimal."

Excessive Vitamin Intake (Specify) (NI-5.9.2)

Definition

Higher intake of one or more vitamins compared to established reference standards or recommendations based on physiological needs

Etiology (Cause/Contributing Risk Factors)

Factors gathered during the nutrition assessment process that contribute to the existence or the maintenance of pathophysiological, psychosocial, situational, developmental, cultural, and/or environmental problems:

- Physiological causes decreasing nutrient needs due to prolonged immobility or chronic renal disease
- Access to foods and supplements in excess of needs, eg, cultural or religious practices; less-than-optimal food and supplements given to pregnant women, older adults, or children
- Food- and nutrition-related knowledge deficit concerning food and supplemental sources of vitamins
- Psychological causes, eg, depression or eating disorders
- Accidental overdose from oral and supplemental forms, enteral or parenteral sources

Signs/Symptoms (Defining Characteristics)

A typical cluster of subjective and objective signs and symptoms gathered during the nutrition assessment process that provide evidence that a problem exists; quantify the problem and describe its severity.

Nutrition Assessment Category	Potential Indicators of This Nutrition Diagnosis (one or more must be present)
Biochemical Data, Medical Tests, and Procedures	Vitamin D: ↑ 25(OH) D, ↑ ionized calcium >5.4 mg/dL (1.35 mmol/L) with ↑ parathyroid hormone, normal or ↑ serum calcium, and ↑ serum phosphorus >2.6 mg/dL (0.84 mmol/L)
	Vitamin K: ↓ prothrombin time or altered INR
	Niacin: ↑ N'methyl-nicotinamide excretion >7.3 µmol/day
	Vitamin B-6: ↑ plasma pyridoxal 5'phosphate >15.7 ng/mL (94 nmol/L)
	Vitamin A: ↑ serum retinol concentration >60 µg/dL (2.09 µmol/L)
	Pantothenic acid: ↑ plasma
	Biotin: ↑ serum
Anthropometric Measurements	Vitamin D: growth retardation

Continued on next page

Excessive Vitamin Intake (Specify) (NI-5.9.2)

Continued from previous page

Nutrition Assessment Category	Potential Indicators of This Nutrition Diagnosis (one or more must be present)
Nutrition-Focused Physical Findings	Vitamin A: changes in the skin and mucous membranes; dry lips (cheilitis); early—dryness of the nasal mucosa and eyes; later—dryness, erythema, scaling and peeling of the skin, hair loss, and nail fragility. Headache, nausea, and vomiting. Infants may have bulging fontanelle; children may develop bone alterations
	Vitamin D: calcification of soft tissues (calcinosis), including the kidney, lungs, heart, and even the tympanic membrane of the ear, which can result in deafness. Headache and nausea. Infants given excessive amounts of vitamin D may have gastrointestinal upset, bone fragility
	Vitamin K: hemolytic anemia in adults or severe jaundice in infants has been noted on rare occasions
	Niacin: histamine release, which causes flushing, aggravation of asthma, or liver disease
Food/Nutrition-Related History	Reports or observations of: • Estimated intake reflecting excessive intake of foods and supplements containing vitamins as compared to estimated requirements, including fortified cereals, meal replacements, vitamin-mineral supplements, other dietary supplements (eg, fish liver oils or capsules), tube feeding, and/or parenteral solutions • Estimated intake > more than Tolerable Upper Limit (UL) for vitamin A based on reference intake standard • Estimated intake more than UL for vitamin D based on reference intake standard • Estimated intake more than UL for niacin based on reference intake standard
Client History	Conditions associated with a diagnosis or treatment, eg, chronic liver or kidney diseases, heart failure, cancer

Arrows used with laboratory values: ↑ represents above reference standard and ↓ represents below reference standard.

Diagnosis

Inadequate* Mineral Intake (Specify) (NI-5.10.1)

Definition

Lower intake of one or more minerals compared to established reference standards or recommendations based on physiological needs

> **Note:** Whenever possible, nutrient intake data should be considered in combination with clinical, biochemical, anthropometric information, medical diagnosis, clinical status, and/or other factors as well as diet to provide a valid assessment of nutritional status based on a totality of the evidence (Institute of Medicine. Dietary Reference Intakes: Applications in Dietary Assessment. Washington, DC: National Academies Press; 2000).

Etiology (Cause/Contributing Risk Factors)

Factors gathered during the nutrition assessment process that contribute to the existence or the maintenance of pathophysiological, psychosocial, situational, developmental, cultural, and/or environmental problems:

- Physiological causes increasing nutrient needs due to prolonged catabolic illness, malabsorption, hyperexcretion, nutrient–drug and nutrient–nutrient interaction, growth and maturation
- Decreased ability to consume sufficient amount of a mineral(s)
- Lack of or limited access to food, eg, economic constraints, restricting food given to older adults and/or children
- Cultural practices that affect ability to access food
- Food- and nutrition-related knowledge deficit concerning food and supplemental sources of minerals
- Misdiagnosis of lactose intolerance/lactase deficiency; perception of conflicting nutrition messages; less than optimal reliance on supplements
- Psychological causes, eg, depression or eating disorders
- Environmental causes, eg, inadequately tested nutrient bioavailability of fortified foods, beverages, and supplements; less than optimal marketing of fortified foods/beverages/supplements as a substitute for natural food source of nutrient(s)

---

*If a synonym for the term "inadequate" is helpful or needed, an approved alternative is "suboptimal."

Inadequate* Mineral Intake (Specify) (NI-5.10.1)

Signs/Symptoms (Defining Characteristics)

A typical cluster of subjective and objective signs and symptoms gathered during the nutrition assessment process that provide evidence that a problem exists; quantify the problem and describe its severity.

Nutrition Assessment Category	Potential Indicators of This Nutrition Diagnosis (one or more must be present)
Biochemical Data, Medical Tests, and Procedures	Calcium: bone mineral content (BMC) ↓ the young adult mean; hypocalciuria, serum 25(OH)D <32 ng/mL ↓ Phosphorus <2.6 mg/dL (0.84 mmol/L) ↓ Ferritin in patient/client with a ↓ mean corpuscular volume (MCV) ↓ Zinc, plasma ↓ Magnesium <1.8 mg/dL (0.7 mmol/L) Iron: ↓ hemoglobin <13 g/L (2 mmol/L) (males); <12 g/L (1.86 mmol/L) (females) Iodine: ↓ urinary excretion <100 µg/L (788 nmol/L) Copper: ↓ serum copper <64 µg/dL (10 µmol/L) ↓ Selenium, plasma ↓ Fluoride, plasma ↓ Manganese, serum ↓ Molybdenum, serum ↓ Boron, serum or plasma
Anthropometric Measurements	Calcium: height loss Iodine: growth abnormalities Chromium: unintentional weight loss
Nutrition-Focused Physical Findings	Calcium: hypertension, acute—hyperactive reflexes, tetany, muscle spasm, irregular heart rhythm Iron: pallor of face, mucosa, pale gums, tachycardia, fatigue Potassium: weakness, constipation, hypoactive reflexes Phosphorous: fatigue, myalgia, ataxia, confusion, parasthesias Zinc: dysgeusia, poor wound healing, skin lesions (buttocks, perianal area, mouth, nose, eyes), alopecia Copper: depigmentation of hair and skin, osteoporosis Selenium: depigmentation of hair and skin Iodine: enlarged thyroid Fluoride: dental caries Manganese: dermatitis

Continued on next page

*If a synonym for the term "inadequate" is helpful or needed, an approved alternative is "suboptimal."

Diagnosis

Inadequate* Mineral Intake (Specify) (NI-5.10.1)

Continued from previous page

Nutrition Assessment Category	Potential Indicators of This Nutrition Diagnosis (one or more must be present)
Food/Nutrition-Related History	Reports or observations of: • Estimated mineral intake from diet less than recommended intake • Food avoidance and/or elimination of whole food group(s) from diet • Lack of interest in food • Less than optimal food choices and/or chronic dieting behavior • Verbalizes inaccurate or incomplete knowledge • Cultural or religious practices that affect intake
Client History	Conditions associated with a diagnosis or treatment, eg, malabsorption as a result of celiac disease, short bowel syndrome, inflammatory bowel disease, or postmenopausal women without estrogen supplementation and increased calcium need, bariatric surgery, parenteral nutrition Polycystic ovary syndrome, premenstrual syndrome, kidney stones, colon polyps Other significant medical diagnoses and therapies Geographic latitude and history of ultraviolet B exposure/use of sunscreen Change in living environment/independence Calcium: obesity Vitamin/mineral deficiency

Arrows used with laboratory values: ↑ represents above reference standard and ↓ represents below reference standard.

*If a synonym for the term "inadequate" is helpful or needed, an approved alternative is "suboptimal."

Diagnosis

Excessive Mineral Intake (Specify) (NI-5.10.2)

Definition

Higher intake of one or more minerals compared to established reference standards or recommendations based on physiological needs

Etiology (Cause/Contributing Risk Factors)

Factors gathered during the nutrition assessment process that contribute to the existence or the maintenance of pathophysiological, psychosocial, situational, developmental, cultural, and/or environmental problems:

- Food- and nutrition-related knowledge deficit concerning food and supplemental sources of minerals
- Unsupported beliefs/attitudes about food, nutrition, and nutrition-related topics
- Food faddism
- Accidental oversupplementation
- Overconsumption of a limited variety of foods
- Lack of knowledge about management of a disorder altering mineral homeostasis
- Lack of knowledge about management of a disease state requiring mineral restriction

Excessive Mineral Intake (Specify) (NI-5.10.2)

Signs/Symptoms (Defining Characteristics)

A typical cluster of subjective and objective signs and symptoms gathered during the nutrition assessment process that provide evidence that a problem exists; quantify the problem and describe its severity.

Nutrition Assessment Category	Potential Indicators of This Nutrition Diagnosis (one or more must be present)
Biochemical Data, Medical Tests, and Procedures	↑ TSH (excessive iodine intake) ↓ HDL (excessive zinc intake) ↑ Serum ferritin and transferrin saturation (iron overload or excessive intake) ↑ Phosphorus, serum ↑ Magnesium, serum ↓ Copper, serum (excessive zinc intake) ↑ Fluoride, plasma ↑ Selenium, serum ↑ Manganese, serum ↑ Molybdenum, serum ↑ Boron, serum or plasma
Anthropometric Measurements	
Nutrition-Focused Physical Findings	Hair and nail changes Extraskeletal calcifications, affecting vasculature or skin Puritis Anorexia GI disturbances Enamel or skeletal fluorosis Central nervous system effects Verbalizes inaccurate or incomplete knowledge Verbalizes unsupported beliefs and attitudes
Food/Nutrition-Related History	Reports or observations of: • Estimated intake containing high amounts of mineral compared to reference intake standard (eg, DRIs)
Client History	Heart failure Kidney disease Liver damage Parenteral nutrition

Arrows used with laboratory values: ↑ represents above reference standard and ↓ represents below reference standard.

Diagnosis

Swallowing Difficulty (NC-1.1)

Definition

Impaired or difficult movement of food and liquid within the oral cavity to the stomach

Etiology (Cause/Contributing Risk Factors)

Factors gathered during the nutrition assessment process that contribute to the existence or the maintenance of pathophysiological, psychosocial, situational, developmental, cultural, and/or environmental problems:

- Mechanical causes, eg, inflammation, surgery, stricture; oral, pharyngeal, or esophageal tumors; prior mechanical ventilation
- Motor causes, eg, neurological or muscular disorders, such as cerebral palsy, stroke, multiple sclerosis, scleroderma; prematurity or altered suck, swallow, or breathe patterns

Signs/Symptoms (Defining Characteristics)

A typical cluster of subjective and objective signs and symptoms gathered during the nutrition assessment process that provide evidence that a problem exists; quantify the problem and describe its severity.

Nutrition Assessment Category	Potential Indicators of This Nutrition Diagnosis (one or more must be present)
Biochemical Data, Medical Tests, and Procedures	Radiological findings, eg, abnormal swallow study
Anthropometric Measurements	
Nutrition-Focused Physical Findings	Evidence of dehydration, eg, dry mucous membranes, poor skin turgor
	Non-normal findings in cranial nerves and (CN VII) muscles of facial expression, (nerve IX) gag reflex, swallow (nerve X) and tongue range of motions (nerve XII), cough reflex, drooling, facial weakness, and ability to perform wet and dry swallow
	Coughing, choking, prolonged chewing, pouching of food, regurgitation, facial expression changes during eating, drooling, noisy wet upper airway sounds, feeling of "food getting stuck," pain while swallowing
Food/Nutrition-Related History	Reports or observations of: • Prolonged feeding time • Decreased estimated food intake • Avoidance of foods • Mealtime resistance
Client History	Conditions associated with a diagnosis or treatment, eg, dysphagia, achalasia
	Repeated upper respiratory infections and/or pneumonia

Biting/Chewing (Masticatory) Difficulty (NC-1.2)

Definition

Impaired ability to bite or chew food in preparation for swallowing

Etiology (Cause/Contributing Risk Factors)

Factors gathered during the nutrition assessment process that contribute to the exience or the maintenance of patho-physiological, psychosocial, situational, developmental, cultural, and/or environmental problems:

- Craniofacial malformations
- Oral surgery
- Neuromuscular dysfunction
- Partial or complete edentulism
- Soft tissue disease (primary or oral manifestations of a systemic disease)
- Xerostomia

Diagnosis

Biting/Chewing (Masticatory) Difficulty (NC-1.2)

Signs/Symptoms (Defining Characteristics)

A typical cluster of subjective and objective signs and symptoms gathered during the nutrition assessment process that provide evidence that a problem exists; quantify the problem and describe its severity.

Nutrition Assessment Category	Potential Indicators of This Nutrition Diagnosis (one or more must be present)
Biochemical Data, Medical Tests, and Procedures	
Anthropometric Measurements	
Nutrition-Focused Physical Findings	Partial or complete edentulism
	Alterations in cranial nerve function (V, VII, IX, X, XII)
	Dry mouth
	Oral lesions interfering with eating ability
	Impaired tongue movement
	Ill-fitting dentures or broken dentures
Food/Nutrition-Related History	Reports or observations of:
	• Decreased estimated food intake
	• Alterations in estimated food intake from usual
	• Decreased estimated intake or avoidance of food difficult to form into a bolus, eg, nuts, whole pieces of meat, poultry, fish, fruits, vegetables
	• Avoidance of foods of age-appropriate texture
	• Spitting food out or prolonged feeding time
Client History	Conditions associated with a diagnosis or treatment, eg, alcoholism; Alzheimer's; head, neck, or pharyngeal cancer; cerebral palsy; cleft lip/palate; oral soft tissue infections (eg, candidiasis, leukoplakia); lack of developmental readiness; oral manifestations of systemic disease (eg, rheumatoid arthritis, lupus, Crohn's disease, penphigus vulgaris, HIV, diabetes)
	Recent major oral surgery
	Wired jaw
	Chemotherapy with oral side effects
	Radiation therapy to oral cavity

Breastfeeding Difficulty (NC-1.3)

Definition

Inability to sustain infant nutrition through breastfeeding

Etiology (Cause/Contributing Risk Factors)

Factors gathered during the nutrition assessment process that contribute to the existence or the maintenance of pathophysiological, psychosocial, situational, developmental, cultural, and/or environmental problems:

- Infant:
  - Difficulty latching on, eg, tight frenulum
  - Poor sucking ability
  - Oral pain
  - Malnutrition/malabsorption
  - Lethargy, sleepiness
  - Irritability
  - Swallowing difficulty
  - Introduction of feeding via bottle or other route that may affect breastfeeding
- Mother:
  - Painful breasts, nipples
  - Breast or nipple abnormality
  - Mastitis
  - Perception of or actual inadequate breastmilk* supply
  - Lack of social or environmental support
  - Cultural practices that affect the ability to breastfeed
  - Introduction of feeding via bottle or other route that may affect breastfeeding

*If a synonym for the term "breastmilk" is helpful or needed, an approved alternative is "human milk."

Breastfeeding Difficulty (NC-1.3)

Signs/Symptoms (Defining Characteristics)

A typical cluster of subjective and objective signs and symptoms gathered during the nutrition assessment process that provide evidence that a problem exists; quantify the problem and describe its severity.

Nutrition Assessment Category	Potential Indicators of This Nutrition Diagnosis (one or more must be present)
Biochemical Data, Medical Tests, and Procedures	Laboratory evidence of dehydration (infant)
	Fewer than reference standard, eg, six wet diapers in 24 hours (infant)
Anthropometric Measurements	Any weight loss or poor weight gain (infant)
Nutrition-Focused Physical Findings	Frenulum abnormality (infant)
	Vomiting or diarrhea (infant)
	Hunger, lack of satiety after feeding (infant)
Food/Nutrition-Related History	Reports or observations of (infant):
	Coughing
	Crying, latching on and off, pounding on breasts
	Decreased feeding frequency/duration, early cessation of feeding, and/or feeding resistance
	Lethargy
	Reports or observations of (mother):
	Small amount of breastmilk when pumping
	Lack of confidence in ability to breastfeed
	Doesn't hear infant swallowing
	Concerns regarding choice to breastfeed/lack of support
	Insufficient knowledge of breastfeeding or infant hunger/satiety signals
	Lack of facilities or accommodations at place of employment or in community for breastfeeding
	Feeding via bottle or other route
Client History	Conditions associated with a diagnosis or treatment (infant), eg, cleft lip/palate, thrush, premature birth, malabsorption, infection
	Conditions associated with a diagnosis or treatment (mother), eg, mastitis, candidiasis, engorgement, history of breast surgery

Diagnosis

Altered Gastrointestinal (GI) Function (NC-1.4)

Definition

Changes in digestion, absorption, or elimination

Etiology (Cause/Contributing Risk Factors)

Factors gathered during the nutrition assessment process that contribute to the existence or the maintenance of pathophysiological, psychosocial, situational, developmental, cultural, and/or environmental problems:

- Alteration in GI tract structure and/or function
- Changes in GI tract motility, eg, gastroparesis
- Compromised exocrine function of related GI organs, eg, pancreas, liver
- Decreased functional length of the GI tract, eg, short-bowel syndrome

Altered Gastrointestinal (GI) Function (NC-1.4)

Signs/Symptoms (Defining Characteristics)

A typical cluster of subjective and objective signs and symptoms gathered during the nutrition assessment process that provide evidence that a problem exists; quantify the problem and describe its severity.

Nutrition Assessment Category	Potential Indicators of This Nutrition Diagnosis (one or more must be present)
Biochemical Data, Medical Tests, and Procedures	Abnormal digestive enzyme and fecal studies
	Abnormal hydrogen breath test, d-xylose test, stool culture, and gastric emptying and/or bowel transit time
	Endoscopic or colonoscopy examination, abdominal scan, biopsy results
	Abnormal pH, sphincter, motility, morphology, or reflux studies
	Abnormal anemia profile
	Abnormal vitamin, mineral, fatty acid, trace element, and PTH results
	Abnormal tissue transglutaminase antibodies (IgA/IgG)
Anthropometric Measurements	Weight loss of ≥5% in 1 month, ≥10% in 6 months
	Growth stunting or failure in children
	Abnormal bone mineral density tests
Nutrition-Focused Physical Findings	Abdominal distension
	Increased (or sometimes decreased) bowel sounds
	Wasting due to malnutrition in severe cases
	Anorexia, nausea, vomiting, diarrhea, steatorrhea, constipation, abdominal pain, reflux, gas, belching, flatus, bloating, fecal incontinence
	Evidence of vitamin and/or mineral deficiency, eg, glossitis, cheilosis, mouth lesions, skin rashes, hair loss
Food/Nutrition-Related History	Reports or observations of: • Avoidance or limitation of estimated total intake or intake of specific foods/food groups due to GI symptoms, eg, bloating, cramping, pain, diarrhea, steatorrhea (greasy, floating, or foul-smelling stools), especially following ingestion of food
Client History	Conditions associated with a diagnosis or treatment, eg, malabsorption, maldigestion, steatorrhea, obstruction, constipation, diverticulitis, Crohn's disease, inflammatory bowel disease, cystic fibrosis, celiac disease, cancers, irritable bowel syndrome, infection, dumping syndrome
	Surgical procedures, eg, esophagectomy, dilatation, fundoplication, gastrectomy, vagotomy, gastric bypass, bowel resections

Diagnosis

Impaired Nutrient Utilization (NC-2.1)

Definition

Changes in ability to metabolize nutrients and bioactive substances

Etiology (Cause/Contributing Risk Factors)

Factors gathered during the nutrition assessment process that contribute to the existence or the maintenance of pathophysiological, psychosocial, situational, developmental, cultural, and/or environmental problems:

- Compromised endocrine function of related GI organs, eg, pancreas, liver, pituitary, parathyroid
- Metabolic disorders, including inborn errors of metabolism
- Medications that affect nutrient metabolism
- Alcohol or drug addiction

Impaired Nutrient Utilization (NC-2.1)

Signs/Symptoms (Defining Characteristics)

A typical cluster of subjective and objective signs and symptoms gathered during the nutrition assessment process that provide evidence that a problem exists; quantify the problem and describe its severity.

Nutrition Assessment Category	Potential Indicators of This Nutrition Diagnosis (one or more must be present)
Biochemical Data, Medical Tests, and Procedures	Abnormal protein, fatty acid, or carbohydrate metabolism profile tests Abnormal liver function tests Abnormal anemia profile Abnormal pituitary hormones (growth hormone [GH], adrenocorticotropic hormone [ACTH], luteinizing hormone [LH], and follicle-stimulating hormone [FSH]) Vitamin and/or mineral deficiency Hypoglycemia, hyperglycemia Abnormal PTH Positive result for urine porphyrins
Anthropometric Measurements	Weight loss of ≥5% in 1 month, ≥10% in 6 months Growth stunting or failure in children Abnormal bone mineral density tests
Nutrition-Focused Physical Findings	Evidence of vitamin and/or mineral deficiency, eg, glossitis, cheilosis, mouth lesions Thin, wasted appearance
Food/Nutrition-Related History	Reports or observations of: • Avoidance or limitation of intake of specific foods/food groups due to physical symptoms • Alcohol or drug use
Client History	Conditions associated with a diagnosis or treatment, eg, cystic fibrosis, celiac disease, Crohn's disease, infection, radiation therapy, inborn errors of metabolism, endocrine disorders, pituitary disorders, renal failure, liver failure, acute or inherited porphyria, short-bowel syndrome

Diagnosis

Altered Nutrition-Related Laboratory Values (Specify) (NC-2.2)

Diagnosis

Definition

Changes in lab values due to body composition, medications, body system changes or genetics, or changes in ability to eliminate byproducts of digestive and metabolic processes

Etiology (Cause/Contributing Risk Factors)

Factors gathered during the nutrition assessment process that contribute to the existence or the maintenance of pathophysiological, psychosocial, situational, developmental, cultural, and/or environmental problems:

- Kidney, liver, cardiac, endocrine, neurologic, and/or pulmonary dysfunction
- Prematurity
- Other organ dysfunction that leads to biochemical changes
- Metabolic disorders, including inborn errors of metabolism

Altered Nutrition-Related Laboratory Values (Specify) (NC-2.2)

Signs/Symptoms (Defining Characteristics)

A typical cluster of subjective and objective signs and symptoms gathered during the nutrition assessment process that provide evidence that a problem exists; quantify the problem and describe its severity.

Nutrition Assessment Category	Potential Indicators of This Nutrition Diagnosis (one or more must be present)
Biochemical Data, Medical Tests, and Procedures	↑ AST, ALT, Total bilirubin, serum ammonia (liver disorders)
	↑ BUN, ↑ Cr, ↑ K, ↑ phosphorus, ↓ glomerular filtration rate (GFR) (kidney disorders)
	Altered pO_2 and pCO_2 (pulmonary disorders)
	↑ Serum lipids
	↑ Plasma glucose and/or Hemoglobin A1C levels
	Inadequate blood glucose control
	↑ Urine microalbumin
	Abnormal protein, fatty acid, or carbohydrate metabolism profile
	Other findings of acute or chronic disorders that are abnormal and of nutritional origin or consequence
Anthropometric Measurements	Rapid weight changes
	Other anthropometric measures that are altered
Nutrition-Focused Physical Findings	Jaundice, edema, ascites, pruritis (liver disorders)
	Edema, shortness of breath (cardiac disorders)
	Blue nail beds, clubbing (pulmonary disorders)
	Anorexia, nausea, vomiting
Food/Nutrition-Related History	Reports or observations of:
	• Estimated intake of foods high in or overall excess intake of protein, potassium, phosphorus, sodium, fluid
	• Estimated intake of micronutrients less than recommendations
	• Food- and nutrition-related knowledge deficit, eg, lack of information, incorrect information, or noncompliance with modified diet
Client History	Conditions associated with a diagnosis or treatment, eg, renal or liver disease, alcoholism, cardiopulmonary disorders, diabetes, inborn errors of metabolism

Arrows used with laboratory values: ↑ represents above reference standard and ↓ represents below reference standard.

Diagnosis

Food–Medication Interaction (Specify) (NC-2.3)

Definition

Undesirable/harmful interaction(s) between food and over-the-counter (OTC) medications, prescribed medications, herbals, botanicals, and/or dietary supplements that diminishes, enhances, or alters the effect of nutrients and/or medications

Etiology (Cause/Contributing Risk Factors)

Factors gathered during the nutrition assessment process that contribute to the existence or the maintenance of pathophysiological, psychosocial, situational, developmental, cultural, and/or environmental problems:

- Combined ingestion or administration of medication and food that results in undesirable/harmful interaction

Signs/Symptoms (Defining Characteristics)

A typical cluster of subjective and objective signs and symptoms gathered during the nutrition assessment process that provide evidence that a problem exists; quantify the problem and describe its severity.

Nutrition Assessment Category	Potential Indicators of This Nutrition Diagnosis (one or more must be present)
Biochemical Data, Medical Tests, and Procedures	Alterations of biochemical tests based on medication effects and patient/client conditions
Anthropometric Measurements	Alterations of anthropometric measurements based on medication effects and patient/client conditions, eg, weight gain and corticosteroids
Nutrition-Focused Physical Findings	Changes in appetite or taste

Food/Nutrition-Related History	Reports or observations of:
	• Intake that is problematic or inconsistent with OTC medications, prescribed drugs, herbals, botanicals, or dietary supplements, such as:
	  ○ Fish oils and prolonged bleeding
	  ○ Coumadin and vitamin K–rich foods
	  ○ High-fat diet while on cholesterol-lowering medications
	  ○ Iron supplements, constipation, and low-fiber diet
	• Intake that does not support replacement or mitigation of OTC medications, prescribed drugs, herbals, botanicals, and dietary supplements effects
	• Multiple drugs (OTC medications, prescribed drugs, herbals, botanicals, or dietary supplements) that are known to have food–medication interactions
	• Medications that require nutrient supplementation that cannot be accomplished via food intake, eg, isoniazid and vitamin B-6

Client History

Underweight (NC-3.1)

Definition

Low body weight compared to established reference standards or recommendations

Etiology (Cause/Contributing Risk Factors)

Factors gathered during the nutrition assessment process that contribute to the existence or the maintenance of pathophysiological, psychosocial, situational, developmental, cultural, and/or environmental problems:

- Disordered eating pattern
- Excessive physical activity
- Unsupported beliefs/attitudes about food, nutrition, and nutrition-related topics
- Inadequate energy intake
- Increased energy needs
- Lack of or limited access to food
- Small for gestational age, intrauterine growth retardation/restriction, and/or lack of progress/appropriate weight gain per day

Underweight (NC-3.1)

Signs/Symptoms (Defining Characteristics)

A typical cluster of subjective and objective signs and symptoms gathered during the nutrition assessment process that provide evidence that a problem exists; quantify the problem and describe its severity.

Nutrition Assessment Category	Potential Indicators of This Nutrition Diagnosis (one or more must be present)
Biochemical Data, Medical Tests, and Procedures	↑ Measured resting metabolic rate (RMR) higher than expected and/or estimated
Anthropometric Measurements	Decreased skinfold thickness and mid-arm muscle circumference BMI <18.5 (adults) BMI for older adults (older than 65 years) <22 Birth to 2 years • Weight for age <5th percentile • Weight for length <5th percentile Ages 2 to 20 years • Weight for stature <5th percentile • BMI <5th percentile • Weight for age <5th percentile
Nutrition-Focused Physical Findings	Decreased muscle mass, muscle wasting (gluteal and temporal) Hunger
Food/Nutrition-Related History	Reports or observations of: • Estimated intake of food less than estimated or measured needs • Limited supply of food in home • Dieting, food faddism • Refusal to eat • Physical activity more than recommended amount • Medications that affect appetite, eg, stimulants for ADHD
Client History	Malnutrition Illness or physical disability Mental illness, dementia, confusion Athlete, dancer, gymnast Vitamin/mineral deficiency

Arrows used with laboratory values: ↑ represents above reference standard and ↓ represents below reference standard.

Diagnosis

Unintended* Weight Loss (NC-3.2)

Definition

Decrease in body weight that is not planned or desired

Note: May not be an appropriate nutrition diagnosis when changes in body weight are due to fluid.

Etiology (Cause/Contributing Risk Factors)

Factors gathered during the nutrition assessment process that contribute to the existence or maintenance of pathophysiological, psychosocial, situational, developmental, cultural, and/or environmental problems:

- Physiological causes increasing nutrient needs, eg, due to prolonged catabolic illness, trauma, malabsorption
- Decreased ability to consume sufficient energy
- Lack of or limited access to food, eg, economic constraints, restricting food given to older adults and/or children
- Cultural practices that affect ability to access food
- Prolonged hospitalization
- Psychological causes such as depression od disordered eating
- Lack of self-feeding ability

*If a synonym for the term "unintended" is helpful or needed, an approved alternative is "involuntary."

Unintended* Weight Loss (NC-3.2)

Signs/Symptoms (Defining Characteristics)

A typical cluster of subjective and objective signs and symptoms gathered during the nutrition assessment process that provide evidence that a problem exists; quantify the problem and describe its severity.

Nutrition Assessment Category	Potential Indicators of This Nutrition Diagnosis (one or more must be present)
Biochemical Data, Medical Tests, and Procedures	
Anthropometric Measurements	Weight loss of ≥5% within 30 days, ≥7.5% in 90 days, or ≥10% in 180 days (adults)
	Not gaining weight as expected; 5% weight loss in 6 months and/or a shift downward in growth percentiles crossing two or more percentile channels on reference growth standard charts (pediatrics)
Nutrition-Focused Physical Findings	Fever
	Decreased senses, ie, smell, taste, vision
	Increased heart rate
	Increased respiratory rate
	Loss of subcutaneous fat and muscle stores
	Change in way clothes fit
	Changes in mental status or function (eg, depression)
Food/Nutrition-Related History	Reports or observations of:
	• Normal or usual estimated intake in face of illness
	• Poor intake, change in eating habits, early satiety, skipped meals
	• Medications associated with weight loss, such as certain antidepressants
Client History	Conditions associated with a diagnosis or treatment, eg, AIDS/HIV, burns, chronic obstructive pulmonary disease, dysphagia, hip/long bone fracture, infection, surgery, trauma, hyperthyroidism (pre- or untreated), some types of cancer or metastatic disease (specify), substance abuse
	Cancer chemotherapy

*If a synonym for the term "unintended" is helpful or needed, an approved alternative is "involuntary."

Overweight/Obesity (NC-3.3)

Definition

Increased adiposity compared to established reference standards or recommendations, ranging from overweight to morbid obesity

Etiology (Cause/Contributing Risk Factors)

Factors gathered during the nutrition assessment process that contribute to the existence or the maintenance of pathophysiological, psychosocial, situational, developmental, cultural, and/or environmental problems:

- Decreased energy needs
- Disordered eating pattern
- Excessive energy intake
- Food- and nutrition-related knowledge deficit
- Not ready for diet/lifestyle change
- Physical inactivity
- Increased psychological/life stress

Signs/Symptoms (Defining Characteristics)

A typical cluster of subjective and objective signs and symptoms gathered during the nutrition assessment process that provide evidence that a problem exists; quantify the problem and describe its severity.

Nutrition Assessment Category	Potential Indicators of This Nutrition Diagnosis (one or more must be present)
Biochemical Data, Medical Tests, and Procedures	↓ Measured resting metabolic rate (RMR) less than expected and/or estimated
Anthropometric Measurements	BMI more than normative standard for age and sex: • Overweight: 25 to 29.9 (adults); 85th to 94th percentiles (pediatrics) • Obese Class I: 30 to 34.9 (adults) • Obese Class II: 35 to 39.9 (adults) • Obese Class III: 40+* (adults) • Obese ≥95th percentile (pediatrics) Waist circumference more than normative standard for age and sex Increased skinfold thickness Body fat percentage >25% for men and >32% for women Weight for height more than normative standard for age and sex
Nutrition-Focused Physical Findings	Increased body adiposity

Continued on next page

Diagnosis

---

*If a synonym for the term "Obese Class III" is helpful or needed, an approved alternative is "morbid obesity."

Overweight/Obesity (NC-3.3)

Continued from previous page

Diagnosis

Nutrition Assessment Category	Potential Indicators of This Nutrition Diagnosis (one or more must be present)
Food/Nutrition-Related History	Reports or observations of: • Overconsumption of high-fat and/or energy-dense food or beverages • Large portions of food (portion size more than twice than recommended) • Estimated excessive energy intake • Infrequent, low-duration, and/or low-intensity physical activity; factors affecting physical activity access • Large amounts of sedentary activities, eg, TV watching, reading, computer use in both leisure and work/school • Uncertainty regarding nutrition-related recommendations • Inability to apply nutrition-related recommendations • Unwillingness or disinterest in applying nutrition-related recommendations • Inability to lose a significant amount of excess weight through conventional weight loss intervention • Medications that impact RMR, eg, midazolam, propranalol, glipizide
Client History	Conditions associated with a diagnosis or treatment, eg, hypothyroidism, metabolic syndrome, eating disorder not otherwise specified, depression Physical disability or limitation History of familial obesity History of childhood obesity History of physical, sexual, or emotional abuse

Arrows used with laboratory values: ↑ represents above reference standard and ↓ represents below reference standard.

Unintended* Weight Gain (NC-3.4)

Definition

Weight gain more than that which is desired or planned

Etiology (Cause/Contributing Risk Factors)

Factors gathered during the nutrition assessment process that contribute to the existence or the maintenance of pathophysiological, psychosocial, situational, developmental, cultural, and/or environmental problems:

- Illnesses or conditions causing unexpected weight gain because of, eg, head trauma, immobility, paralysis or related condition, Cushing's syndrome, hypothyroidism, other endocrine disorders
- Chronic use of medications known to cause weight gain, such as use of certain antidepressants, antipsychotics, corticosteroids, certain HIV medications
- Condition leading to excessive fluid weight gains
- Not ready for diet/lifestyle change

---

*If a synonym for the term "unintended" is helpful or needed, an approved alternative is "involuntary."

Unintended* Weight Gain (NC-3.4)

Signs/Symptoms (Defining Characteristics)

A typical cluster of subjective and objective signs and symptoms gathered during the nutrition assessment process that provide evidence that a problem exists; quantify the problem and describe its severity.

Diagnosis

Nutrition Assessment Category	Potential Indicators of This Nutrition Diagnosis (one or more must be present)
Biochemical Data, Medical Tests, and Procedures	↓ Serum albumin ↓ Sodium, serum ↑ Fasting serum lipid levels ↑ Fasting glucose levels Fluctuating hormone levels ↑ Cortisol ↑ Growth hormone ↑ Thyroid stimulating hormone ↓ Thyroxine (T4)
Anthropometric Measurements	Increased weight; any increase in weight more than planned or desired Weight gain of >5% within 30 days, >7.5% in 90 days, or >10% in 180 days (adults)
Nutrition-Focused Physical Findings	Fat accumulation, excessive subcutaneous fat stores, noticeable change in body fat distribution Extreme hunger with or without palpitations, tremor, and sweating Edema Shortness of breath Muscle weakness Fatigue
Food/Nutrition-Related History	Reports or observations of: • Estimated intake inconsistent with estimated or measured energy needs • Changes in recent estimated food intake level • Fluid administration more than requirements • Use of alcohol or narcotics • Medications associated with increased appetite • Physical inactivity or change in physical activity level
Client History	Conditions associated with a diagnosis or treatment of asthma, psychiatric illnesses, rheumatic conditions, Cushing's syndrome, obesity, Prader-Willi syndrome, Down syndrome, spina bifida, hypothyroidism, pituitary conditions

Arrows used with laboratory values: ↑ represents above reference standard and ↓ represents below reference standard.

*If a synonym for the term "unintended" is helpful or needed, an approved alternative is "involuntary."

Growth Rate Below Expected (NC-3.5)

Definition

Rate of growth or growth velocity slower than expected or weight gain that is suboptimal in comparison with goal or reference standard

Etiology (Cause/Contributing Risk Factors)

Factors gathered during the nutrition assessment process that contribute to the existence of or the maintenance of pathophysiological, psychosocial, situational, developmental, cultural, and/or environmental problems:

- Physiological impetus for increased nutrient needs (eg, critical illness or trauma; pregnancy; metabolic illness, eg, type 1 diabetes; malabsorption)
- Decreased ability to consume sufficient energy
- Lack of or limited access to food
- Psychological causes such as depression or disordered eating
- Limited food acceptance
- Food and nutrition-related knowledge deficit
- Unsupported beliefs/attitudes about food, nutrition, and nutrition-related topics
- Small for gestational age, intrauterine growth restriction/retardation, lack of appropriate weight gain, hyperemesis gravidarum

Growth Rate Below Expected (NC-3.5)

Signs/Symptoms (Defining Characteristics)

A typical cluster of subjective and objective signs and symptoms gathered during the nutrition assessment process that provide evidence that a problem exists; quantify the problem and describe its severity.

Nutrition Assessment Category	Potential Indicators of This Nutrition Diagnosis (one or more must be present)
Biochemical Data, Medical Tests, and Procedures	Positive urine ketones, ↑ fasting (or postprandial) glucose level Fluctuating hormone levels during pregnancy Zinc deficiency Iron deficiency Abnormal protein, fatty acid, or carbohydrate metabolism profile
Anthropometric Measurements	Weight-for-age decrease in two or more percentile channels Weight-gain velocity less than expected based on established reference standard and/or guideline Length- or height-for-age decrease in two or more percentile channels Length- or height-gain velocity less than expected based on established reference standard and/or guideline
Nutrition-Focused Physical Findings	Decreased muscle mass, muscle wasting (gluteal and temporal) Hunger Decreased fat mass
Food/Nutrition-Related History	Reports or observations of: • Estimated energy intake inconsistent with estimated or measured needs • Restricted fluids decreasing ability to meet nutritional needs • Difficulty breastfeeding, eg, poor latch • Limited food acceptance, eg, not progressing to foods as expected or recommended • Medications associated with decreased appetite or weight loss • Use of alcohol or narcotics during pregnancy • Increase in physical activity levels • Normal or usual intake in presence of illness • Poor intake, change in eating habits, early satiety, or skipped meals
Client History	Conditions associated with a diagnosis or treatment impacting growth, including AIDS/HIV, burns, pulmonary disease, dysphagia, long bone fracture, infection, surgery, trauma, hyperthyroid, hypothyroid, substance abuse, some types of cancer or metastatic disease, inborn errors of metabolism Food insecurity

Arrows used with laboratory values: ↑ represents above reference standard and ↓ represents below reference standard.

Diagnosis

Starvation Related Malnutrition (Undernutrition) (NC-4.1.1)

Definition

Inadequate intake of protein and/or energy over a period of time sufficient to result in loss of fat and/or muscle mass without apparent inflammation and in the context of environmental and/or social circumstances. Non severe (moderate) and Severe starvation-related malnutrition characteristics are included here:

Note: There is an ongoing international effort to harmonize the definitions of adult malnutrition.[1] At present, the eNCPT malnutrition indicator criteria provided reflect the malnutrition clinical characteristics (MCC) Academy/ASPEN Adult Malnutrition Consensus Statement.[2] Three additional validated nutrition assessment approaches, the Subjective Global Assessment, the Patient Generated Subjective Global Assessment, and the Mini-Nutritional Assessment Long Form, to identify malnutrition are also in a chart that follows the MCC and may be used to identify malnutrition.

The Academy/ASPEN Adult Malnutrition Consensus Statement recommends a minimum of two clinical characteristics or indicators be present for a diagnosis of malnutrition. For additional information please visit the Academy's webpage at http://www.eatrightpro.org/resources/practice/practice-resources/malnutrition.

Etiology (Cause/Contributing Risk Factors)

Factors gathered during the nutrition assessment process that contribute to the existence or the maintenance of pathophysiological, psychosocial, situational, developmental, cultural, and/or environmental problems:

- Alteration in gastrointestinal tract structure and/or function
- Lack of or limited access to food, eg, economic constraints, restricting food given to older adults, neglect or abuse, recent immigration/refugee from and/or to poorly resourced or war-torn countries
- Cultural or religious practices that affect the ability to access food
- Food- and nutrition-related knowledge deficit concerning amount of energy and amount and type of dietary protein
- Behavioral/psychological causes, eg, depression or eating disorders
- Oral health limitations
- Impaired sensory perception impacting food consumption

Signs/Symptoms (Defining Characteristics)

A typical cluster of subjective and objective signs and symptoms gathered during the nutrition assessment process that provide evidence that a problem exists; quantify the problem and describe its severity.

Nutrition Assessment Category	Potential Indicators of This Nutrition Diagnosis (one or more must be present)
Biochemical Data, Medical Tests, and Procedures	

Continued on next page

Starvation Related Malnutrition (Undernutrition) (NC-4.1.1)

Diagnosis

Continued from previous page

Nutrition Assessment Category	Potential Indicators of This Nutrition Diagnosis (one or more must be present)
Anthropometric Measurements	Malnutrition can occur at any weight/BMI • Inadequate maternal weight gain • Non severe (moderate) malnutrition: unintentional weight loss of 20% in 1 year, 10% in 6 months, 7.5% in 3 months, or 5% in 1 month (adults) • Severe malnutrition: unintentional weight loss of >20% in 1 year, >10% in 6 months, >7.5% in 3 months, or >5% in 1 month (adults)
Nutrition-Focused Physical Findings	Non severe (moderate) malnutrition • Mild loss of subcutaneous fat, eg, orbital, triceps, fat overlying the ribs • Mild muscle loss, eg, wasting of the temples (temporalis muscle), clavicles (pectoralis and deltoids), shoulders (deltoids), interosseous muscles, scapula (latissimus dorsi, trapezius, deltoids), thigh (quadriceps), and calf (gastrocnemius) • Mild localized or generalized fluid accumulation (extremities, vulvar/scrotal, ascites) Severe malnutrition • Severe loss of subcutaneous fat, eg, orbital, triceps, fat overlying the ribs • Severe muscle loss, eg, wasting of the temples (temporalis muscle), clavicles (pectoralis and deltoids), shoulders (deltoids), interosseous muscles, scapula (latissimus dorsi, trapezius, deltoids), thigh (quadriceps), and calf (gastrocnemius) • Severe localized or generalized fluid accumulation (extremities, vulvar/scrotal, ascites)
Food/Nutrition-Related History	Reports or observations of: Non severe (moderate) malnutrition • Estimated energy intake <75% of estimated energy requirement for ≥3 months Severe malnutrition • Estimated energy intake <50% of estimated energy requirement for ≥1 month • Measurably reduced changes in handgrip strength or other functional indicators

Note: Handgrip strength in adults: norms are device dependent; can identify presence of malnutrition but not quantify the degree of the deficit; may not be able to perform on certain patients. Please refer to the Academy/ASPEN Adult and Pediatric Malnutrition Consensus Statements for further information.

Continued on next page

Starvation Related Malnutrition (Undernutrition) (NC-4.1.1)

Continued from previous page

Nutrition Assessment Category	Potential Indicators of This Nutrition Diagnosis (one or more must be present)
Client History	Reports or observations of the following: • Anorexia nervosa, benign esophageal stricture, substance abuse, physical abuse, neglect, poverty, frailty, and anything that results in limited access to food (associated with malnutrition in the context of environmental and social circumstances) • Pre-existing medical diagnosis of malnutrition • Genetic or acquired conditions: cerebral palsy, cystic fibrosis, seizure disorders, metabolic disease, IBD

Diagnosis

Starvation Related Malnutrition (Undernutrition) (NC-4.1.1)

Diagnosis

Nutrition Assessment Tools for Identifying Malnutrition				
Assessment Parameter	SGA	PG-SGA	MNA-LF	MCC
Name/Author/Year	Detsky et al. (1987)[4]	Ottery 2015 http://pt-global.org/[18]	Guigoz et al. (1994) http://mna-olderadults.com/[19,20]	Academy/ASPEN Consensus Statement 2012[2]
Weight loss/BMI±	X	X	X	X
Dietary intake±	X	X	X	X
GI symptoms	X	X		
Comorbidity		X	X	
Metabolic demand		X		
Functional capacity±	X		X	X
Fluid status (edema/ascites)	X	X		X
Fat stores±	X	X	Mid-arm circumference, calf circumference	X
Muscle stores±	X	X		X
Neuropsychological			X	
Method of categorization	Rating: SGA A (well nourished) SGA B (mild-moderate malnutrition) SGA C (severe malnutrition)	Rating: SGA A/B/C (assessed per SGA) Scores for triaging nutrition interventions	Numerical score: No nutritional risk Risk of malnutrition Malnourished	2 or more characteristics demonstrated out of 6 identifies malnutrition Severity defined by specific thresholds
Validated: Setting	Acute Rehabilitation Community Residential aged care	Acute	Acute Rehabilitation Community Long-term care	
Validated: Patient Group	Surgery Geriatric Oncology Renal	Oncology Renal Stroke	Geriatric	
Validated: Ages	Adults of all ages	Adults of all ages	Adults >65 years	

± Parameters that most influence the rating

Chronic Disease or Condition Related Malnutrition (Undernutrition) (NC-4.1.2)

Definition

Inadequate intake of protein and/or energy over a period of time sufficient to result in loss of fat and/or muscle mass with apparent mild to moderate inflammation and in the context of chronic illness or condition. Non severe (moderate) and Severe chronic disease or condition related malnutrition characteristics are included here.

> **Note:** There is an ongoing international effort to harmonize the definitions of adult malnutrition.[1] At present, the eNCPT malnutrition indicator criteria provided reflect the malnutrition clinical characteristics (MCC) Academy/ASPEN Adult Malnutrition Consensus Statement.[2] Three additional validated nutrition assessment approaches, the Subjective Global Assessment, the Patient Generated Subjective Global Assessment, and the Mini-Nutritional Assessment Long Form, to identify malnutrition are also in a chart that follows the MCC and may be used to identify malnutrition.
>
> The Academy/ASPEN Adult Malnutrition Consensus Statement recommends a minimum of two clinical characteristics or indicators be present for a diagnosis of malnutrition. For additional information please visit the Academy's webpage at http://www.eatrightpro.org/resources/practice/practice-resources/malnutrition.

Etiology (Cause/Contributing Risk Factors)

Factors gathered during the nutrition assessment process that contribute to the existence or maintenance of pathophysiological, psychosocial, situational, developmental, cultural, and/or environmental problems:

- Physiological causes increasing nutrient needs due to illness or condition
- Physiological causes resulting in anorexia or diminished intake
- Alteration in gastrointestinal tract structure and/or function

Chronic Disease or Condition Related Malnutrition (Undernutrition) (NC-4.1.2)

Diagnosis

Signs/Symptoms (Defining Characteristics)

A typical cluster of subjective and objective signs and symptoms gathered during the nutrition assessment process that provide evidence that a problem exists; quantify the problem and describe its severity.

Nutrition Assessment Category	Potential Indicators of This Nutrition Diagnosis (one or more must be present)
Biochemical Data, Medical Tests, and Procedures	
Anthropometric Measurements	Malnutrition can occur at any weight/BMI • Inadequate maternal weight gain • Non severe (moderate) malnutrition: unintentional weight loss of 20% in 1 year, 10% in 6 months, 7.5% in 3 months, or 5% in 1 month (adults) • Severe malnutrition: unintentional weight loss of >20% in 1 year, >10% in 6 months, >7.5% in 3 months, or >5% in 1 month (adults)
Nutrition-Focused Physical Findings	Non severe (moderate) malnutrition • Mild loss of subcutaneous fat, eg, orbital, triceps, fat overlying the ribs • Mild muscle loss, eg, wasting of the temples (temporalis muscle), clavicles (pectoralis and deltoids), shoulders (deltoids), interosseous muscles, scapula (latissimus dorsi, trapezius, deltoids), thigh (quadriceps), and calf (gastrocnemius) • Mild localized or generalized fluid accumulation (extremities, vulvar/scrotal, ascites) Severe malnutrition • Severe loss of subcutaneous fat, eg, orbital, triceps, fat overlying the ribs • Severe muscle loss, eg, wasting of the temples (temporalis muscle), clavicles (pectoralis and deltoids), shoulders (deltoids), interosseous muscles, scapula (latissimus dorsi, trapezius, deltoids), thigh (quadriceps), and calf (gastrocnemius) • Severe localized or generalized fluid accumulation (extremities, vulvar/scrotal, ascites)
Food/Nutrition-Related History	Reports or observations of: Non severe (moderate) malnutrition • Estimated energy intake <75% of estimated energy requirement for ≥1 month Severe malnutrition • Estimated energy intake <75% of estimated energy requirement for ≥1 month • Measurably reduced changes in handgrip strength or other functional indicators

Continued on next page

Chronic Disease or Condition Related Malnutrition (Undernutrition) (NC-4.1.2)

Continued from previous page

Nutrition Assessment Category	Potential Indicators of This Nutrition Diagnosis (one or more must be present)

Note: Handgrip strength in adults: norms are device dependent; can identify presence of malnutrition but not quantify the degree of the deficit; may not be able to perform on certain patients. Please refer to the Academy/ASPEN Adult Malnutrition Consensus Statement for further information.

Client History	Reports or observations of the following, for example:

- Organ failure, malignancies, rheumatoid diseases, gastrointestinal diseases, sarcopenic obesity, malabsorptive syndromes, and other etiologies, including but not limited to diabetes, congestive heart failure, chronic kidney disease, and chronic obstructive pulmonary disease (associated with malnutrition in the context of chronic disease/condition)
- Pre-existing medical diagnosis of malnutrition disease/condition.
- Genetic or acquired conditions: Cerebral Palsy, cystic fibrosis, seizure disorders, metabolic disease, IBD

Note: In the past, hepatic transport protein measures (eg, albumin and prealbumin) were used as indicators of malnutrition. See the Evidence Analysis Library questions on this topic at https://www.andeal.org/topic.cfm?cat=4302. Accessed April 3, 2017.

Diagnosis

Chronic Disease or Condition Related Malnutrition (Undernutrition) (NC-4.1.2)

Diagnosis

Nutrition Assessment Tools for Identifying Malnutrition				
Assessment Parameter	SGA	PG-SGA	MNA-LF	MCC
Name/Author/Year	Detsky et al. (1987)[4]	Ottery 2015 http://pt-global.org/[18]	Guigoz et al. (1994) http://mna-olderadults.com/[19,20]	Academy/ASPEN Consensus Statement 2012[2]
Weight loss/BMI±	X	X	X	X
Dietary intake±	X	X	X	X
GI symptoms	X	X		
Comorbidity		X	X	
Metabolic demand		X		
Functional capacity±	X	X	X	X
Fluid status (edema/ascites)	X	X		X
Fat stores±	X	X	Mid-arm circumference, calf circumference	X
Muscle stores±	X	X		X
Neuropsychological			X	
Method of categorization	Rating: SGA A (well nourished) SGA B (mild-moderate malnutrition) SGA C (severe malnutrition)	Rating: SGA A/B/C (assessed per SGA) Scores for triaging nutrition interventions	Numerical score: No nutritional risk Risk of malnutrition Malnourished	2 or more characteristics demonstrated out of 6 identifies malnutrition Severity defined by specific thresholds
Validated: Setting	Acute Rehabilitation Community Residential aged care	Acute	Acute Rehabilitation Community Long-term care	
Validated: Patient Group	Surgery Geriatric Oncology Renal	Oncology Renal Stroke	Geriatric	
Validated: Ages	Adults of all ages	Adults of all ages	Adults >65 years	

± Parameters that most influence the rating

Acute Disease or Injury Related Malnutrition (Undernutrition) (NC-4.1.3)

Definition

Inadequate intake of protein and/or energy resulting in loss of fat and/or muscle mass with apparent marked inflammatory response and in the context of acute illness or injury. Non severe (moderate) and Severe acute disease or injury related malnutrition characteristics are included here.

Note: There is an ongoing international effort to harmonize the definitions of adult malnutrition.[1] At present, the eNCPT malnutrition indicator criteria provided reflect the malnutrition clinical characteristics (MCC) Academy/ASPEN Adult Malnutrition Consensus Statement.[2] Three additional validated nutrition assessment approaches, the Subjective Global Assessment, the Patient Generated Subjective Global Assessment, and the Mini-Nutritional Assessment Long Form, to identify malnutrition are also in a chart that follows the MCC and may be used to identify malnutrition.

The Academy/ASPEN Adult Malnutrition Consensus Statement recommends a minimum of two clinical characteristics or indicators be present for a diagnosis of malnutrition. For additional information please visit the Academy's webpage at http://www.eatrightpro.org/resources/practice/practice-resources/malnutrition.

Etiology (Cause/Contributing Risk Factors)

Factors gathered during the nutrition assessment process that contribute to the existence or maintenance of pathophysiological, psychosocial, situational, developmental, cultural, and/or environmental problems:

- Physiological causes increasing nutrient needs due to acute illness or acute injury/trauma
- Physiological causes resulting in anorexia or diminished intake
- Alteration in gastrointestinal tract structure and/or function
- Food- and nutrition-related knowledge deficit concerning amount of energy and amount and type of dietary protein

Diagnosis

Acute Disease or Injury Related Malnutrition (Undernutrition) (NC-4.1.3)

Diagnosis

Signs/Symptoms (Defining Characteristics)

A typical cluster of subjective and objective signs and symptoms gathered during the nutrition assessment process that provide evidence that a problem exists; quantify the problem and describe its severity.

Nutrition Assessment Category	Potential Indicators of This Nutrition Diagnosis (one or more must be present)
Biochemical Data, Medical Tests, and Procedures	
Anthropometric Measurements	Malnutrition can occur at any weight/BMI • Inadequate maternal weight gain • Non severe (moderate) malnutrition: unintentional weight loss of 7.5% in 3 months, 5% in 1 month, or 1%–2% in 1 week • Severe malnutrition: unintentional weight loss of >7.5% in 3 months, >5% in 1 month, or >2% in 1 week
Nutrition-Focused Physical Findings	Non severe (moderate) malnutrition • Mild loss of subcutaneous fat, eg, orbital, triceps, fat overlying the ribs • Mild muscle loss, eg, wasting of the temples (temporalis muscle), clavicles (pectoralis and deltoids), shoulders (deltoids), interosseous muscles, scapula (latissimus dorsi, trapezius, deltoids), thigh (quadriceps), and calf (gastrocnemius) • Mild localized or generalized fluid accumulation (extremities, vulvar/scrotal, ascites) Severe malnutrition • Moderate loss of subcutaneous fat, eg, orbital, triceps, fat overlying the ribs • Moderate muscle loss, eg, wasting of the temples (temporalis muscle), clavicles (pectoralis and deltoids), shoulders (deltoids), interosseous muscles, scapula (latissimus dorsi, trapezius, deltoids), thigh (quadriceps), and calf (gastrocnemius) • Moderate to severe localized or generalized fluid accumulation (extremities, vulvar/scrotal, ascites)

Continued on next page

Acute Disease or Injury Related Malnutrition (Undernutrition) (NC-4.1.3)

Continued from previous page

Nutrition Assessment Category	Potential Indicators of This Nutrition Diagnosis (one or more must be present)
Food/Nutrition-Related History	Reports or observations of: Non severe (moderate) malnutrition • Estimated energy intake <75% of estimated energy requirement for >7 days Severe malnutrition • Estimated energy intake <50% of estimated energy requirement for ≥ 5 days • Measurably reduced changes in handgrip strength or other functional indicators

Note: Handgrip strength in adults: norms are device dependent; can identify presence of malnutrition but not quantify the degree of the deficit; may not be able to perform on certain patients. Please refer to the Academy/ASPEN Adult Malnutrition Consensus Statement for further information.

Client History	Reports or observations of the following: • Major infections, eg, sepsis, pneumonia, peritonitis, wound infections; major burns; trauma; closed head injury; acute lung injury; adult respiratory distress syndrome; selected major surgeries (associated with malnutrition in the context of acute injury/illness) • Pre-existing medical diagnosis of malnutrition

Note: In the past, hepatic transport protein measures (eg albumin and prealbumin) were used as indicators of malnutrition. See the Evidence Analysis Library questions on this topic at https://www. andevidencelibrary.com/topic. cfm?cat=4302. Accessed April 3, 2017.

Diagnosis

Acute Disease or Injury Related Malnutrition (Undernutrition) (NC-4.1.3)

Diagnosis

Nutrition Assessment Tools for Identifying Malnutrition				
Assessment Parameter	**SGA**	**PG-SGA**	**MNA-LF**	**MCC**
Name/Author/Year	Detsky et al. (1987)[4]	Ottery 2015 http://pt-global.org/[18]	Guigoz et al. (1994) http://mna-olderadults.com/[19,20]	Academy/ASPEN Consensus Statement 2012[2]
Weight loss/BMI±	X	X	X	X
Dietary intake±	X	X	X	X
GI symptoms	X	X		
Comorbidity		X	X	
Metabolic demand		X		
Functional capacity±	X	X	X	X
Fluid status (edema/ascites)	X	X		X
Fat stores±	X	X	Mid-arm circumference, calf	X
Muscle stores±	X	X	Circumference	X
Neuropsychological			X	
Method of categorization	Rating: SGA A (well nourished) SGA B (mild-moderate malnutrition) SGA C (severe malnutrition)	Rating: SGA A/B/C (assessed per SGA) Scores for triaging nutrition interventions	Numerical score: No nutritional risk Risk of malnutrition Malnourished	2 or more characteristics demonstrated out of 6 identifies malnutrition Severity defined by specific thresholds
Validated: Setting	Acute Rehabilitation Community Residential aged care	Acute	Acute Rehabilitation Community Long-term care	
Validated: Patient Group	Surgery Geriatric Oncology Renal	Oncology Renal Stroke	Geriatric	
Validated: Ages	Adults of all ages	Adults of all ages	Adults >65 years	

± Parameters that most influence the rating

Non Illness Related Pediatric Malnutrition (Undernutrition) (NC-4.1.4)

Definition

Inadequate nutrient intake due to environmental or behavioral factors which may negatively affect growth, development, and/or other outcomes

Note: The Academy/ASPEN Pediatric Malnutrition Consensus Statement recommends specific indicators when only one indicator is present and additional indicators when two or more indicators are present for a diagnosis of malnutrition.

For additional information, please reference this publication and visit the Academy's webpage at http://www.eatright-pro.org/resources/practice/practice-resources/malnutrition.

Etiology (Cause/Contributing Risk Factors)

Factors gathered during the nutrition assessment process that contribute to the existence or the maintenance of pathophysiological, psychosocial, situational, developmental, cultural, and/or environmental problems:

- Lack of or limited access to food, eg, economic constraints, restricting food/feedings given to children, neglect or abuse, adoption/immigration/refugee from or in poorly resourced or war-torn countries
- Interruptions of or intolerance to feedings
- Social, economic, behavioral, cultural, or religious practices that affect the ability to access food

Diagnosis

Non Illness Related Pediatric Malnutrition (Undernutrition) (NC-4.1.4)

Signs/Symptoms (Defining Characteristics)

A typical cluster of subjective and objective signs and symptoms gathered during the nutrition assessment process that provide evidence that a problem exists; quantify the problem and describe its severity.

Nutrition Assessment Category	Potential Indicators of This Nutrition Diagnosis (one or more must be present)
Biochemical Data, Medical Tests, and Procedures	
Anthropometric Measurements	When a single data point is available:

Mild malnutrition
- −1 to −1.9 weight for length z score
- −1 to −1.9 body mass index for age z score
- −1 to −1.9 mid-upper arm circumference z score

Moderate malnutrition
- −2 to −2.9 weight for length z score
- −2 to −2.9 body mass index for age z score
- −2 to −2.9 mid-upper arm circumference z score

Severe malnutrition
- −3 weight for length z score or below
- −3 body mass index for age z score or below
- −3 for length/height for age z score or below
- −3 mid-upper arm circumference z score or below

Note: For further information on z score data interpretation, refer to http://www.who.int/childgrowth/training/module_c_interpreting_indicators.pdf?ua=1.

Continued on next page

Non Illness Related Pediatric Malnutrition (Undernutrition) (NC-4.1.4)

Continued from previous page

Nutrition Assessment Category	Potential Indicators of This Nutrition Diagnosis (one or more must be present)
Anthropometric Measurements (cont.)	When two or more data points are available, the following additional indicators may then be assessed: Mild malnutrition • <75% of the norm for expected weight gain velocity (<2 years of age) • 5% usual body weight loss (2–20 years of age) • Decline of 1 z score in weight for length or BMI for age z score Moderate malnutrition • <50% of the norm for expected weight gain velocity (<2 years of age) • 7.5% usual body weight loss (2–20 y of age) • Decline of 2 z score in weight for length or BMI for age z score Severe malnutrition • <25% of the norm for expected weight gain velocity (<2 years of age) • 10% usual body weight loss (2–20 yearsof age) • Decline of 3 z score in weight for length or BMI for age z score
Note: Proxy measures described in the Academy/ASPEN Pediatric Malnutrition Consensus Statement can be used when typical anthropometric measures cannot be obtained.	
Nutrition-Focused Physical Findings	Stagnation in Tanner staging Moderate malnutrition • Mild loss of subcutaneous fat, eg, orbital, triceps, fat overlying the ribs • Mild muscle loss, eg, wasting of the temples (temporalis muscle), clavicles (pectoralis and deltoids), shoulders (deltoids), interosseous muscles, scapula (latissimus dorsi, trapezius, deltoids), thigh (quadriceps), and calf (gastrocnemius) • Mild localized or generalized fluid accumulation (extremities, vulvar/scrotal, ascites) Severe malnutrition • Severe loss of subcutaneous fat, eg, orbital, triceps, fat overlying the ribs • Severe muscle loss, eg, wasting of the temples (temporalis muscle), clavicles (pectoralis and deltoids), shoulders (deltoids), interosseous muscles, scapula (latissimus dorsi, trapezius, deltoids), thigh (quadriceps), and calf (gastrocnemius) • Severe localized or generalized fluid accumulation (extremities, vulvar/scrotal, ascites)

Continued on next page

CLINICAL DOMAIN—MALNUTRITION DISORDERS

Non Illness Related Pediatric Malnutrition (Undernutrition) (NC-4.1.4)

Continued from previous page

Nutrition Assessment Category	Potential Indicators of This Nutrition Diagnosis (one or more must be present)
Food/Nutrition-Related History	Reports or observations of: • Change in functional indicators, eg, handgrip strength or other measures of physical activity and/or strength

Note: Handgrip strength in children >6 years of age: norms are device dependent; can identify presence of malnutrition but not quantify the degree of the deficit; may not be able to perform on certain patients. Please refer to the Academy/ASPEN Pediatric Malnutrition Consensus Statement for further information.

When two or more data points are available:

Mild malnutrition
• Inadequate nutrient intake of 51% to 75% estimated energy/protein need

Moderate malnutrition
• Inadequate nutrient intake of 26% to 50% estimated energy/protein need

Severe malnutrition
• Inadequate nutrient intake of ≤25% estimated energy/protein need

Client History

Reports or observations of the following:
• Anorexia nervosa, abuse, neglect, poverty, frailty, and anything that results in limited access to food (associated with malnutrition in the context of environmental and social circumstances)
• Existing medical diagnosis of malnutrition

Note: In the past, hepatic transport protein measures (eg, albumin and prealbumin) were used as indicators of malnutrition. See the Evidence Analysis Library questions on this topic at https://www.andeal.org/topic.cfm?cat=4302. Accessed April 3, 2017.

Illness Related Pediatric Malnutrition (Undernutrition) (NC-4.1.5)

Definition

Nutrient deficit or imbalance due to disease or injury which may negatively affect growth, development, and/or other outcomes

> **Note:** The Academy/ASPEN Pediatric Malnutrition Consensus Statement recommends specific indicators when only one indicator is present and additional indicators when two or more indicators are present for diagnosis of malnutrition.
>
> For additional information, please reference these publications and, visit the Academy's Web page at: http://www.eat-rightpro.org/resources/practice/practice-resources/malnutrition

Etiology (Cause/Contributing Risk Factors)

Factors gathered during the nutrition assessment process that contribute to the existence or the maintenance of pathophysiological, psychosocial, situational, developmental, cultural, and/or environmental problems:

- Physiological causes increasing nutrient needs due to prematurity, genetic/congenital disorders, illness, injury, or trauma
- Inadequate intake related to anorexia or feeding intolerance
- Alteration in gastrointestinal tract structure and/or function
- Altered utilization of nutrients
- Psychological causes, eg, depression or eating disorders

Diagnosis

Illness Related Pediatric Malnutrition (Undernutrition) (NC-4.1.5)

Diagnosis

Signs/Symptoms (Defining Characteristics)

A typical cluster of subjective and objective signs and symptoms gathered during the nutrition assessment process that provide evidence that a problem exists; quantify the problem and describe its severity.

Nutrition Assessment Category	Potential Indicators of This Nutrition Diagnosis (one or more must be present)
Biochemical Data, Medical Tests, and Procedures	
Anthropometric Measurements	When a single data point is available:
	Mild malnutrition
	• −1 to −1.9 weight for length *z* score
	• −1 to −1.9 body mass index for age *z* score
	• −1 to −1.9 mid-upper arm circumference *z* score
	Moderate malnutrition
	• −2 to −2.9 weight for length *z* score
	• −2 to −2.9 body mass index for age *z* score
	• −2 to −2.9 mid-upper arm circumference *z* score
	Severe malnutrition
	• −3 weight for length *z* score or below
	• −3 body mass index for age *z* score or below
	• −3 for length/height for age *z* score or below
	• −3 mid-upper arm circumference *z* score or below

Note: For further information on *z* score data interpretation refer to: http://www.who.int/childgrowth/training/module_c_interpreting_indicators.pdf?ua=1.

Continued on next page

Illness Related Pediatric Malnutrition (Undernutrition) (NC-4.1.5)

Continued from previous page

Nutrition Assessment Category	Potential Indicators of This Nutrition Diagnosis (one or more must be present)
Anthropometric Measurements (cont.)	When two or more data points are available the following additional indicators may then be assessed Mild malnutrition • <75% of the norm for expected weight gain velocity (<2 years of age) • 5% usual body weight loss (2–20 years of age) • Decline of 1 *z* score in weight for length or BMI for age *z* score Moderate malnutrition • <50% of the norm for expected weight gain velocity (<2 years of age) • 7.5% usual body weight loss (2–20 years of age) • Decline of 2 *z* score in weight for length or BMI for age *z* score Severe malnutrition • <25% of the norm for expected weight gain velocity (<2 years of age) • 10% usual body weight loss (2–20 years of age) • Decline of 3 *z* score in weight for length or BMI for age *z* score

Note: Proxy measures described in the Academy/ASPEN Pediatric Malnutrition Consensus Statement can be used when typical anthropometric measures cannot be obtained.

Nutrition-Focused Physical Findings	Stagnation in Tanner staging Moderate malnutrition • Mild loss of subcutaneous fat, eg, orbital, triceps, fat overlying the ribs • Mild muscle loss, eg, wasting of the temples (temporalis muscle), clavicles (pectoralis and deltoids), shoulders (deltoids), interosseous muscles, scapula (latissimus dorsi, trapezius, deltoids), thigh (quadriceps), and calf (gastrocnemius) • Mild localized or generalized fluid accumulation (extremities, vulvar/scrotal, ascites) Severe malnutrition • Severe loss of subcutaneous fat, eg, orbital, triceps, fat overlying the ribs • Severe muscle loss, eg, wasting of the temples (temporalis muscle), clavicles (pectoralis and deltoids), shoulders (deltoids), interosseous muscles, scapula (latissimus dorsi, trapezius, deltoids), thigh (quadriceps), and calf (gastrocnemius) • Severe localized or generalized fluid accumulation (extremities, vulvar/scrotal, ascites)

Diagnosis

Continued on next page

Illness Related Pediatric Malnutrition (Undernutrition) (NC-4.1.5)

Continued from previous page

Diagnosis

Nutrition Assessment Category	Potential Indicators of This Nutrition Diagnosis (one or more must be present)
Food/Nutrition-Related History	Reports or observations of: • Change in functional indicators, eg, handgrip strength or other measures of physical activity and/or strength

Note: Handgrip strength in children >6 years of age: norms are device dependent; can identify presence of malnutrition but not quantify the degree of the deficit; may not be able to perform on certain patients. Please refer to the Academy/ASPEN Pediatric Malnutrition Consensus Statement for further information.

	When two or more data points are available Mild malnutrition • Inadequate nutrient intake of 51% to 75% estimated energy/protein need Moderate malnutrition • Inadequate nutrient intake of 26% to 50% estimated energy/protein need Severe malnutrition • Inadequate nutrient intake of ≤25% estimated energy/protein need
Client History	Reports or observations of the following: • Organ failure, malignancies, rheumatoid diseases, gastrointestinal diseases, growth failure, malabsorptive syndromes, and other etiologies including but not limited to congenital birth defects or genetic anomalies such as spinal muscular atrophy • Sepsis, pneumonia, peritonitis, and wound infections, burns, trauma, closed head injury, acute lung injury, respiratory distress syndrome, and surgeries • Existing medical diagnosis of malnutrition • History of prematurity, congenital birth defects (cardiac/renal/gastrointestinal/neurological/pulmonary) • Genetic or acquired conditions: cerebral palsy, cystic fibrosis, seizure disorders, metabolic disease, irritable bowel syndrome • Feeding difficulty, food allergy, eosinophilic enteritis

Note: In the past, hepatic transport protein measures (eg albumin and prealbumin) were used as indicators of malnutrition. See the Evidence Analysis Library questions on this topic at https://www. andevidencelibrary.com/topic.cfm?cat=4302. Accessed April 3, 2017.

Food- and Nutrition-Related Knowledge Deficit* (NB-1.1)

Definition

Incomplete or inaccurate knowledge about food, nutrition, or nutrition-related information and guidelines

Etiology (Cause/Contributing Risk Factors)

Factors gathered during the nutrition assessment process that contribute to the existence or the maintenance of pathophysiological, psychosocial, situational, developmental, cultural, and/or environmental problems:

- Unsupported beliefs/attitudes about food, nutrition, and nutrition-related topics
- Lack of prior nutrition-related education
- Lack of understanding of infant/child cues to indicate hunger
- Cultural beliefs that affect ability to learn/apply information
- Impaired cognitive ability, including learning disabilities, neurological or sensory impairment, and/or dementia
- Prior exposure to incorrect information
- Unwilling or disinterested in learning/applying information
- Uncertain how to apply nutrition information

Diagnosis

*If a synonym for the term "Food- and nutrition-related knowledge deficit" is helpful or needed, an approved alternative is "Limited food and nutrition related knowledge."

Food- and Nutrition-Related Knowledge Deficit* (NB-1.1)

Signs/Symptoms (Defining Characteristics)

A typical cluster of subjective and objective signs and symptoms gathered during the nutrition assessment process that provide evidence that a problem exists; quantify the problem and describe its severity.

Nutrition Assessment Category	Potential Indicators of This Nutrition Diagnosis (one or more must be present)
Biochemical Data, Medical Tests, and Procedures	
Anthropometric Measurements	
Nutrition-Focused Physical Findings	
Food/Nutrition-Related History	Patient/client: • Verbalizes inaccurate or incomplete information • Provides inaccurate or incomplete written response to questionnaire/written tool or is unable to read written tool • No prior knowledge of need for food- and nutrition-related recommendations • No prior education provided on how to apply food and nutrition related information • Demonstrates inability to apply food- and nutrition-related information, eg, select food based on nutrition therapy or prepare infant feeding as instructed • Relates concerns about previous attempts to learn information • Verbalizes unwillingness or disinterest in learning information
Client History	Conditions associated with a diagnosis or treatment New medical diagnosis or change in existing diagnosis or condition Ethnic or cultural related issues impacting application of information

*If a synonym for the term "Food- and nutrition-related knowledge deficit" is helpful or needed, an approved alternative is "Limited food and nutrition related knowledge."

Diagnosis

Not Ready for Diet/Lifestyle Change (NB-1.3)

Definition

Lack of perceived value of nutrition-related behavior change compared to costs (consequences or effort required to make changes); conflict with personal value system; preceding event, condition or cause to behavior change.

Etiology (Cause/Contributing Risk Factors)

Factors gathered during the nutrition assessment process that contribute to the existence or the maintenance of pathophysiological, psychosocial, situational, developmental, cultural, and/or environmental problems:

- Unsupported beliefs/attitudes about food, nutrition, and nutrition-related topics
- Impaired cognitive ability, including learning disabilities, neurological or sensory impairment, and/or dementia
- Lack of social support for implementing changes
- Denial of need to change
- Perception that time, interpersonal, or financial constraints prevent changes
- Unwilling or disinterested in learning/applying information
- Lack of self-efficacy for making change or demoralization from previous failures at change

Signs/Symptoms (Defining Characteristics)

A typical cluster of subjective and objective signs and symptoms gathered during the nutrition assessment process that provide evidence that a problem exists; quantify the problem and describe its severity.

Nutrition Assessment Category	Potential Indicators of This Nutrition Diagnosis (one or more must be present)
Biochemical Data, Medical Tests, and Procedures	
Anthropometric Measurements	
Nutrition-Focused Physical Findings	Negative body language, eg, frowning, lack of eye contact, defensive posture, lack of focus, fidgeting
Note: Body language varies by culture.	
Food/Nutrition-Related History	Reports or observations of: • Denial of need for food- and nutrition-related changes • Inability to understand required changes • Failure to keep appointments/schedule follow-up appointments or engage in counseling • Previous failures to effectively change target behavior • Defensiveness, hostility, or resistance to change • Lack of efficacy to make change or to overcome barriers to change • Factors affecting physical activity access
Client History	

Disordered Eating Pattern (NB-1.5)

Definition

Beliefs, attitudes, thoughts, and behaviors related to food, eating, and weight management, including classic eating disorders as well as less severe, similar conditions, that negatively impact health.

Note: May not be an appropriate nutrition diagnosis for individuals with Limited food acceptance NI-2.11.

Etiology (Cause/Contributing Risk Factors)

Factors gathered during the nutrition assessment process that contribute to the existence or the maintenance of pathophysiological, psychosocial, situational, developmental, cultural, and/or environmental problems:

- Familial, societal, biological/genetic, and/or environmental-related obsessive desire to be thin
- Weight regulation/preoccupation significantly influences self-esteem

Diagnosis

Disordered Eating Pattern (NB-1.5)

Signs/Symptoms (Defining Characteristics)

A typical cluster of subjective and objective signs and symptoms gathered during the nutrition assessment process that provide evidence that a problem exists; quantify the problem and describe its severity.

Nutrition Assessment Category	Potential Indicators of This Nutrition Diagnosis (one or more must be present)
Biochemical Data, Medical Tests, and Procedures	↓ Cholesterol, abnormal lipid profiles, hypoglycemia, hypokalemia (anorexia nervosa [AN])
	Hypokalemia and hypochloremic alkalosis (bulimia nervosa [BN])
	Hyponatremia, hypothyroid, elevated BUN (AN)
	Urine positive for ketones (AN)
Anthropometric Measurements	BMI <17.5, arrested growth and development, failure to gain weight during period of expected growth, weight less than 85% of expected (AN)
	BMI >29 (eating disorder not otherwise specified [EDNOS])
	Significant weight fluctuation (BN)
Nutrition-Focused Physical Findings	Severely depleted adipose and somatic protein stores (AN)
	Lanugo hair formation on face and trunk; brittle, listless hair; cyanosis of hands and feet, dry skin
	Normal or excess adipose and normal somatic protein stores (BN, EDNOS)
	Damaged tooth enamel (BN)
	Enlarged parotid glands (BN)
	Peripheral edema (BN)
	Skeletal muscle loss (AN)
	Low body temperature
	Inability to concentrate (AN)
	Positive Russell's Sign (BN) callous on back of hand from self-induced vomiting
	Bradycardia (heart rate <60 beats/min), hypotension (systolic <90 mm Hg), and orthostatic hypotension (AN)
	Self-induced vomiting, diarrhea, bloating, constipation, and flatulence (BN); always cold (AN)
	Muscle weakness, fatigue, dehydration (AN, BN)
	Denial of hunger (AN)

Continued on next page

Disordered Eating Pattern (NB-1.5)

Continued from previous page

Food/Nutrition-Related History	Reports or observations of:
	• Avoidance of food or energy-containing beverages (AN, BN)
	• Avoidance of social events at which food is served
	• Fear of foods or dysfunctional thoughts regarding food or food experiences (AN, BN)
	• Food and weight preoccupation (AN, BN)
	• Knowledgeable about current diet fad (AN, BN, EDNOS)
	• Fasting (AN, BN)
	• Estimated intake of larger quantity of food in a defined time period, a sense of lack of control over eating (BN, EDNOS)
	• Excessive physical activity (AN, BN, EDNOS)
	• Eating much more rapidly than normal until feeling uncomfortably full; consuming large amounts of food when not feeling physically hungry; eating alone because of embarrassment; feeling very guilty after overeating (EDNOS)
	• Eating in private (AN, BN)
	• Irrational thoughts about food's effect on the body (AN, BN, EDNOS)
	• Pattern of chronic dieting
	• Excessive reliance on nutrition terming and preoccupation with nutrient content of foods
	• Inflexibility with food selection
	• Misuse of laxatives, enemas, diuretics, stimulants, and/or metabolic enhancers (AN, BN)
	• Excessive use of condiments and food mixing
Client History	Diagnosis, eg, anorexia nervosa, bulimia nervosa, binge eating, eating disorder not otherwise specified, amenorrhea
	History of mood and anxiety disorders (eg, depression, obsessive–compulsive disorder [OCD]), personality disorders, substance abuse disorders
	Family history of eating disorder, depression, OCD, anxiety disorders (AN, BN)
	Irritability, depression (AN, BN)
	Anemia
	Leukopenia
	Cardiac arrhythmias, bradycardia (AN, BN)

Arrows used with laboratory values: ↑ represents above reference standard and ↓ represents below reference standard.

Limited Adherence to Nutrition-Related Recommendations (NB-1.6)

Definition

Lack of nutrition-related changes as per intervention agreed on by patient/client

Etiology (Cause/Contributing Risk Factors)

Factors gathered during the nutrition assessment process that contribute to the existence or the maintenance of pathophysiological, psychosocial, situational, developmental, cultural, and/or environmental problems:

- Lack of social support for implementing changes
- Lack of value for behavior change or competing values
- Lack of confidence in ability to change
- Perception that lack of resources (eg, time, financial, or interpersonal) prevent changes
- Previous lack of success in making health-related changes
- Food and nutrition-related knowledge deficit concerning how to make nutrition-related changes
- Unwilling or disinterested in applying/learning information
- Unsupported beliefs or attitudes about food or nutrition-related topics

Limited Adherence to Nutrition-Related Recommendations (NB-1.6)

Signs/Symptoms (Defining Characteristics)

A typical cluster of subjective and objective signs and symptoms gathered during the nutrition assessment process that provide evidence that a problem exists; quantify the problem and describe its severity.

Nutrition Assessment Category	Potential Indicators of This Nutrition Diagnosis (one or more must be present)
Biochemical Data, Medical Tests, and Procedures	Expected laboratory outcomes are not achieved
Anthropometric Measurements	Expected anthropometric outcomes are not achieved
Nutrition-Focused Physical Findings	Negative body language, eg, frowning, lack of eye contact, fidgeting, defensive posture, crying

Note: Body language varies by culture.

Food/Nutrition-Related History	Reports or observations of: • Expected food/nutrition-related outcomes are not achieved • Inability to recall changes agreed upon • Failure to complete any agreed upon homework • Lack of compliance or inconsistent compliance with plan • Failure to keep appointments or schedule follow-up appointments • Lack of appreciation of the importance of making recommended nutrition-related changes • Uncertainty as to how to consistently apply food/nutrition information • Verbalizes frustration with attempts to apply food/nutrition information • Verbalizes previous failures to effectively change target behavior • Presence of a lack of self-efficacy or confidence to make changes • Noting internal and/or external barriers to change
Client History	Lack of social and/or familial support

Undesirable Food Choices* (NB-1.7)

Definition

Food and/or beverage choices that are inconsistent with dietary reference intake standards (eg, Dietary Reference Intakes), national food guidelines (eg, US Dietary Guidelines, MyPlate), diet quality index standards (eg, Healthy Eating Index) or as defined in the nutrition prescription

Etiology (Cause/Contributing Risk Factors)

Factors gathered during the nutrition assessment process that contribute to the existence or the maintenance of pathophysiological, psychosocial, situational, developmental, cultural, and/or environmental problems:

- Lack of prior exposure to accurate nutrition-related information
- Cultural practices that affect the ability to learn/apply information
- Impaired cognitive ability, including learning disabilities, neurological or sensory impairment, and/or dementia
- High level of fatigue or other side effect of medical, surgical, or radiological therapy
- Lack of or limited access to recommended foods
- Perception that lack of resources (eg, time, financial, or interpersonal) prevent selection of food choices consistent with recommendations
- Food allergies and aversions impeding food choices consistent with guidelines
- Lack of motivation and/or readiness to apply or support systems change
- Unwilling or disinterested in learning/applying information
- Psychological causes such as depression or disordered eating

*If a synonym for the term "Undesirable food choices" is helpful or needed, an approved alternative is "Unbalanced diet."

Undesirable Food Choices* (NB-1.7)

Signs/Symptoms (Defining Characteristics)

A typical cluster of subjective and objective signs and symptoms gathered during the nutrition assessment process that provide evidence that a problem exists; quantify the problem and describe its severity.

Nutrition Assessment Category	Potential Indicators of This Nutrition Diagnosis (one or more must be present)
Biochemical Data, Medical Tests, and Procedures	↑ Lipid panel
Anthropometric Measurements	
Nutrition-Focused Physical Findings	Findings consistent with vitamin/mineral deficiency or excess
Food/Nutrition-Related History	Reports or observations of: • Estimated intake inconsistent with dietary reference intake standards (eg, DRIs), national food guidelines (eg, US Dietary Guidelines, MyPlate), diet quality index standards (eg, Healthy Eating Index), or nutrition prescription • Inaccurate or incomplete understanding of the guidelines • Inability to apply guideline information • Inability to select (eg, access), or unwillingness or disinterest in selecting, food consistent with the guidelines
Client History	Conditions associated with a diagnosis or treatment, eg, mental illness

Arrows used with laboratory values: ↑ represents above reference standard and ↓ represents below reference standard.

*If a synonym for the term "Undesirable food choices" is helpful or needed, an approved alternative is "Unbalanced diet."

Physical Inactivity* (NB-2.1)

Definition

Low level of activity or sedentary behavior to the extent that it reduces energy expenditure and impacts health.

Etiology (Cause/Contributing Risk Factors)

Factors gathered during the nutrition assessment process that contribute to the existence or the maintenance of pathophysiological, psychosocial, situational, developmental, cultural, and/or environmental problems:

- Unsupported beliefs/attitudes about physical activity
- Injury, lifestyle change, condition (eg, advanced stages of cardiovascular disease, obesity, kidney disease), physical disability, or limitation that reduces physical activity or activities of daily living
- Food and nutrition-related knowledge deficit concerning health benefits of physical activity
- Lack of prior exposure to accurate nutrition-related information
- Lack of role models, eg, for children
- Lack of social support for implementing changes
- Lack of or limited access to safe exercise environment and/or equipment
- Lack of value for behavior change or competing values
- Time constraints
- Financial constraints that may prevent sufficient level of activity (eg, cost of equipment or shoes or club membership to gain access)

---

*If a synonym for the term "Physical inactivity" is helpful or needed, an approved alternative is "Limited physical activity."

Physical Inactivity* (NB-2.1)

Signs/Symptoms (Defining Characteristics)

A typical cluster of subjective and objective signs and symptoms gathered during the nutrition assessment process that provide evidence that a problem exists; quantify the problem and describe its severity.

Nutrition Assessment Category	Potential Indicators of This Nutrition Diagnosis (one or more must be present)
Biochemical Data, Medical Tests, and Procedures	
Anthropometric Measurements	Obesity: BMI >30 (adults); BMI >95th percentile (pediatrics >3 years)
Nutrition-Focused Physical Findings	Excessive subcutaneous fat and low muscle mass
Food/Nutrition-Related History	Reports or observations of: • Infrequent, low-duration, and/or low-intensity physical activity • Large amounts of sedentary activities, eg, TV watching, reading, computer use in both leisure and work/school • Low level of nonexercise activity thermogenesis (NEAT) expended by physical activities other than planned exercise, eg, sitting, standing, walking, fidgeting • Low cardiorespiratory fitness and/or low muscle strength • Medications that cause somnolence and decreased cognition • Factors affecting physical activity access
Client History	Medical diagnoses that may be associated with or result in decreased activity, eg, arthritis, chronic fatigue syndrome, morbid obesity, knee surgery Psychological diagnosis, eg, depression, anxiety disorders

*If a synonym for the term "Physical inactivity" is helpful or needed, an approved alternative is "Limited physical activity."

Excessive Physical Activity (NB-2.2)

Definition

Involuntary or voluntary physical activity or movement that interferes with energy needs, growth, or exceeds that which is necessary to achieve optimal health.

Etiology (Cause/Contributing Risk Factors)

Factors gathered during the nutrition assessment process that contribute to the existence or maintenance of patho-physiological, psychosocial, situational, developmental, cultural, and/or environmental problems:

- Disordered eating
- Irrational beliefs/attitudes about food, nutrition, and fitness
- "Addictive" behaviors/personality

Diagnosis

BEHAVIORAL–ENVIRONMENTAL DOMAIN—PHYSICAL ACTIVITY AND FUNCTION

Excessive Physical Activity (NB-2.2)

Signs/Symptoms (Defining Characteristics)

A typical cluster of subjective and objective signs and symptoms gathered during the nutrition assessment process that provide evidence that a problem exists; quantify the problem and describe its severity.

Nutrition Assessment Category	Potential Indicators of This Nutrition Diagnosis (one or more must be present)
Biochemical Data, Medical Tests, and Procedures	↑ Liver enzymes, eg, LDH, AST Altered micronutrient status, eg, ↓ serum ferritin, zinc, and insulin-like growth factor-binding protein ↑ Hematocrit Possibly ↑ cortisol levels
Anthropometric Measurements	Weight loss, arrested growth and development, failure to gain weight during period of expected growth (related usually to disordered eating)
Nutrition-Focused Physical Findings	Depleted adipose and somatic protein stores (related usually to disordered eating) Chronic muscle soreness
Food/Nutrition-Related History	Reports or observations of: • Continued/repeated high levels of exercise exceeding levels necessary to improve health and/or athletic performance • Exercise daily without rest/rehabilitation days • Exercise while injured/sick • Forsaking family, job, social responsibilities to exercise • Overtraining
Client History	Conditions associated with a diagnosis or treatment, eg, anorexia nervosa, bulimia nervosa, binge eating, eating disorder not otherwise specified, amenorrhea, stress fractures Chronic fatigue Evidence of addictive, obsessive, or compulsive tendencies Suppressed immune function Frequent and/or prolonged injuries and/or illnesses

Arrows used with laboratory values: ↑ represents above reference standard and ↓ represents below reference standard.

Diagnosis

Inability* to Manage Self-Care (NB-2.3)

Definition

Lack of capacity or unwillingness to implement methods to support healthful food- and nutrition-related behavior

Etiology (Cause/Contributing Risk Factors)

Factors gathered during the nutrition assessment process that contribute to the existence or the maintenance of pathophysiological, psychosocial, situational, developmental, cultural, and/or environmental problems:

- Food- and nutrition-related knowledge deficit concerning self-care
- Lack of social support for implementing changes
- Lack of developmental readiness to perform self-management tasks, eg, pediatrics
- Lack of value for behavior change or competing values
- Perception that lack of resources (eg, time, financial, or interpersonal) prevent self-care
- Cultural practices that affect ability to manage self-care
- Impaired cognitive ability, including learning disabilities, neurological or sensory impairment, and/or dementia
- Prior exposure to incompatible information
- Not ready for diet/lifestyle change
- Unwilling or disinterested in learning/applying information
- Lack of or limited access to self-management tools or decision guides

Diagnosis

---

*If a synonym for the term "Inability to manage self-care" is helpful or needed, an approved alternative is "Limited ability to manage self-care."

Inability* to Manage Self-Care (NB-2.3)

Signs/Symptoms (Defining Characteristics)

A typical cluster of subjective and objective signs and symptoms gathered during the nutrition assessment process that provide evidence that a problem exists; quantify the problem and describe its severity.

Nutrition Assessment Category	Potential Indicators of This Nutrition Diagnosis (one or more must be present)
Biochemical Data, Medical Tests, and Procedures	
Anthropometric Measurements	
Nutrition-Focused Physical Findings	
Food/Nutrition-Related History	Reports or observations of: • Inability to interpret data or self-management tools • Embarrassment or anger regarding need for self-monitoring • Uncertainty regarding changes could/should be made in response to data in self-monitoring records
Client History	Diagnoses that are associated with self-management, eg, diabetes mellitus, obesity, cardiovascular disease, renal or liver disease
	Conditions associated with a diagnosis or treatment, eg, cognitive or emotional impairment
	New medical diagnosis or change in existing diagnosis or condition

*If a synonym for the term "Inability to manage self-care" is helpful or needed, an approved alternative is "Limited ability to manage self-care."

Intake of Unsafe Food (NB-3.1)

Definition

Intake of food and/or fluids intentionally or unintentionally contaminated with toxins, poisonous products, infectious agents, microbial agents, additives, allergens, and/or agents of bioterrorism

Etiology (Cause/Contributing Risk Factors)

Factors gathered during the nutrition assessment process that contribute to the existence or the maintenance of pathophysiological, psychosocial, situational, developmental, cultural, and/or environmental problems:

- Food and nutrition-related knowledge deficit concerning potentially unsafe food
- Lack of knowledge about proper food/feeding (infant and enteral formula or breastmilk*) storage, and preparation
- Exposure to contaminated water or food, eg, community outbreak of illness documented by surveillance and/or response agency
- Mental illness, confusion, or altered awareness
- Lack of or limited access to food storage equipment/facilities, eg, refrigerator
- Lack of or limited access to safe food supply, eg, inadequate markets with safe, uncontaminated food

Diagnosis

---

*If a synonym for the term "breastmilk" is helpful or needed, an approved alternative is "human milk."

Intake of Unsafe Food (NB-3.1)

Signs/Symptoms (Defining Characteristics)

A typical cluster of subjective and objective signs and symptoms gathered during the nutrition assessment process that provide evidence that a problem exists; quantify the problem and describe its severity.

Nutrition Assessment Category	Potential Indicators of This Nutrition Diagnosis (one or more must be present)
Biochemical Data, Medical Tests, and Procedures	Positive stool culture for infectious causes, such as listeria, salmonella, hepatitis A, E. coli, cyclospora Toxicology reports for drugs, medicinals, poisons in blood or food samples
Anthropometric Measurements	
Nutrition-Focused Physical Findings	Evidence of dehydration, eg, dry mucous membranes, damaged tissues Diarrhea, cramping, bloating, fever, nausea, vomiting, vision problems, chills, dizziness, headache
Food/Nutrition-Related History	Reports or observations of: • Fish suspected to contain mercury (pregnant and lactating women) • Nonfood items (pregnant and lactating women) • Raw eggs, unpasteurized milk products, soft cheeses, undercooked meats (infants, children, immunocompromised persons, pregnant and lactating women, and older adults) • Wild plants, berries, mushrooms • Unsafely stored and prepared foods or products (enteral and infant formula, breastmilk) • Mislabeled or unlabeled foods • Verbalizes inaccurate or incomplete knowledge
Client History	Conditions associated with a diagnosis or treatment, eg, foodborne illness such as bacterial, viral, or parasitic infection, mental illness, dementia Poisoning by drugs, medicinals, and biological substances Poisoning from poisonous foodstuffs and poisonous plants Cardiac, neurologic, respiratory changes

Diagnosis

Limited Access to Food (NB-3.2)

Definition

Diminished ability to acquire a sufficient quantity and variety of healthful food based on dietary reference intake standards (eg, Dietary Reference Intakes), national food guidelines (eg, US Dietary Guidelines, MyPlate), or as defined in the nutrition prescription

Etiology (Cause/Contributing Risk Factors)

Factors gathered during the nutrition assessment process that contribute to the existence or the maintenance of pathophysiological, psychosocial, situational, developmental, cultural, and/or environmental problems:

- Caregiver intentionally or unintentionally not providing access to food, eg, unmet needs for food or eating assistance, excess of poor nutritional quality food, abuse/neglect
- Community and geographical constraints for shopping and transportation
- Food and nutrition-related knowledge deficit concerning sufficient quantity or variety of culturally appropriate healthful food
- Lack of financial resources or lack of access to financial resources to purchase a sufficient quantity or variety of culturally appropriate healthful foods
- Lack of food planning, purchasing, and preparation skills
- Limited, absent, or lack of participation in community supplemental food or other programs, eg, food pantries, emergency kitchens, or shelters
- Failure to participate in federal food programs, eg, WIC, National School Breakfast/Lunch Program, food stamps
- Schools lacking nutrition/wellness policies or application of policies ensuring convenient, appetizing, competitively priced culturally appropriate healthful foods at meals, snacks, and school-sponsored activities
- Physical or psychological limitations that diminish ability to shop, eg, walking, sight, mental/emotional health
- Limitation to food because of concerns about weight or aging
- Factors contributing to a contaminated food supply

Limited Access to Food (NB-3.2)

Diagnosis

Signs/Symptoms (Defining Characteristics)

A typical cluster of subjective and objective signs and symptoms gathered during the nutrition assessment process that provide evidence that a problem exists; quantify the problem and describe its severity.

Nutrition Assessment Category	Potential Indicators of This Nutrition Diagnosis (one or more must be present)
Biochemical Data, Medical Tests, and Procedures	Indicators of macronutrient or vitamin/mineral status as indicated by biochemical findings
Anthropometric Measurements	Growth failure based on reference growth standards, eg, National Center for Health Statistics (NCHS)
	Underweight: BMI <18.5 (adults)
	Unintentional weight loss: >10% in 6 months, >5% in 1 month (adults); any unintentional weight loss in children
	Overweight/obesity: BMI >25 (adults); >95th percentile (pediatrics)
Nutrition-Focused Physical Findings	Findings consistent with vitamin/mineral deficiency
	Hunger
Food/Nutrition-Related History	Reports or observations of:
	• Food faddism or unsupported beliefs and attitudes of patient/client
	• Belief that aging can be slowed by dietary limitations and extreme exercise
	• Estimated inadequate intake of food and/or specific nutrients
	• Limited supply of food in home
	• Limited variety of foods
	• Lack of resources for food
	• Lack of transportation or other community constraints limiting availability of food
	• Lack of knowledge or skills on how to use food
	• Lack of knowledge or skills on how to apply and/or participate in food assistance programs
	• Behaviors consistent with food insecurity (eg, skipping meals; buying low-cost food items; changes in eating patterns, rituals, or customs)
	• Lack of knowledge on how to identify, store, or prepare safe food
	• Conditions that contribute to food contamination
	• Fasting pattern
Client History	Malnutrition, vitamin/mineral deficiency
	Illness or physical disability
	Conditions associated with a diagnosis or treatment, eg, mental illness, dementia
	Lack of suitable support systems

No Nutrition Diagnosis at This Time (NO-1.1)

Definition

Absence of a current nutrition problem warranting a nutrition intervention. This determination results from a nutrition assessment

Note: This nutrition diagnostic term is not appropriate if additional information for the nutrition assessment is needed or pending.

Etiology (Cause/Contributing Risk Factors)

Factors gathered during the nutrition assessment process that contribute to the existence or the maintenance of pathophysiological, psychosocial, situational, developmental, cultural, and/or environmental problems:

- Not applicable

Signs/Symptoms (Defining Characteristics)

A typical cluster of subjective and objective signs and symptoms gathered during the nutrition assessment process that provide evidence that a problem exists; quantify the problem and describe its severity.

Nutrition Assessment Category	Potential Indicators of This Nutrition Diagnosis (one or more must be present)
Biochemical Data, Medical Tests, and Procedures	Not applicable
Anthropometric Measurements	Not applicable
Nutrition-Focused Physical Findings	Not applicable
Food/Nutrition-Related History	Not applicable
Client History	Conditions associated with a diagnosis or treatment, eg, palliative/end-of-life care

Diagnosis

SNAPSHOT   NCP Step 3: Nutrition Intervention

Purpose: The purpose of nutrition intervention is to resolve or improve the identified nutrition diagnosis(es) or nutrition problem(s) by planning and implementing appropriate interventions. Nutrition interventions are selected and tailored to the needs of the individual patient/client*, family, group, community, or population.

Determining a nutrition intervention: The nutrition diagnosis and its etiology drive the selection of a nutrition intervention. Nutrition intervention strategies are selected to change nutritional intake, nutrition-related knowledge or behavior, access to supportive care and services; or environmental conditions, organizational processes, and public environmental conditions, organizational processes, and public policies that impact the nutrition problem. Nutrition intervention goals provide the basis for monitoring progress and measuring outcomes.

Terminology for nutrition intervention is organized in 5 domains (categories):

Food and/or Nutrient Delivery	Nutrition Education	Nutrition Counseling	Coordination of Nutrition Care	Population Based Nutrition Action
Individualized approach for food/nutrient provision	A formal process to instruct or train a patient/client in a skill or to impart knowledge to help patients/clients voluntarily manage or modify food, nutrition, and physical activity choices and behavior to maintain or improve health	A supportive process, characterized by a collaborative counselor–patient relationship, to establish food, nutrition, and physical activity priorities, goals, and individualized action plans that acknowledge and foster responsibility for self-care to treat an existing condition and promote health	Consultation with, referral to, or coordination of nutrition care with other health care providers, institutions, or agencies that can assist in treating or managing nutrition-related problems	Interventions designed to improve the nutritional well-being of a population

Use of nutrition intervention terminology: Nutrition intervention is accomplished in two distinct and interrelated steps: planning and implementing.

Planning the nutrition intervention involves:
- prioritizing nutrition diagnoses
- consulting the Academy's Evidence-Based Nutrition Practice Guidelines, other practice guidelines, and sources of recommendations

> **Note:** The evidence-based nutrition practice guideline topics can be accessed from the Projects tab.

- determining patient-/client-focused or population-level expected outcomes for each nutrition diagnosis
- conferring with patient/client/caregivers or others
- defining a nutrition intervention plan and related strategies
- defining time and frequency of care
- identifying resources needed.

Implementation is the action phase and involves:
- communication of the nutrition care plan
- carrying out the plan.

Critical Thinking Skills
- Setting goals and prioritizing
- Defining the nutrition prescription or basic plan
- Making interdisciplinary connections
- Initiating behavioral and other nutrition interventions
- Matching nutrition intervention strategies with patient/client's, community's, or population's needs, nutrition diagnosis, and values
- Choosing from among alternatives to determine a course of action
- Specifying the time and frequency of care

For more information, sign in as a subscriber at https://ncpt.webauthor.com.

Intervention

---

*Patient/client refers to individuals, groups, populations, family members, and/or caregivers.

Each term is designated with an alphanumeric NCPT hierarchical code, followed by a five-digit (eg, 99999) Academy SNOMED CT/LOINC unique identifier (ANDUID). Neither should be used in nutrition documentation. The ANDUID is for data tracking purposes in electronic health records.

	NCPT Code	ANDUID
Nutrition Prescription (NP)	NP-1.1	10794

The patient/client's individual recommended dietary intake of energy and/or selected foods or nutrients based on current reference standards and dietary guidelines and the patient/client's health and nutrition diagnosis (specify).

FOOD AND/OR NUTRIENT DELIVERY (ND)

Individualized approach for food /nutrient provision.

Meals and Snacks (1)

Regular eating episode (meal); food served between regular meals (snack).

	NCPT Code	ANDUID
❏ General/healthful diet	ND-1.1	10489
❏ Modify composition of meals/snacks	ND-1.2	10828
❏ Texture modified diet (1)	ND-1.2.1	10829
❏ Easy to chew diet	ND-1.2.1.1	10914
❏ Mechanically altered diet	ND-1.2.1.2	10915
❏ Pureed diet	ND-1.2.1.3	10916
❏ Liquid consistency-thin liquids	ND-1.2.1.4	10865
❏ Liquid consistency-nectar thick liquids	ND-1.2.1.5	10866
❏ Liquid consistency-honey thick liquids	ND-1.2.1.6	10867
❏ Liquid consistency-spoon thick liquids	ND-1.2.1.7	10868
❏ Energy modified diet (2)	ND-1.2.2	10830
❏ Increased energy diet	ND-1.2.2.1	10935
❏ Decreased energy diet	ND-1.2.2.2	10936
❏ Protein modified diet (3)	ND-1.2.3	10831
❏ Consistent protein diet	ND-1.2.3.1	10896
❏ Increased protein diet	ND-1.2.3.2	10972
❏ Decreased protein diet	ND-1.2.3.3	10973
❏ Decreased gluten diet	ND-1.2.3.5	11000
❏ Gluten free diet	ND-1.2.3.5.1	11027
❏ Carbohydrate modified diet (4)	ND-1.2.4	10832
❏ Consistent carbohydrate diet	ND-1.2.4.1	10860
❏ Increased carbohydrate diet	ND-1.2.4.2	10930
❏ Increased complex carbohydrate diet	ND-1.2.4.2.1	11972
❏ Increased simple carbohydrate diet	ND-1.2.4.2.2	11973

Meals and Snacks (1) (continued)

	NCPT Code	ANDUID
❏ Decreased carbohydrate diet	ND-1.2.4.3	10931
❏ Decreased complex carbohydrate diet	ND-1.2.4.3.1	11974
❏ Decreased simple carbohydrate diet	ND-1.2.4.3.2	11975
❏ Lactose modified diet	ND-1.2.4.5	10862
❏ Fat modified diet (5)	ND-1.2.5	10833
❏ Increased fat diet	ND-1.2.5.1	10937
❏ Decreased fat diet	ND-1.2.5.2	10938
❏ Fiber modified diet (7)	ND-1.2.7	10834
❏ Increased fiber diet	ND-1.2.7.1	10945
❏ Decreased fiber diet	ND-1.2.7.2	10946
❏ Fluid modified diet (8)	ND-1.2.8	10835
❏ Increased fluid diet	ND-1.2.8.1	10874
❏ Fluid restricted diet	ND-1.2.8.2	10873
❏ Clear liquid diet	ND-1.2.8.3	10876
❏ Full liquid diet	ND-1.2.8.4	10877
❏ Diets modified for specific foods or ingredients (9)	ND-1.2.9	10836
❏ Mineral modified diet (11)	ND-1.2.11	10838
❏ Calcium modified diet	ND-1.2.11.1	10879
❏ Increased calcium diet	ND-1.2.11.1.1	10953
❏ Decreased calcium diet	ND-1.2.11.1.2	10954
❏ Iron modified diet	ND-1.2.11.3	10886
❏ Increased iron diet	ND-1.2.11.3.1	10960
❏ Decreased iron diet	ND-1.2.11.3.2	10961
❏ Potassium modified diet	ND-1.2.11.5	10891
❏ Increased potassium diet	ND-1.2.11.5.1	10966
❏ Decreased potassium diet	ND-1.2.11.5.2	10967
❏ Phosphorus modified diet	ND-1.2.11.6	10890
❏ Increased phosphorus diet	ND-1.2.11.6.1	10964
❏ Decreased phosphorus diet	ND-1.2.11.6.2	10965
❏ Sodium modified diet	ND-1.2.11.7	10893
❏ Increased sodium diet	ND-1.2.11.7.1	10968
❏ Decreased sodium diet	ND-1.2.11.7.2	10969

Intervention

	NCPT Code	ANDUID

Enteral and Parenteral Nutrition (2)

Nutrition provided through the GI tract via tube, catheter, or stoma (enteral) or intravenously, centrally, or peripherally (parenteral).

Enteral Nutrition (2.1)

Nutrition provided through the GI tract.

	NCPT Code	ANDUID
❏ Modify composition of enteral nutrition	ND-2.1.1	10503
❏ Modify concentration of enteral nutrition	ND-2.1.2	10502
❏ Modify rate of enteral nutrition	ND-2.1.3	10500
❏ Modify volume of enteral nutrition	ND-2.1.4	10501
❏ Modify schedule of enteral nutrition	ND-2.1.5	10504
❏ Modify route of enteral nutrition	ND-2.1.6	10792
❏ Insert enteral feeding tube	ND-2.1.7	10497
❏ Enteral nutrition site care	ND-2.1.8	10498
❏ Feeding tube flush	ND-2.1.9	10499

Parenteral Nutrition/IV Fluids (2.2)

Nutrition and fluids provided intravenously.

	NCPT Code	ANDUID
❏ Modify composition of parenteral nutrition	ND-2.2.1	10511
❏ Modify concentration of parenteral nutrition	ND-2.2.2	10510
❏ Modify rate of parenteral nutrition	ND-2.2.3	10509
❏ Modify volume of parenteral nutrition	ND-2.2.4	11141
❏ Modify schedule of parenteral nutrition	ND-2.2.5	10512
❏ Modify route of parenteral nutrition	ND-2.2.6	10793
❏ Parenteral nutrition site care	ND-2.2.7	10507
❏ IV fluid delivery	ND-2.2.8	10508

Nutrition Supplement Therapy (3)

Medical Food Supplement Therapy (3.1)

Commercial or prepared foods or beverages intended to supplement energy, protein, carbohydrate, fiber, and/or fat intake.

	NCPT Code	ANDUID
❏ Commercial beverage	ND-3.1.1	10515
❏ Modified beverage	ND-3.1.3	10517

Bioactive Substance Management (3.3)

Addition or change in provision of bioactive substances.

	NCPT Code	ANDUID
❏ Psyllium	ND-3.3.4	10817
❏ Glucan	ND-3.3.5	10563
❏ Alcohol	ND-3.3.7	10565
❏ Caffeine	ND-3.3.8	10566
❏ Other	ND-3.3.9	10567

(specify) _____

Feeding Assistance (4)

Accommodation or assistance in eating.

	NCPT Code	ANDUID
❏ Adaptive eating device	ND-4.1	10808
❏ Feeding position	ND-4.2	10570
❏ Meal set-up	ND-4.3	10571
❏ Mouth care	ND-4.4	10572
❏ Menu selection assistance	ND-4.5	10809
❏ Other	ND-4.6	10573

(specify) _____

NUTRITION EDUCATION (E)

Formal process to instruct or train patients/clients in a skill or to impart knowledge to help patients/clients voluntarily manage or modify food, nutrition, and physical activity choices and behavior to maintain or improve health.

Nutrition Education—Content (1)

Instruction or training intended to lead to nutrition-related knowledge.

	NCPT Code	ANDUID
❏ Purpose of the nutrition education	E-1.1	10588
❏ Priority modifications	E-1.2	10589
❏ Survival information	E-1.3	10590
❏ Nutrition relationship to health/disease	E-1.4	10591
❏ Recommended modifications	E-1.5	10592
❏ Other or related topics	E-1.6	10593
❏ Other	E-1.7	10594

(specify) _____

	NCPT Code	ANDUID
❏ Physical activity guidance	E-1.8	12012

Nutrition Education—Application (2)

Instruction or training leading to nutrition-related result interpretation or skills.

	NCPT Code	ANDUID
❏ Result interpretation	E-2.1	10596
❏ Skill development	E-2.2	10597
❏ Other	E-2.3	10598

(specify) _____

Intervention

	NCPT Code	ANDUID

NUTRITION COUNSELING (C)

A supportive process, characterized by a collaborative counselor–patient/client relationship to establish food, nutrition, and physical activity priorities, goals, and individualized action plans that acknowledge and foster responsibility for self-care to treat an existing condition and promote health.

Theoretical Basis/Approach (1)

The theories or models used to design and implement an intervention.

	NCPT Code	ANDUID
❏ Cognitive–behavioral theory	C-1.1	10601
❏ Health belief model	C-1.2	10602
❏ Social learning theory	C-1.3	10603
❏ Transtheoretical model/stages of change	C-1.4	10604
❏ Other	C-1.5	10605

(specify) _____

Strategies (2)

Selectively applied evidence-based methods or plans of action designed to achieve a particular goal.

	NCPT Code	ANDUID
❏ Motivational interviewing	C-2.1	10607
❏ Goal setting	C-2.2	10608
❏ Self-monitoring	C-2.3	10609
❏ Problem solving	C-2.4	10610
❏ Social support	C-2.5	10611
❏ Stress management	C-2.6	10612
❏ Stimulus control	C-2.7	10613
❏ Cognitive restructuring	C-2.8	10614
❏ Relapse prevention	C-2.9	10615
❏ Rewards/contingency management	C-2.10	10616
❏ Other	C-2.11	10617

(specify) _____

COORDINATION OF NUTRITION CARE BY A NUTRITION PROFESSIONAL (RC)

Consultation with, referral to, or coordination of nutrition care with other providers, institutions, or agencies that can assist in treating or managing nutrition-related problems.

Collaboration and Referral of Nutrition Care (1)

Facilitating services with other professionals, institutions, or agencies during nutrition care.

	NCPT Code	ANDUID
❏ Team meeting	RC-1.1	10620
❏ Referral to RDN with different expertise	RC-1.2	10621
❏ Collaboration with other providers	RC-1.4	10812

Discharge and Transfer of Nutrition Care to New Setting or Provider (2)

Discharge planning and transfer of nutrition care from one level or location of care to another.

	NCPT Code	ANDUID
❏ Discharge and transfer to other providers	RC-2.1	10813
❏ Discharge and transfer to community agencies/programs	RC-2.2	10814
❏ Discharge and transfer to another nutrition professional	RC-2.3	10627

Note: This Abridged Nutrition Care Process Reference Terminology (NCPT) Student Manual does not include terms from the fifth domain, Population Based Nutrition Action. See the full edition at http://ncpt.webauthor.com.

Nutrition Prescription (NP-1.1)

Definition

The patient/client's recommended dietary intake of energy and/or selected foods or nutrients based on current reference standards and dietary guidelines and the patient/client's health condition and nutrition diagnosis

Purpose

To communicate the nutrition professional's diet/nutrition recommendation based on a nutrition assessment

Indicators

- Recommended general, healthful diet
- Recommended modified diet
  - Recommended texture modification (specify, eg, mechanically altered, pureed)
  - Recommended liquid consistency modification (specify, eg, thin, nectar thick, honey thick, spoon thick)
  - Recommended energy/nutrient modification
  - Energy modification (specify, eg, calories, kcal, or kJ/day)
  - Recommended protein modification (specify, eg, g/day; g/kg/day; percent of calories, kcal, or kJ)
  - Recommended carbohydrate modification
    - Carbohydrate controlled diet (specify, eg, distribution)
    - Amount (specify, eg, g/day; g/kg/min; percent of calories, kcal, or kJ)
    - Other (specify, eg, no concentrated sweets)
  - Recommended fat modification (specify, eg, g/day; g/kg/day; percent of calories, kcal, or kJ)
    - Recommended monounsaturated fat level (specify, eg, g/day; percent of calories, kcal, or kJ)
    - Recommended polyunsaturated fat level (specify, eg, g/day; percent of calories, kcal, or kJ)
    - Recommended saturated fat level (specify, eg, g/day; percent of calories, kcal, or kJ)
    - Recommended trans fat level (specify, eg, g/day; percent of calories, kcal, or kJ)
  - Recommended cholesterol intake (specify, eg, mg/day)
  - Recommended fiber level (specify, eg, type, g/day, g/1,000 calories/kcal/kJ/day)
  - Recommended fluid level (specify, eg, oz or mL/day, mL/kg/day, mL per calories/kcal/kJ expended, mL/ m^2/day, mL output)
    - Clear liquid
    - Full liquid
  - Recommended modifications for specific foods or ingredients
  - Recommended vitamin intake
    - Vitamin A (specify form, µg or RE, frequency)
    - Niacin (specify form, mg, frequency)
    - Vitamin C (mg/day, frequency)
    - Vitamin B6 (specify form, mg, frequency)
    - Vitamin D (specify form, µg or IU, frequency)
    - Folate (specify form, µg, frequency)
    - Vitamin E (specify form, mg or IU, frequency)
    - Vitamin B12 (µg, frequency)

Nutrition Prescription (NP-1.1)

- Vitamin K (µg, frequency)
- Pantothenic acid (mg, frequency)
- Thiamin (mg, frequency)
- Biotin (µg, frequency)
- Riboflavin (mg, frequency)
- Multivitamin (yes/no, specify dose, frequency)
- Recommended mineral intake
  - Calcium (specify form, mg, frequency)
  - Molybdenum (µg, frequency)
  - Copper (µg or mg, frequency)
  - Boron (mg, frequency)
  - Fluoride (mg, frequency)
  - Cobalt (µg, frequency)
  - Iodine (µg, frequency)
  - Selenium (specify form, µg, frequency)
  - Iron (specify form, mg, frequency)
  - Zinc (mg, frequency)
  - Magnesium (mg, frequency)
  - Potassium (specify form, g or mg, frequency)
  - Phosphorus (mg, frequency)
  - Sodium (mg or g, frequency)
  - Sulfate (g or mmol, frequency)
  - Chloride (mg, frequency)
  - Manganese (mg, frequency)
  - Chromium (specify form, µg, frequency)
  - Multi-mineral (yes/no, specify dose, frequency)
  - Multi-trace element (yes/no, specify dose, frequency)
  - Recommended enteral nutrition order (specify, eg, formula, rate/schedule)
  - Tube feeding modulars (specify, eg, carbohydrate, protein, fat, fiber)
- Recommended parenteral nutrition order (specify, eg, solution, rate, access)
- Recommended level of bioactive substances (specify, eg, substance, amount)
- Recommended food intake
  - Grain group intake (specify, eg, servings, exchanges, amounts)
  - Fruit and vegetable intake (specify, eg, servings, exchanges, amounts)
  - Meat, poultry, fish, eggs, beans, nut intake (specify, eg, servings, exchanges, amounts)
  - Milk and milk product intake (specify, eg, servings, exchanges, amounts)
  - Fat intake (specify, eg, type, servings, exchanges, amounts)

Note: The nutrition prescription can be used as a comparative standard for nutrition assessment and nutrition monitoring and evaluation.

Intervention

Meals and Snacks (ND-1)

Definition

Meals are defined as regular eating episodes that may include a variety of foods consisting of grains and/or starches, meat and/or meat alternatives, fruits and vegetables, and milk or milk products. A snack is defined as food served between regular meals

Details of Intervention

A typical intervention might be further described with the following details. Nutrition and dietetics practitioners recommend, implement, or order nutrition interventions, and the action(s) may be to initiate, modify or discontinue a nutrition intervention(s):

- General/healthful diet
- Modify composition of meals/snacks
  - Texture modified diet
    - Easy to chew diet
    - Mechanically altered diet
    - Pureed diet
    - Liquid consistency-thin liquids
    - Liquid consistency-nectar thick liquids
    - Liquid consistency-honey thick liquids
    - Liquid consistency-spoon thick liquids
  - Energy modified diet
    - Increased energy diet
    - Decreased energy diet
  - Protein modified diet
    - Consistent protein diet
    - Increased protein diet
    - Decreased protein diet
    - Decreased casein diet
    - Decreased gluten diet
      - ➤ Gluten free diet
    - Amino acid modified diet
    - Arginine modified diet
      - ➤ Increased arginine diet
      - ➤ Decreased arginine diet
    - Glutamine modified diet
      - ➤ Increased glutamine diet
      - ➤ Decreased glutamine diet
    - Histidine modified diet
      - ➤ Increased histidine diet
      - ➤ Decreased histidine diet
    - Increased homocysteine diet

Meals and Snacks (ND-1)

- Isoleucine modified diet
  - Increased isoleucine diet
  - Decreased isoleucine diet
- Leucine modified diet
  - Increased leucine diet
  - Decreased leucine diet
- Lysine modified diet
  - Increased lysine diet
  - Decreased lysine diet
- Methionine modified diet
  - Increased methionine diet
  - Decreased methionine diet
- Phenylalanine modified diet
  - Increased phenylalanine diet
  - Decreased phenylalanine diet
- Threonine modified diet
  - Increased threonine diet
  - Decreased threonine diet
- Tryptophan modified diet
  - Increased tryptophan diet
  - Decreased tryptophan diet
- Decreased tyramine diet
- Tyrosine modified diet
  - Increased tyrosine diet
  - Decreased tyrosine diet
- Valine modified diet
  - Increased valine diet
  - Decreased valine diet

○ Carbohydrate modified diet
  - Consistent carbohydrate diet
  - Increased carbohydrate diet
    - Increased complex carbohydrate diet
    - Increased simple carbohydrate diet
  - Decreased carbohydrate diet
    - Decreased complex carbohydrate diet
    - Decreased simple carbohydrate diet
  - Galactose modified diet
    - Increased galactose diet
    - Decreased galactose diet

Meals and Snacks (ND-1)

Intervention

- Lactose modified diet
  - Increased lactose diet
  - Decreased lactose diet
- Fructose modified diet
  - Increased fructose diet
  - Decreased fructose diet
- Fat modified diet
  - Increased fat diet
  - Decreased fat diet
  - Monounsaturated fat modified diet
    - Increased monounsaturated fat diet
    - Decreased monounsaturated fat diet
  - Polyunsaturated fat modified diet
    - Increased polyunsaturated fat diet
      - Increased linoleic acid diet
    - Decreased polyunsaturated fat diet
      - Decreased linoleic acid diet
  - Saturated fat modified diet
    - Decreased saturated fat diet
  - Trans fat modified diet
    - Decreased trans fat modified diet
  - Omega 3 fatty acid modified diet
    - Increased omega 3 fatty acid diet
      - Increased alpha linolenic acid diet
      - Increased eicosapentanenoic acid diet
      - Increased docosahexaenoic acid
    - Decreased omega 3 fatty acid diet
      - Decreased alpha linolenic acid diet
      - Decreased eicosapentanenoic acid diet
      - Decreased docosahexaenoic acid
  - Medium chain triglyceride modified diet
    - Increased medium chain triglyceride diet
    - Decreased medium chain triglyceride diet
- Cholesterol modified diet
  - Decreased cholesterol diet
- Fiber modified diet
  - Increased fiber diet
  - Decreased fiber diet

Meals and Snacks (ND-1)

- Soluble fiber modified diet
  - Increased soluble fiber diet
  - Decreased soluble fiber diet
- Insoluble fiber modified diet
  - Increased insoluble fiber diet
  - Decreased insoluble fiber diet
- Fluid modified diet
  - Increased fluid diet
  - Fluid restricted diet
  - Clear liquid diet
  - Full liquid diet
- Diets modified for specific foods or ingredients
- Vitamin modified diet
  - Vitamin A modified diet
    - Increased vitamin A diet
    - Decreased vitamin A diet
  - Vitamin C modified diet
    - Increased vitamin C diet
    - Decreased vitamin C diet
  - Vitamin D modified diet
    - Increased vitamin D diet
    - Decreased vitamin D diet
  - Vitamin E modified diet
    - Increased vitamin E diet
    - Decreased vitamin E diet
  - Vitamin K modified diet
    - Increased vitamin K diet
    - Decreased vitamin K diet
  - Thiamine modified diet
    - Increased thiamine diet
    - Decreased thiamine diet
  - Riboflavin modified diet
    - Increased riboflavin diet
    - Decreased riboflavin diet
  - Niacin modified diet
    - Increased niacin diet
    - Decreased niacin diet

Meals and Snacks (ND-1)

Intervention

- Folic acid modified diet
  - ➤ Increased folic acid diet
  - ➤ Decreased folic acid diet
- Vitamin B6 modified diet
  - ➤ Increased vitamin B6 diet
  - ➤ Decreased vitamin B6 diet
- Vitamin B12 modified diet
  - ➤ Increased vitamin B12 diet
  - ➤ Decreased vitamin B12 diet
- Pantothenic acid modified diet
  - ➤ Increased pantothenic acid diet
  - ➤ Decreased pantothenic acid diet
- Biotin modified diet
  - ➤ Increased biotin diet
  - ➤ Decreased biotin diet
- Mineral modified diet
  - Calcium modified diet
    - ➤ Increased calcium diet
    - ➤ Decreased calcium diet
  - Chloride modified diet
  - Iron modified diet
    - ➤ Increased iron diet
    - ➤ Decreased iron diet
  - Magnesium modified diet
    - ➤ Increased magnesium diet
    - ➤ Decreased magnesium diet
  - Potassium modified diet
    - ➤ Increased potassium diet
    - ➤ Decreased potassium diet
  - Phosphorus modified diet
    - ➤ Increased phosphorus diet
    - ➤ Decreased phosphorus diet
  - Sodium modified diet
    - ➤ Increased sodium diet
    - ➤ Decreased sodium diet
  - Zinc modified diet
    - ➤ Increased zinc diet
    - ➤ Decreased zinc diet

Meals and Snacks (ND-1)

- Sulfur modified diet
- Fluoride modified diet
- Copper modified diet
  - Increased copper diet
  - Decreased copper diet
- Iodine modified diet
  - Increased iodine diet
  - Decreased iodine diet
- Selenium modified diet
- Manganese modified diet
- Chromium modified diet
  - Increased chromium diet
- Molybdenum modified diet
- Boron modified diet
- Cobalt modified diet
- Modify schedule of food/fluids (eg, timing of foods/fluids, number of meals)
  - Modify schedule of intake to limit fasting
- Specific food/beverages or groups
  - Fruit modified diet
  - Vegetable modified diet
    - Starchy vegetable modified diet
    - Bean and pea modified diet
  - Grain modified diet
    - Diet modified for uncooked food starch
  - Protein food modified diet
    - Diet with foods modified to be low in protein
    - Diet modified for egg
      - Raw egg free diet
- Other, specify

Meals and Snacks (ND-1)

Typically Used With the Following

Nutrition Diagnostic Terminology Used in PES Statements	Common Examples (not intended to be inclusive)
Nutrition Diagnoses	Increased energy expenditure (NI-1.1)
	Inadequate energy intake (NI-1.2)
	Inadequate oral intake (NI-2.1)
	Excessive fat intake (NI-5.5.2)
	Excessive carbohydrate intake (NI-5.8.2)
	Inconsistent carbohydrate intake (NI-5.8.4)
	Biting/chewing (masticatory) difficulty (NC-1.2)
	Growth rate below expected (NC-3.5)
	Limited access to food (NB-3.2)
	Underweight (NC-3.1)
Etiology	Lack of access to healthful food choices, eg, current food access, food provided by caregiver
	Physiological causes, eg, increased energy needs due to increased activity level, metabolic change, malabsorption, growth, extreme weakness, critical illness
	Psychological causes, eg, disordered eating
	Neurological causes, eg, difficulty chewing, swallowing
	Food and nutrition knowledge deficit regarding foods patient/client is consuming

Continued on next page

Intervention

Meals and Snacks (ND-1)

Continued from previous page

Nutrition Diagnostic Terminology Used in PES Statements	Common Examples (not intended to be inclusive)
Signs and Symptoms	Biochemical Data, Medical Tests and Procedures • Serum cholesterol level • Hemoglobin A1C results Anthropometric Measurements • Weight change Nutrition-Focused Physical Findings • Dental caries • Diarrhea • Evidence of muscle and/or fat wasting • Hunger Food/Nutrition-Related History • Cultural or religious practices that do not support modified food/nutrition intake • Changes in physical activity • Intake of less than optimal foods • Food- and nutrition-related knowledge deficit concerning appropriate amount or timing of carbohydrate intake Client History • Conditions associated with diagnosis or treatment, eg, surgery, trauma, sepsis, diabetes mellitus, inborn errors of metabolism, digestive enzyme deficiency, obesity • Chronic use of medications that increase or decrease nutrient requirements or impair nutrient metabolism

Other Considerations (eg, patient/client negotiation, patient/client needs and desires, and readiness to change):
• Compliance skills and abilities
• Economic concerns with purchasing food and/or special food items
• Willingness/ability to change behavior to comply with diet
• Ability to prepare food
• Availability/access to a qualified practitioner for follow-up and monitoring

Intervention

Enteral Nutrition (ND-2.1)

Definition

Nutrition provided through the gastrointestinal (GI) tract via tube, catheter, or stoma that delivers nutrients distal to the oral cavity

Details of Intervention

A typical intervention might be further described with the following details. Nutrition and dietetics practitioners recommend, implement, or order nutrition interventions, and the action(s) may be to initiate, modify, or discontinue a nutrition intervention(s):

- Modify composition of enteral nutrition (eg, formula name or description; special additives, including supplemental fat, carbohydrate, protein, or fiber)
- Modify concentration of enteral nutrition (eg, calories/kcal/kJ per mL)
- Modify rate of enteral nutrition (eg, mL/hour)
- Modify volume of enteral nutrition (eg, mL/day, mL/feeding)
- Modify schedule of enteral nutrition (eg, number of hours per 24 hours, continuous, intermittent, bolus)
- Modify route of enteral nutrition (eg, nasoentric, oroenteric, percutaneous, or surgical access with gastric, duodenal, or jejunal placement)
- Insert enteral feeding tube
- Enteral nutrition site care (eg, change dressings and provide enteral feeding tube site care)
- Feeding tube flush (eg, type, volume mL/flush, frequency)

Note: Related nutrition interventions, eg, checking gastric residual volume or elevating the head of the bed, are documented using Coordination of Nutrition Care.

Enteral Nutrition (ND-2.1)

Typically Used With the Following

Nutrition Diagnostic Terminology Used in PES Statements	Common Examples (not intended to be inclusive)
Nutrition Diagnoses	Swallowing difficulty (NC-1.1)
	Altered GI function (NC-1.4)
	Inadequate oral intake (NI-2.1)
	Increased nutrient needs (NI-5.1)
	Inadequate protein-energy intake (NI-5.2)
	Inadequate protein intake (NI-5.6.1)
	Inadequate enteral nutrition infusion (NI-2.3)
Etiology	Altered gastrointestinal tract function, inability to absorb nutrients
	Inability to chew/swallow
	Decreased ability to consume sufficient energy, eg, increased nutrient needs due to catabolic illness
	Respiratory or other critical illness requiring mechanical ventilation
	Disease process or complication of therapy which results in excess fluid loss or retention (eg, CHF, liver failure, renal failure)
Signs and Symptoms	Anthropometric Measurements
	• Weight loss
	• Growth failure
	• Insufficient maternal weight gain
	Nutrition-Focused Physical Findings
	• Obvious muscle and/or fat wasting
	• Poor skin turgor (tenting)
	• Fluid retention (edema)
	Food/Nutrition-Related History
	• Intake < 75% of requirements (insufficient intake)
	• Existing or expected inadequate intake for 7 to 14 days
	Client History
	• Aspiration
	• Coma

Other Considerations (eg, patient/client negotiation, patient/client needs and desires, and readiness to change):
- End-of-life issues, ethical considerations, patient/client rights, and family/caregiver issues
- Other nutrient intake (oral, parenteral nutrition), medications containing energy
- Enteral formulary composition and product availability
- Availability/access to a qualified practitioner for follow-up and monitoring
- Economic constraints that limit availability of food/enteral products

Parenteral Nutrition/IV Fluids (ND-2.2)

Definition

Administration of nutrients and fluids intravenously, centrally (delivered into a large-diameter vein, usually the superior vena cava adjacent to the right atrium), or peripherally (delivered into a peripheral vein, usually of the hand or forearm)

Details of Intervention

A typical intervention might be further described with the following details. Nutrition and dietetics practitioners recommend, implement, or order nutrition interventions, and the action(s) may be to initiate, modify, or discontinue a nutrition intervention(s):

- Modify composition of parenteral nutrition (formula or description)
- Modify concentration of parenteral nutrition (eg, percent, grams of solute per mL)
- Modify rate of parenteral nutrition (eg, mL/hour)
- Modify volume of parenteral nutrition
- Modify schedule of parenteral nutrition (eg, hours, timing, taper schedule)
- Modify route of parenteral nutrition (eg, peripheral, central, and/or type of catheter)
- Parenteral nutrition site care (eg, change dressings and provide line care for parenteral access)
- IV fluid delivery (eg, type; amount mL/day, mL/hour, mL with medications)

Parenteral Nutrition/IV Fluids (ND-2.2)

Typically Used With the Following

Nutrition Diagnostic Terminology Used in PES Statements	Common Examples (not intended to be inclusive)
Nutrition Diagnoses	Altered GI function (NC-1.4)
	Inadequate parenteral nutrition infusion (NI-2.7)
	Impaired nutrient utilization (NC-2.1)
Etiology	Altered gastrointestinal tract function, inability to absorb nutrients, or excessive loss of nutrients (eg, severe vomiting, diarrhea, high fistula output)
	Decreased functional length of GI tract
	Bowel obstruction
Signs and Symptoms	Anthropometric Measurements
	• Unintentional weight loss
	• Growth failure
	• Insufficient maternal weight gain
	Nutrition-Focused Physical Findings
	• Obvious muscle and/or fat wasting
	• Poor skin turgor (tenting)
	• Fluid retention (edema, ascites)
	• Diarrhea
	• Vomiting
	Food/Nutrition-Related History
	• Intake < requirements (insufficient intake)
	• Existing or expected inadequate intake for 7 to 14 days
	Client History
	• Malabsorption, maldigestion
	• Emesis
	• Diffuse peritonitis, intestinal obstruction, paralytic ileus, gastrointestinal ischemia, perforated viscus, short-bowel syndrome

Other Considerations (eg, patient/client negotiation, patient/client needs and desires, and readiness to change):
- End-of-life issues, ethical considerations, patient/client rights, and family/caregiver issues
- Other nutrient intake (oral, enteral nutrition)
- Parenteral formulary composition and product availability
- Availability/access to a qualified practitioner for follow-up and monitoring
- Economic constraints that limit availability of parenteral products

Intervention

Medical Food Supplement Therapy (ND-3.1)

Definition

Commercial or prepared foods or beverages intended to supplement energy, protein, carbohydrate, fiber, and/or fat intake that may also contribute to vitamin and mineral intake

Details of Intervention

A typical intervention might be further described with the following details. Nutrition and dietetics practitioners recommend, implement, or order nutrition interventions, and the action(s) may be to initiate, modify, or discontinue a nutrition intervention(s):

- Commercial (prepackaged) beverage
- Commercial (prepackaged) food
- Modified (prepared) beverage
- Modified (prepared) food
- Purpose (eg, to supplement energy, protein, carbohydrate, fiber, and/or fat intake)

Intervention

Medical Food Supplement Therapy (ND-3.1)

Typically Used With the Following

Nutrition Diagnostic Terminology Used in PES Statements	Common Examples (not intended to be inclusive)
Nutrition Diagnoses	Inadequate oral intake (NI-2.1)
	Inadequate fluid intake (NI-3.1)
	Increased nutrient needs (NI-5.1)
	Malnutrition (undernutrition) (NC-4.1)
	Growth rate below expected (NC-3.5)
Etiology	Neurologic deficit (stroke)
	Difficulty chewing or swallowing
	Food allergies or intolerance
	Altered GI function
	Disease or treatment-related anorexia (eg, cancer, infection, medication side effects)
	Small for gestational age, intrauterine growth restriction, lack of appropriate weight gain, hyperemesis gravidarum
	Inborn errors of metabolism
Signs and Symptoms	Anthropometric Measurements
	• Delayed growth
	• Unintended weight loss
	Nutrition-Focused Physical Findings
	• Obvious muscle and/or fat wasting
	• Poor skin turgor (tenting)
	Food/Nutrition-Related History
	• Insufficient usual intake
	• Insufficient macro- and/or micronutrient intake
	Client History
	• Diagnosis consistent with elevated nutrient needs
	• Potential for repletion of nutritional status
	• Oral/facial trauma

Other Considerations (eg, patient/client negotiation, patient/client needs and desires, and readiness to change):
- Appetite sufficient to take medical food supplements
- System constraints that prevent meeting the client's preferences for specific flavors, textures, foods, and the timing of feedings
- Economic concerns and product/food availability
- Ability to procure medical food supplement
- Access to medical food supplement storage

Intervention

Bioactive Substance Management (ND-3.3)

Definition

Addition or change in provision of bioactive substances (eg, plant stanol and sterol esters, psyllium, food additives, other bioactive substances)

Details of Intervention

A typical intervention might be further described with the following details. Nutrition and dietetics practitioners recommend, implement, or order nutrition interventions, and the action(s) may be to initiate, modify, or discontinue a nutrition intervention(s):

- Plant stanol esters (specif,y eg, form, frequency)
- Plant sterol esters (specify, eg, form, frequency)
- Soy protein (specify, eg, form, frequency)
- Psyllium (specify, eg, form, frequency)
- ß-glucan (specify, eg, form, frequency)
- Food additives (those thought to have an impact on a patient/client's health) (specify, eg, amount, form, frequency)
- Alcohol (specify, eg, oz/mL, form, frequency)
- Caffeine (specify, eg, mg, oz/mL, form, frequency)
- Other substance (for which there is evidence of bioactivity) (specify, eg, amount, form, frequency)

Bioactive Substance Management (ND-3.3)

Typically Used With the Following

Nutrition Diagnostic Terminology Used in PES Statements	Common Examples (not intended to be inclusive)
Nutrition Diagnoses	Inadequate bioactive substance intake (NI-4.1)
	Excessive bioactive substance intake (NI-4.2)
	Excessive alcohol intake (NI-4.3)
	Predicted food–medication interaction (NC-2.4)
	Food- and nutrition-related knowledge deficit (NB-1.1)
	Undesirable food choices (NB-1.7)
Etiology	Food- and nutrition-related knowledge deficit concerning recommended bioactive substance intake
	Lack of or limited access to food that contains a bioactive substance
	Contamination, misname, mislabel or lack of labeling, misuse, recent brand change, recent dose increase, recent formulation change of substance consumed
	Combined ingestion or administration of medication and food that results in undesirable/harmful interaction
	Adverse side effect related to bioactive substance
Signs and Symptoms	Food/Nutrition-Related History • Nutrient intake analysis reveals bioactive substance intake more or less than recommended • Intake reveals consumption of food additive to which the patient/client is sensitive or intolerant Client History • Medical diagnosis associated with increased bioactive substance need

Other Considerations (eg, patient/client negotiation, patient/client needs and desires, and readiness to change):

- Emerging scientific evidence to support the use of bioactive supplements in specific populations, specific medical conditions, and/or with medical treatments
- Availability of a qualified practitioner with additional education/training in the use of bioactive supplements in practice

Intervention

Feeding Assistance (ND-4)

Definition

Accommodation or assistance designed to restore the patient/client's ability to eat independently, support adequate nutrient intake, and reduce the incidence of unplanned weight loss and dehydration

Details of Intervention

A typical intervention might be further described with the following details. Nutrition and dietetics practitioners recommend, implement, or order nutrition interventions, and the action(s) may be to initiate, modify, or discontinue a nutrition intervention(s):

- Adaptive eating devices (equipment or utensils) (eg, specify)
- Feeding position (eg, specify patient/client position in relationship to eating or degree angle for enteral feeding)
- Meal set-up (eg, specify actions to make food accessible for consumption)
- Mouth care (eg, specify treatment to promote oral health and hygiene)
- Menu selection assistance (yes/no)
- Other (specify)

Feeding Assistance (ND-4)

Typically Used With the Following

Nutrition Diagnostic Terminology Used in PES Statements	Common Examples (not intended to be inclusive)
Nutrition Diagnoses	Inadequate energy intake (NI-1.2)
	Inadequate oral intake (NI-2.1)
	Inadequate enteral nutrition infusion (NI-2.3)
	Unintended weight loss (NC-3.2)
	Self-feeding difficulty (NB-2.6)
Etiology	Physical disability
	Poor food/nutrient intake
	Neurological issues, eg, decreased memory, concentration problems
Signs and Symptoms	Anthropometric Measurements
	• Weight loss
	Food/Nutrition-Related History
	• Dropping the utensils or food
	Client History
	• Conditions associated with a diagnosis or treatment, eg,cerebral palsy, stroke, dementia
	• History of aspiration or conditions which increase risk of aspiration
	• Refusal to use prescribed adaptive eating devices or follow prescribed positioning techniques

Other Considerations (eg, patient/client negotiation, patient/client needs and desires, and readiness to change):
- Acceptance of feeding assistance/feeding devices
- Poor environment to foster adequate intake
- Lack of individual to provide assistance at meal time
- Lack of training in methods of feeding assistance
- Lack of available physical therapy, occupational therapy, or speech therapy evaluations
- Ability to understand the reasoning behind the recommendations and then want to make personal changes
- Lack of assistance when translation of menu items is needed

Nutrition Education—Content (E-1)

Definition

Instruction or training intended to lead to nutrition-related knowledge

Note: This reference sheet only refers to patient/client nutrition education. Please use Nutrition Counseling (C) for documentation of the Theoretical Basis/Approach (C-1) and Strategies (C-2) used for patient/client behavior change.

Details of Intervention

A typical intervention might be further described with the following details. Nutrition and dietetics practitioners recommend, implement, or order nutrition interventions, and the action(s) may be to initiate, modify, or discontinue a nutrition intervention(s):

- Purpose (eg, prevention, disease management) of the nutrition education
- Priority modifications (eg, issue of most concern to patient/client's health and well-being)
- Survival information (minimum necessary nutrition modifications until patient/client can return for more nutrition education)
- Nutrition relationship to health/disease
- Recommended modifications (eg, explain multiple nutrition prescription recommendations)
- Other or related topics (eg, saturated and trans fatty acid intake versus total fat intake, menu planning, food purchasing)
- Other (specify)
- Physical activity guidance (instruction or training intended to lead to physical activity related knowledge and change)

Intervention

Nutrition Education—Content (E-1)

Typically Used With the Following

Nutrition Diagnostic Terminology Used in PES Statements	Common Examples (not intended to be inclusive)
Nutrition Diagnoses	Predicted food–medication interaction (NC-2.4)
	Underweight (NC-3.1)
	Overweight/obesity (NC-3.3)
	Food- and nutrition-related knowledge deficit (NB-1.1)
	Unsupported beliefs/attitudes about food- or nutrition-related topics (NB-1.2)
	Self-monitoring deficit (NB-1.4)
	Disordered eating pattern (NB-1.5)
	Limited adherence to nutrition-related recommendations (NB-1.6)
	Physical inactivity (NB-2.1)
	Excessive physical activity (NB-2.2)
	Poor nutrition quality of life (NB-2.5)
	Altered nutrition-related laboratory values (NC-2.2)
	Other: Any diagnoses related to inadequate, excessive, or inconsistent intake
Etiology	Knowledge deficit related to newly diagnosed medical condition and/or nutrition problem
	Medical or surgical procedure requiring modified diet
	Prior exposure to incorrect information
Signs and Symptoms	Food/Nutrition-Related History
	• Unable to explain purpose of the nutrition prescription or rationale for nutrition prescription in relationship to disease/health
	• Expresses need for additional information or clarification of education or additional time to learn information
	• Unable to select appropriate foods or supplements
	• Unable to choose appropriate timing, volume, or preparation/handling of foods
	• Uncertain of physical activity (type and frequency)
	• Unable to distinguish legitimate from false information
	Biochemical Data, Medical Tests and Procedures
	• Laboratory data indicating nutrition education warranted

Intervention

Nutrition Education—Content (E-1)

Other Considerations (eg, patient/client negotiation, patient/client needs and desires, and readiness to change):

- Met with several providers in one day and is unable or unwilling to receive more nutrition education at this time
- Profile reflects complicated situation warranting additional education/instruction
- Being discharged from the hospital
- Caregiver unavailable at time of nutrition education
- Baseline knowledge
- Learning style
- Other education and learning needs (eg, new medication or other treatment administration)
- Diminished literacy, including ability to read, write, or comprehend information and/or language barrier
- Potential for referral to RDN with different expertise
- Promote patient-defined health goals and outcomes
- Counseling needed for the unmotivated or precontemplative patient/client

Intervention

Nutrition Education—Application (E-2)

Definition

Instruction or training intended to lead to nutrition-related result interpretation or skills

Note: This reference sheet only refers to patient/client nutrition education. Please use Nutrition Counseling (C) for documentation of the Theoretical Basis/Approach (C-1) and Strategies (C-2) used for patient/client behavior change.

Details of Intervention

A typical intervention might be further described with the following details. Nutrition and dietetics practitioners recommend, implement, or order nutrition interventions, and the action(s) may be to initiate, modify, or discontinue a nutrition intervention(s):

- Result interpretation (eg, engage in training on medical or other results to coincide with nutrition prescription, such as distribution of carbohydrate throughout the day based on blood glucose monitoring results or heart rate during physical activity)
- Skill development (eg, glucometer use, home tube feeding and feeding pump training, cooking skills/preparation, physical activity equipment)
- Other (specify)

Typically Used With the Following

Nutrition Diagnostic Terminology Used in PES Statements	Common Examples (not intended to be inclusive)
Nutrition Diagnoses	Food- and nutrition-related knowledge deficit (NB-1.1)
	Unsupported beliefs/attitudes about food- or nutrition-related topics (NB-1.2)
	Self-monitoring deficit (NB-1.4)
	Disordered eating pattern (NB-1.5)
	Physical inactivity (NB-2.1)
	Altered nutrition-related laboratory values (NC-2.2)
	Other: Any diagnoses related to inadequate, excessive, or inconsistent intake
Etiology	Deficient understanding of how to interpret nutrition-related results
	Exposure to incorrect food and nutrition application information
	Lack of self-management skills
Signs and Symptoms	Food/Nutrition-Related History
	• Expresses desire to apply nutrition information
	• Food and nutrient intake tracking incomplete
	Biochemical Data, Medical Tests, and Procedures
	• Laboratory data indicating nutrition education warranted

Nutrition Education—Application (E-2)

Other Considerations (eg, patient/client negotiation, patient/client needs and desires, and readiness to change)

- Profile reflects complicated situation warranting additional education/instruction
- Increased or decreased capacity and willingness to learn information
- Quality of life may be enhanced with in-depth nutrition education and understanding
- Baseline knowledge
- Lifestyle factors
- Education approaches that enhance skill transfer
- Diminished literacy, including ability to read, write, or comprehend information and/or language barrier

Intervention

Theoretical Basis/Approach (C-1)

Definition

The theories or models used to design and implement an intervention. Theories and theoretical models consist of principles, constructs, and variables, which offer systematic explanations of the human behavior change process. Behavior change theories and models provide a research-based rationale for designing and tailoring nutrition interventions to achieve the desired effect. A theoretical framework for curriculum and treatment protocols, it guides determination of: (1) what information patients/clients need at different points in the behavior change process, (2) what tools and strategies may be best applied to facilitate behavior change, and (3) outcome measures to assess effectiveness in interventions or components of interventions

Application Guidance

One or more of the following theories or theoretical models may influence a practitioner's counseling style or approach. Practitioners are asked to identify those theories (C-1) that most influence the intervention being documented. An intervention might also incorporate tools and strategies derived from a variety of behavior change theories and models. The practitioner is also asked to indicate which strategies (C-2) they used in a particular intervention session

Details of Intervention

A typical intervention might be further described with the following details. Nutrition and dietetics practitioners recommend, implement, or order nutrition interventions and the action(s) may be to initiate, modify, or discontinue a nutrition intervention(s):

The following theories and models have proven valuable in providing a theoretical framework for evidence-based individual and interpersonal level nutrition interventions. Other theories may be useful for community level interventions (eg, Community Organization, Diffusion of Innovations, Communication Theory).

- Cognitive-behavioral theory
- Health belief model
- Social learning theory
- Transtheoretical model/stages of change

Additional information regarding each of the above theories and models can be found within this reference sheet.

Intervention

Theoretical Basis/Approach (C-1)

Typically Used With the Following

Nutrition Diagnostic Terminology Used in PES Statements	Common Examples (not intended to be inclusive)
Nutrition Diagnoses	Overweight/obesity (NC-3.3)
	Unsupported beliefs/attitudes about food or nutrition-related topics (NB-1.2)
	Not ready for diet/lifestyle change (NB-1.3)
	Self-monitoring deficit (NB-1.4)
	Disordered eating pattern (NB-1.5)
	Limited adherence to nutrition-related recommendations (NB-1.6)
	Undesirable food choices (NB-1.7)
	Physical inactivity (NB-2.1)
	Excessive physical activity (NB-2.2)
	Inability to manage self care (NB-2.3)
	Poor nutrition quality of life (NB-2.5)
	Other: Any diagnoses related to inadequate, excessive, or inconsistent intake
Etiology	New medical diagnosis
	Unsupported beliefs/attitudes about food, nutrition, and nutrition-related topics
	Lack of value for behavior change, competing values
	Cultural/religious practices that interfere with implementation of the nutrition prescription
	Lack of efficacy to make changes or to overcome barriers to change
	Lack of focus/attention to detail, difficulty with time management and/or organization
	Perception that time, interpersonal, or financial constraints prevent change
	Prior exposure to incorrect or incompatible information
	Not ready for diet/lifestyle change
	Lack of caretaker or social support for implementing changes
	High level of fatigue or other side effect of medical condition

Continued on next page

Intervention

Theoretical Basis/Approach (C-1)

Continued from previous page

Nutrition Diagnostic Terminology Used in PES Statements	Common Examples (not intended to be inclusive)
Signs and Symptoms (Defining Characteristics)	Food/Nutrition-Related History • Frustration with nutrition and/or physical activity recommendations • Previous failures to effectively change target behavior • Defensiveness, hostility, or resistance to change • Sense of lack of control of eating • Inability to apply food- and nutrition-related information/guidelines • Inability to change food- and nutrition-related behavior • Absent or incomplete self-monitoring records • Inability to problem solve/self-manage • Irrational thoughts about self and effects of food intake • Unrealistic expectations • Inflexibility with food selection • Evidence of excessive, inadequate, or inconsistent intake related to needs

Other Considerations (eg, patient/client negotiation, patient/client needs and desires, and readiness to change):
- Lifestyle factors
- Language barrier
- Educational level
- Culture
- Socioeconomic status

Intervention

Theoretical Basis/Approach
Cognitive-Behavioral Theory (C-1.1)

Description

Cognitive-Behavioral Theory (CBT) is based on the assumption that all behavior is learned and is directly related to internal factors (eg, thoughts and thinking patterns) and external factors (eg, environmental stimulus and reinforcement) that are related to the problem behaviors. Application involves use of both cognitive and behavioral change strategies to effect behavior change

Implication for Counseling Interventions

CBT, derived from an educational model, is based on the assumption that most emotional and behavioral reactions are learned and can be unlearned. The goal of CBT is to facilitate client identification of cognitions and behaviors that lead to less-than-optimal eating or exercise habits and replace these with more rational thoughts and actions. The process is:

- Goal directed
- Process oriented
- Facilitated through a variety of problem-solving tools

Behavioral and cognitive techniques to modify eating and exercise habits are taught for continuous application by the patient/client. Practitioners implement Cognitive-Behavioral Theory by partnering with clients to study their current environment to:

- Identify determinants or antecedents to behavior that contribute to less than optimal eating/exercise
- Identify resultant behavior (eg, overeating, vomiting)
- Analyze consequences of this behavior (cognitions, positive and negative reinforcers and punishments, eg, decreased anxiety, feeling overfull, losing or gaining weight)
- Make specific goals to modify the environment/cognitions to reduce target behaviors

Cognitive and behavioral strategies used to promote change in diet and physical activity may include:

- Goal setting
- Self-monitoring
- Problem solving
- Social support
- Stress management
- Stimulus control
- Cognitive restructuring
- Relapse prevention
- Rewards/contingency management

Intervention

Theoretical Basis/Approach
Health Belief Model (C-1.2)

Description

The Health Belief Model (HBM) is a psychological model that focuses on an individual's attitudes and beliefs to attempt to explain and predict health behaviors. The HBM is based on the assumption that an individual will be motivated to take health-related action if that person (1) feels that a negative health condition (eg, diabetes) can be avoided or managed, (2) has a positive expectation that by taking a recommended action, he or she will avoid negative health consequences (eg, good blood glucose control will preserve eye sight), and (3) believes he or she can successfully perform a recommended health action (eg, I can use carbohydrate counting and control my diet. I can engage in regular physical activity).

Implication for Counseling Interventions

The HBM is particularly helpful to practitioners planning interventions targeted to individuals with clinical nutrition-related risk factors, such as diabetes, high blood cholesterol, and/or hypertension. The six major constructs of the model have been found to be important in impacting an individual's motivation to take health-related action. The following table provides definitions and application guidance for the key constructs of the theory. Motivational interviewing strategies may be appropriate to address perceived susceptibility, severity, benefits, and barriers. Behavioral strategies are most appropriate once the patient/client begins to take action to modify his or her diet and/or physical activity.

These six constructs are useful components in designing behavior change programs. It is important for the practitioner to understand the patient's perception of the health threat and potential benefits of treatment. According to the HBM, an asymptomatic person with diabetes may not be compliant with his or her treatment regimen if he or she does not:

- Believe that he or she has diabetes (susceptibility)
- Believe that diabetes will seriously impact his or her life (perceived seriousness)
- Believe that following the carbohydrate controlled diet will decrease the negative effects of diabetes (perceived benefits)
- Believe that the effort to follow the diet is worth the benefit to be gained (perceived barriers)
- Have stimulus to initiate action (cue to action)
- Have confidence in his or her ability to achieve success (self-efficacy)

Theoretical Basis/Approach
Health Belief Model (C-1.2)

Intervention

Construct	Definition	Strategies
Perceived Susceptibility	Client's belief or opinion of the personal threat a health condition represents for them; client opinion regarding whether they have the condition (eg, diabetes or hypertension) or their chance of getting the disease or condition	• Educate on disease/condition risk factors • Tailor information to the client • Ask client if they think they are at risk or have the disease/condition • Guided discussions • Motivational interviewing (express empathy, open-ended questions, reflective listening, affirming, summarizing, and eliciting self-motivation statements)
Perceived Severity	Client's belief about the impact a particular health threat will have on them and their lifestyle	• Educate on consequences of the disease/condition; show graphs, statistics • Elicit client response • Discuss potential impact on client's lifestyle • Motivational interviewing
Perceived Benefits and Barriers	Client's belief regarding benefits they will derive from taking nutrition-related action; perceived benefits versus barriers—client's perception of whether benefits will outweigh the sacrifices and efforts involved in behavior change	• Clearly define benefits of nutrition therapy and physical activity • Role models, testimonials • Explore ambivalence and barriers • Imagine the future • Explore successes • Summarize and affirm the positive
Cues to Action	Internal or external triggers that motivate or stimulate action	• How-to education • Incentive programs • Link current symptoms to disease/condition • Discuss media information • Reminder phone calls/mailings • Social support
Self-Efficacy	Client confidence in their ability to successfully accomplish the necessary action	• Skill training/demonstration • Introduce alternatives and choices • Behavior contracting; small, incremental goals • Coaching, verbal reinforcement

Theoretical Basis/Approach
Social Learning Theory (C-1.3)

Description

Social Learning Theory, also known as Social Cognitive Theory, provides a framework for understanding, predicting, and changing behavior. The theory identifies a dynamic, reciprocal relationship between environment, the person, and behavior. The person can be both an agent for change and a responder to change. It emphasizes the importance of observing and modeling behaviors, attitudes, and emotional reactions of others. Determinants of behavior include goals, outcome expectations, and self-efficacy. Reinforcements increase or decrease the likelihood that the behavior will be repeated (1).

Implication for Counseling Interventions

Social learning theory is rich in concepts applicable to nutrition counseling. The following table provides definitions and application guidance for the key concepts of the theory.

Concept	Definition	Strategies
Reciprocal Determinism	A person's ability to change a behavior is influenced by characteristics within the person (eg, beliefs), the environment, and the behavior itself (eg, difficulty doing the behavior). All three interact to influence if the behavior change will happen	• Consider multiple behavior change strategies targeting motivation, action, the individual and the environment: • Motivational interviewing • Social support • Stimulus control • Demonstration • Skill development training/coaching
Behavioral Capability	The knowledge and skills that are needed for a person to change behavior	• Comprehensive education • Demonstration • Skill development training/coaching
Expectations	For a person to do a behavior, they must believe that the behavior will result in outcomes important to them	• Motivational interviewing • Model positive outcomes of diet/exercise
Self-Efficacy	Confidence in ability to take action and persist in action	• Break task down to component parts • Demonstration/modeling • Skill development training/coaching • Reinforcement • Small, incremental goals/behavioral contracting
Observational Learning	When a person learns how to do a behavior by watching credible others do the same behavior	• Demonstrations • Role modeling • Group problem-solving sessions
Reinforcement	Response to a behavior that will either increase or decrease the likelihood that the behavior will be repeated	• Affirm accomplishments • Encourage self-reward/self-reinforcement • Incentives for process components of change (eg, keeping a food diary or physical activity log)

Intervention

Theoretical Basis/Approach Transtheoretical Model/Stages of Change (C-1.4)

Definition

A theoretical model of intentional health behavior change that describes a sequence of cognitive (attitudes and intentions) and behavioral steps people take in successful behavior change. The model, developed by Prochaska and DiClemente, is composed of a core concept known as Stages of Change, a series of independent variables, the Processes of Change, and outcome measures including decision balance and self-efficacy. The model has been used to guide development of effective interventions for a variety of health behaviors.

Implication for Counseling Interventions

One of the defining characteristics of this model is that it describes behavior change not as a discrete event (eg, today I am going to stop overeating) but as something that occurs in stages over time. The five stages reflect an individual's attitudes, intentions, and behavior related to the change of a specific behavior and include the following:

- Precontemplation—no recognition of need for change; no intention to take action within the next 6 months
- Contemplation—recognition of need to change; intends to take action within the next 6 months
- Preparation—intends to take action in the next 30 days and has taken some behavioral steps in that direction
- Action—has made changes in target behavior for less than 6 months
- Maintenance—has changed target behavior for more than 6 months

Determination of a patient/client stage of change is relatively simple, involving a few questions regarding intentions and current diet. One of the appealing aspects of the theory is that the Process of Change construct describes cognitive and behavioral activities or strategies, which may be applied at various stages to move a person forward through the stages of change. This movement is not always linear, and patients can cycle in and out of various stages. The model has been used to effectively tailor interventions to the needs of clients at various stages. Knowing a patient/client's stage of change can help a practitioner determine:

- Whether intervention now is appropriate
- The type and content of intervention to use (motivational versus action oriented)
- Appropriate and timely questions about past efforts, pros and cons of change, obstacles, challenges, and potential strategies
- The amount of time to spend with the patient/client

The following table provides guidance for applying the stages and processes of change to the adoption of healthful diets.

This theoretical basis/approach has also been used with regard to physical activity.

Theoretical Basis/Approach Transtheoretical Model/Stages of Change (C-1.4)

		Table 3: General Guidelines for Applying Stages and Processes of Change to Adoption of Diets	
State of Readiness	**Key Strategies for Moving to Next Stage**	**Treatment Dos at This Stage**	**Treatment Don'ts at This Stage**
Precontemplation	Increased information and awareness, emotional acceptance	Provide personalized information Allow patient/client to express emotions about his or her disease or about the need to make dietary changes	Do not assume client has knowledge or expect that providing information will automatically lead to behavior change Do not ignore patient/client's emotional adjustment to the need for dietary change, which could override ability to process relevant information.
Contemplation	Increased confidence in one's ability to adopt recommended behaviors	Discuss and resolve barriers to dietary change. Encourage support networks Give positive feedback about a patient/client's abilities Help to clarify ambivalence about adopting behavior and emphasize expected benefits.	Do not ignore the potential impact of family members and others on patient/client's ability to comply Do not be alarmed by or critical of a patient/client's ambivalence
Preparation	Resolution of ambivalence, firm commitment, and specific action plan	Encourage patient/client to set specific, achievable goals (eg, use 1% milk instead of whole milk) Reinforce small changes that client may have already achieved	Do not recommend general behavior changes (eg, "Eat less fat") Do not refer to small changes as "not good enough"
Action	Behavioral skill training and social support	Refer to education program for self-management skills Provide self-help materials	Do not refer patient/client to information-only classes
Maintenance	Problem-solving skills and social and environmental support	Encourage patient/client to anticipate and plan for potential difficulties (eg, maintaining dietary changes on vacation) Collect information about local resources (eg, support groups, shopping guides) Encourage patient/client to "recycle" if he or she has a lapse or relapse Recommend more challenging dietary changes if patient/client is motivated	Do not assume that initial action means permanent change Do not be discouraged or judgmental about a lapse or relapse

Source: Kristal AR, Glanz K, Curry S, Patterson RE. How can stages of change be best used in dietary interventions? *J Am Diet Assoc.* 1999;99:683.

Prochaska recommends the following strategies, which target motivation, be used in the early stages of change: consciousness raising, dramatic relief (eg, emotional arousal via role playing or personal testimonials), environmental reevaluation (eg, empathy training and family interactions), social liberation (eg, advocacy, empowerment) and self-reevaluation (eg, value clarification, healthy role models, and imagery). These strategies are very consistent with motivational interviewing techniques. In the later stages of change, behavioral strategies are most appropriate.

Strategies (C-2)

Definition

An evidence-based method or plan of action designed to achieve a particular goal. Application of behavior change theories in nutrition practice has provided practitioners with a collection of evidence-based strategies to promote behavior change. Some strategies target change in motivation and intention to change, and others target behavior change. Nutrition and dietetics practitioners selectively apply strategies based on patient/client goals and objectives and their personal counseling philosophy and skill

Application Guidance

An intervention typically incorporates tools and strategies derived from a variety of behavior change theories and models. The practitioner is asked to indicate which Strategies (C-2) he or she used in a particular intervention session along with the Theories (C-1) that most influence the intervention being documented.

Details of Intervention

A typical intervention might be further described with the following details. Nutrition and dietetics practitioners recommend, implement, or order nutrition interventions and the action(s) may be to initiate, modify or discontinue a nutrition intervention(s):

The following strategies have proven valuable in providing effective nutrition-related (eg. nutrition therapy, physical activity) behavior change:

- Motivational interviewing
- Goal setting
- Self-monitoring
- Problem solving
- Social support
- Stress management
- Stimulus control
- Cognitive restructuring
- Relapse prevention
- Rewards/contingency management
- Other (specify)

Additional information regarding each of the above strategies can be found within this reference sheet.

Strategies (C-2)

Typically Used With the Following

Nutrition Diagnostic Terminology Used in PES Statements	Common Examples (not intended to be inclusive)
Nutrition Diagnoses	Overweight/obesity (NC-3.3)
	Unsupported beliefs/attitudes about food or nutrition-related topics (NB-1.2)
	Not ready for diet/lifestyle change (NB-1.3)
	Self-monitoring deficit (NB-1.4)
	Disordered eating pattern (NB-1.5)
	Limited adherence to nutrition-related recommendations (NB-1.6)
	Undesirable food choices (NB-1.7)
	Physical inactivity (NB-2.1)
	Excessive physical activity (NB-2.2)
	Inability to manage self care (NB-2.3)
	Poor nutrition quality of life (NB-2.5)
	Other: Any diagnoses related to inadequate, excessive, or inconsistent intake
Etiology	New medical diagnosis
	Unsupported beliefs/attitudes about food, nutrition, and nutrition-related topics
	Lack of value for behavior change, competing values
	Cultural/religious practices that interfere with implementation of the nutrition prescription
	Lack of efficacy to make changes or to overcome barriers to change
	Lack of focus/attention to detail, difficulty with time management and/or organization
	Perception that time, interpersonal, or financial constraints prevent change
	Prior exposure to incorrect or incompatible information
	Not ready for diet/lifestyle change
	Lack of caretaker or social support for implementing changes
	High level of fatigue or other side effect of medical condition

Intervention

Continued on next page

Strategies (C-2)

Continued from previous page

Intervention

Nutrition Diagnostic Terminology Used in PES Statements	Common Examples (not intended to be inclusive)
Signs and Symptoms (Defining Characteristics)	Food/Nutrition-Related History • Frustration with nutrition and/or physical activity recommendations • Previous failures to effectively change target behavior • Defensiveness, hostility, or resistance to change • Sense of lack of control of eating • Inability to apply food- and nutrition-related information/guidelines • Inability to change food- and nutrition-related behavior • Absent or incomplete self-monitoring records • Inability to problem solve/self-manage • Irrational thoughts about self and effects of food intake • Unrealistic expectations • Inflexibility with food selection • Evidence of excessive, inadequate, or inconsistent intake related to needs

Other Considerations (eg, patient/client negotiation, patient/client needs and desires, and readiness to change):
• Lifestyle factors
• Language barrier
• Educational level
• Culture
• Socioeconomic status

Strategy: Motivational Interviewing (C-2.1)

Strategy Descriptions and Application Guidance

Strategy	Description	Implementation Tips
Motivational Interviewing (MI)	A directive, client-centered counseling style for eliciting behavior change by helping patients/clients to explore and resolve ambivalence (1). The approach involves selective response to patient/client speech in a way that helps the patient/client resolve ambivalence and move toward change. The four guiding principles that underlie this counseling approach include: • Express empathy • Develop discrepancy • Roll with resistance • Support self-efficacy The following specific practitioner behaviors are characteristic of the MI style (2): • Expressing acceptance and affirmation • Eliciting and selectively reinforcing the patient/client's own self-motivational statements, expressions of problem recognition, concern, desire, intention to change, and ability to change • Monitoring the patient/client's degree of readiness to change, and ensuring that jumping ahead of the client does not generate resistance • Affirming the patient/client's freedom of choice and self-direction The source of motivation is presumed to reside within the patient/client, and the counselor encourages the patient/client to explore ambivalence, motivation, and possibilities to change, so it is the client who chooses what to change and determines the change plan and strategy MI is an evidence-based counseling strategy which builds on Carl Rogers's client-centered counseling model, Prochaska and DiClemente's transtheoretical model of change, Milton Rokeach's human values theory, and Daryl Bern's theory of self-perception	Tone of counseling: • Partnership • Nonjudgmental • Empathetic/supportive/encouraging • Nonconfrontational • Quiet and eliciting The patient/client does most of the talking, and the counselor guides the patient/client to explore and resolve ambivalence by: • Asking open-ended questions • Listening reflectively • Summarizing • Affirming • Eliciting self-motivational statements • Shared agenda setting/decision making • Allowing clients to interpret information • Rolling with resistance, rather than confronting • Building discrepancy • Eliciting "change talk" • Negotiating a change plan MI is best applied in situations when a patient/client is not ready, is unwilling, or is ambivalent about changing his or her diet or lifestyle MI integrates well with the readiness to change model to move individuals from the early stages to the action stage of change MI is a major paradigm change from the problem solving oriented counseling frequently employed by practitioners MI is not a set of techniques that can be learned quickly, but a style or approach to counseling

Intervention

Strategy: Goal Setting (C-2.2)

Strategy Descriptions and Application Guidance

Strategy	Description	Implementation Tips
Goal Setting	A collaborative activity between the patient/client and the practitioner in which the patient/client decides from all potential activity recommendations what changes he or she will expend effort to implement.	Appropriate for patients/clients ready to make dietary and physical activity changes
		Coach on goal setting skills
		Document and track progress toward short-term and long-term goals
		Probe patient/client about pros and cons of proposed goals
		Assist patient/client in gaining the knowledge and skills necessary to succeed
		Encourage strategies to build confidence (discuss realistic steps and start with easily achievable goals)
		Aid clients in building a supportive environment
		Celebrate successes

Intervention

Strategy: Self-Monitoring (C-2.3)

Strategy Descriptions and Application Guidance

Strategy	Description	Implementation Tips
Self-Monitoring	A technique that involves keeping a detailed record of behaviors that influence diet and/or weight and may include: • What, when, how much eaten • Activities during eating • Emotions and cognitions related to meals/snacks • Frequency, duration, and intensity of exercise • Target nutrient content of foods consumed (eg, calories/kcal/kJ, fat, fiber) • Event, thoughts about event, emotional response, behavioral response • Negative self-talk, replacement thoughts • Blood glucose, blood pressure Self-monitoring is associated with improved treatment outcomes	Provide rationale and instructions for self-monitoring Review and identify patterns Assist with problem solving and goal setting Celebrate successes The amount of feedback required typically diminishes as patient/client skill improves

Intervention

Strategy: Problem Solving (C-2.4)

Strategy Descriptions and Application Guidance

Strategy	Description	Implementation Tips
Problem Solving	Techniques that are taught to assist patients/clients in identifying barriers to achieving goals, identifying and implementing solutions, and evaluating the effectiveness of the solutions (2)	Work collaboratively with patient/client to: • Define the problem • Brainstorm solutions • Weigh pros/cons of potential solutions • Select/implement strategy • Evaluate outcomes • Adjust strategy

Intervention

Strategy: Social Support (C-2.5)

Strategy Descriptions and Application Guidance

Strategy	Description	Implementation Tips
Social Support	Increased availability of social support for dietary and physical activity behavior change. Social support may be generated among an individual's family, church, school, coworkers, health club, or community	A food and nutrition professional may assist a patient/client by: • Establishing a collaborative relationship • Identifying family/community support • Assisting patients/clients in developing assertiveness skills • Using modeling, skill training, respondent and operant conditioning • Conducting education in a group • Encouraging family involvement

Intervention

Strategy: Stress Management (C-2.6)

Strategy Descriptions and Application Guidance

Strategy	Description	Implementation Tips
Stress Management	Reaction to stress can cause some patients/clients to lose their appetite and others to overeat. Food and nutrition professionals are particularly interested in management of stressful situations, which result in less-than-optimal eating behaviors	Two approaches may be used to manage stress: One focuses on changing the environment, and the other focuses on modifying the patient/client's response to stress. Environmental-focused strategies may include: • Guidance on planning ahead • Use of time management skills • Developing a support system • Building skills to prepare quick and healthful meals and incorporate exercise • Guidance on eating on the run Emotion-focused strategies may include: • Use of positive self-talk • Building assertiveness in expressing eating desires • Setting realistic goals • Learning to deal appropriately with emotion-driven eating cravings • Relaxation exercises

Intervention

Strategy: Stimulus Control (C-2.7)

Strategy Descriptions and Application Guidance

Strategy	Description	Implementation Tips
Stimulus Control	Identifying and modifying social or environmental cues or triggers to act, which encourage undesirable behaviors relevant to diet and exercise. In accordance with operant conditioning principles, attention is given to reinforcement and rewards	Review of self-monitoring records with patients/clients may help to identify triggers for undesirable eating Assist client in identifying ways to modify the environment to eliminate triggers. This may include things such as: • Keeping food out of sight • Removing high sugar/high fat snacks from the house • Bringing lunch to work • Establishing a rule—no eating in the car • Helping patient/client establish criteria for rewards for desirable behavior • Ensuring that reward (reinforcement) is received only if criteria are met

Intervention

Strategy: Cognitive Restructuring (C-2.8)

Strategy Descriptions and Application Guidance

Strategy	Description	Implementation Tips
Cognitive Restructuring	Techniques used to increase patient/client's awareness of their perceptions of themselves and their beliefs related to diet, weight, and weight loss expectations	Self-monitoring and techniques such as the ABC Technique of Irrational Beliefs may help patients/clients to become more aware of thoughts that interfere in their ability to meet behavioral goals Help patients/clients replace dysfunctional thoughts with more rationale ones: • Challenge shoulds, oughts, musts • Decatastrophize expected outcomes • Confront faulty self-perceptions • Decenter by envisioning other perspectives • Coach patients/clients on replacing negative self-talk with more positive, empowering, and affirming statements

Intervention

Strategy: Relapse Prevention (C-2.9)

Strategy Descriptions and Application Guidance

Strategy	Description	Implementation Tips
Relapse Prevention	Techniques used to help patients/clients prepare to address high-risk situations for relapse with appropriate strategies and thinking. Incorporates both cognitive and behavioral strategies to enhance long-term behavior change outcomes	Assist patients/clients: • Assess if external circumstances are contributing to lapse, eg, loss of job or support system • Identify high-risk situations for slips • Analyze reactions to slips • Acquire knowledge and skills necessary to address high-risk situations • Gain confidence in their ability to succeed in high-risk situations

Intervention

Strategy: Rewards/Contingency Management (C-2.10)

Strategy Descriptions and Application Guidance

Strategy	Description	Implementation Tips
Rewards/Contingency Management	A systematic process by which behaviors can be changed through the use of rewards for specific actions. Rewards may be derived from the patient/client or the provider	Provide rewards for desired behaviors, eg, attendance, diet progress, consistent self-monitoring, physical activity
		Rewards can be monetary, prizes, parking space, gift certificates
		Assist clients in determining rewards for achievement
		Ensure that rewards are not received if progress is not made

Intervention

Collaboration and Referral of Nutrition Care (RC-1)

Definition

Facilitating services or interventions with other professionals, institutions, or agencies on behalf of the patient/client prior to discharge from nutrition care

Details of Intervention

A typical intervention might be further described with the following details. Nutrition and dietetics practitioners recommend, implement, or order nutrition interventions, and the action(s) may be to initiate, modify, or discontinue a nutrition intervention(s):

- Team meeting (Holding a team meeting to develop a comprehensive plan of care)
- Referral to nutrition and dietetics practitioner with different expertise (A referral for care by other nutrition and dietetics practitioners who provide different expertise)
- Collaborate with other nutrition and dietetics practitioners (Collaboration by nutrition and dietetics practitioner with other nutrition and dietetics practitioners)
- Collaborate with other providers (Collaboration with others such as a physician, dentist, physical therapist, social worker, occupational therapist, speech therapist, nurse, pharmacist, or other specialist dietitian)
- Referral to other provider (Refer to others such as a physician, dentist, physical therapist, social worker, occupational therapist, speech therapist, nurse, pharmacist, or other specialist nutrition and dietetics practitioner)
- Referral to community agencies/programs (Refer to an appropriate agency/program [eg, home-delivered meals], assistance programs for women, infants, and children [eg, WIC], food assistance programs [eg, food pantry, soup kitchen, food stamps], housing assistance, shelters, rehabilitation, physical and mental disability programs, education, training, or employment programs)

Typically Used With the Following

Nutrition Diagnostic Terminology Used in PES Statements	Common Examples (not intended to be inclusive)
Nutrition Diagnoses	Inadequate oral intake (NI-2.1)
	Altered nutrition-related laboratory values (NC-2.2)
	Underweight (NC-3.1)
	Unintended weight loss (NC-3.2)
	Excessive alcohol intake (NI-4.3)
	Overweight/obesity (NC-3.3)
	Physical inactivity (NB-2.1)
	Food–medication interaction (NC-2.3)
	Self-feeding difficulty (NB-2.6)
	Limited access to food (NB-3.2)

Continued on next page

Intervention

Collaboration and Referral
of Nutrition Care (RC-1)

Continued from previous page

Intervention

Nutrition Diagnostic Terminology Used in PES Statements	Common Examples (not intended to be inclusive)
Etiology	Physical disability with impaired feeding ability, other impairments related to activities of daily living
	Mental disability
	Growth and development issues
	Nutrient drug interactions
	Transportation issues
	Food acceptance issues
	Developmental issues
	Economic considerations impacting food/nutrient intake
Signs and Symptoms	Anthropometric Measurements
	• Weight loss
	• Unacceptable growth rates compared to standard growth charts
	Food/Nutrition-Related History
	• Inability to procure food
	• Lack of access to food sources
	• Lack of food preparation skills
	Nutrition-Focused Physical Findings
	Skin breakdown and poor wound healing
	• Client History
	• Anorexia nervosa

Other Considerations (eg, patient/client negotiation, patient/client needs and desires, and readiness to change)
- Availability of services related to patient/client needs (specialty dietitians, clinical pharmacists, speech pathologists, nurse practitioners, etc)
- Anticipated duration of health care encounter/hospital or long-term care discharge
- Resources available for care
- Availability of or access to government medical programs (eg, Medicare/Medicaid, health care exchanges, insurance guidelines, and restrictions)
- Availability of or access to food assistance program (eg, food stamp programs, guidelines, and regulations)

Discharge and Transfer of Nutrition Care to a New Setting or Provider (RC-2)

Definition

Discharge planning and transfer of nutrition care from one level or location of care to another

Details of Intervention

A typical intervention might be further described with the following details. Nutrition and dietetics practitioners recommend, implement, or order nutrition interventions and the action(s) may be to initiate, modify or discontinue a nutrition intervention(s):

- Discharge and transfer to other providers (a referral to others such as a physician, dentist, physical therapist, social worker, occupational therapist, speech therapist, nurse, or pharmacist)

- Discharge and transfer to community agencies/programs (a referral to a community agency/program [eg, home-delivered meals] assistance programs for women, infants, and children [eg, WIC], food assistance programs [eg, food pantry, soup kitchen, food stamps], housing assistance, shelters, rehabilitation, physical and mental disability programs, education, training, or employment programs)

- Discharge and transfer to another nutrition and dietetics practitioner (transfer of nutrition care to another nutrition and dietetics practitioner)

Intervention

Discharge and Transfer of Nutrition Care to a New Setting or Provider (RC-2)

Typically Used With the Following

Intervention

Nutrition Diagnostic Terminology Used in PES Statements	Common Examples (not intended to be inclusive)
Nutrition Diagnoses	Inadequate oral intake (NI-2.1)
	Imbalance of nutrients (NI-5.4)
	Food–medication interaction (NC-2.3)
	Underweight (NC-3.1)
	Overweight/obesity (NC-3.3)
	Impaired ability to prepare foods/meals (NB-2.4)
	Self-feeding difficulty (NB-2.6)
Etiology	Long-term insufficient intake mandating home enteral or parenteral nutrition
	Growth and development considerations requiring intervention in a new setting
Signs and Symptoms	Biochemical Data, Medical Tests, and Procedures
	• Abnormal lab values
	Anthropometric Measurements
	• Less than optimal weight status
	• Continuing weight gain or loss
	Food/Nutrition-Related History
	• Less than optimal dietary practices
	• Unsupported beliefs and attitudes
	Client History
	• Treatment failure
	• Readmission

Other Considerations (eg, patient/client negotiation, patient/client needs and desires, and readiness to change):
- Availability of discharge planning services, options for care
- Preferences for the level and location of care
- Resources available for care
- Availability of or access to government medical programs (eg, Medicare/Medicaid, health care exchanges), insurance guidelines and restrictions
- Health literacy
- Ability to implement treatment at home
- Availability of or access to food assistance programs (eg, food stamp program, guidelines, and regulations)

SNAPSHOT   NCP Step 4:
Nutrition Monitoring and Evaluation

Purpose: The purpose of nutrition monitoring and evaluation is to determine and measure the amount of progress made for the nutrition intervention and whether the nutrition related goals/expected outcomes are being met. The aim is to promote more uniformity within the dietetics profession in assessing the effectiveness of nutrition intervention.

Determining what to measure for nutrition monitoring and evaluation: Practitioners should select nutrition care indicators that will reflect a change as a result of nutrition care. The monitoring and evaluation phase should be considered during the assessment phase while determining the Nutrition Diagnosis and the Nutrition Intervention. Additional factors to consider are the medical diagnosis, health care outcome goals, nutrition quality management goals, practice setting, patient/client* population, and disease state and/or severity.

Terminology for nutrition monitoring and evaluation is organized in 4 domains (categories):

Food/Nutrition-Related History Outcomes	Anthropometric Measurement Outcomes	Biochemical Data, Medical Tests, and Procedure Outcomes	Nutrition-Focused Physical Finding Outcomes
Food and nutrient intake, food and nutrient administration, medication, complementary/alternative medicine use, knowledge/beliefs, food and supplies availability, physical activity, and nutrition quality of life	Height, weight, body mass index (BMI), growth pattern indices/percentile ranks, and weight history	Lab data (eg, electrolytes, glucose) and tests (eg, gastric emptying time, resting metabolic rate)	Physical appearance, muscle and fat wasting, swallow function, appetite, and affect

Note: While the domains, classes, and terms for nutrition assessment and nutrition monitoring and evaluation are combined, there are no nutrition care outcomes associated with the domain titled Client History. Items from this domain are used for nutrition assessment and reassessment only and do not change as a result of nutrition intervention.

Collection and use of nutrition monitoring and evaluation outcome data: This step consists of three components: monitoring, measuring, and evaluating the changes in nutrition care indicators. Practitioners monitor by providing evidence that the nutrition intervention is or is not changing the patient/client's behavior or status. They measure outcomes by collecting data on the appropriate nutrition outcome indicator(s). Finally, nutrition and dietetics practitioners compare the current findings with previous status, nutrition intervention goals, and/or reference standards (ie, criteria) and evaluate the overall impact of the nutrition intervention on the patient/client's health outcomes. The use of standardized indicators and criteria increases the validity and reliability of outcome data collection. All these procedures facilitate electronic charting and aggregation of data for reporting outcomes of the nutrition and dietetics practitioner's interventions for patient/client care.

Critical Thinking Skills

- Selecting appropriate indicators/measures
- Using appropriate reference standards for comparison
- Defining where patient/client is in terms of expected outcomes
- Explaining a variance from expected outcomes
- Determining factors that help or hinder progress
- Deciding between discharge and continuation of nutrition care

For more information, sign in as a subscriber at: https://ncpt.webauthor.com.

---

*Patient/client refers to individuals, groups, populations, family members, and/or caregivers.

Nutrition Assessment Matrix

Food/Nutrition-Related Nutrition Diagnostic Terminology

Parameter (not all-inclusive)	Nutrition Diagnostic Terminology		Nutrition Assessment and/or ME Code	
Food and Nutrient Intake				
Expected food/nutrition related outcomes are not achieved	NB-1.6		FH-5.1.1	FH-8.1.1
Excess intake of energy from energy dense or high fat foods/beverages	NI-1.3 NI-2.2	NC-3.6	FH-1.2.1.1 FH-1.2.1 FH-1.5.1	CS-1.1.1 CS-2.1.1
Restriction or omission of energy dense foods	NI-1.2 NC-3.5		FH-1.2.1.1 FH-1.3.1 FH-1.6.1	CS-1.1.1 CS-2.1.1
Highly variable calorie intake	NI-2.2		FH-1.1.1.1	
Insufficient intake of energy	NI-1.2 NI-1.4 NI-2.1 NI-5.2 NI-5.7.1 NC-3.1	NC-3.5 NC-4.1.1 NC-4.1.2 NC-4.1.3 NC-4.1.4 NC-4.1.5	FH-1.1.1.1 FH-2.1.5	CS-1.1.1
Intake inconsistent with estimated, measured, or recommended needs	NI-1.4 NI-1.5 NI-2.2 NI-2.5 NI-2.6 NI-2.9 NI-2.10	NI-5.11.1 NB-1.4 NC-3.1 NC-3.4 NC-3.5 NC-3.6	FH-1.1 FH-1.2 FH-1.3 FH-1.4 FH-1.5	FH-1.6 CS-1 CS-2 CS-3 CS-4
Excess intake of fluid	NI-3.2	NC-2.2	FH-1.2.1	CS-3.1.1
Insufficient intake of fluid	NI-3.1	NC-3.5	FH-1.2.1	CS-3.1.1
Changes in recent food intake	NC-1.2 NC-3.2	NC-3.4	FH-1.2.2	
Excess intake of foods without available vitamins	NI-5.1	NI-5.9.1	FH-1.6.1	CS-4.1
Excess intake of fortified foods and supplements containing vitamins	NI-5.9.2		FH-1.6.1	CS-4.1
Food group/nutrient imbalance	NB-1.2		FH-1.2.2.1 FH-1.2.2.4	FH-1.2.2.5
Food additive intolerance	NI-4.2		FH-1.4.2.4	

Parameter (not all-inclusive)	Nutrition Diagnostic Terminology		Nutrition Assessment and/or ME Code	
Food variety, limited	NI-2.1	NB-3.2	FH-1.2.2.4	FH-1.2.2.5
	NC-3.5			
Insufficient intake of foods/food groups and nutrients	NI-2.11	NB-2.4	FH-1.2.2	
	NI-5.9.1	NB-3.2		
	NI-5.1	NC-1.1		
	NI-5.2	NC-1.2		
	NI-5.10.1	NC-3.1		
	NI-5.11.1	NC-3.5		
Normal intake of food in the face of illness	NC-3.2	NC-3.5	FH-1.2.2	CH-2.1
Mother with small amount of milk when pumping	NC-1.3		FH-7.1.4	
Enteral or parenteral nutrition therapy	NI-5.6.3	NI-5.7.1	FH-1.3	
Enteral or parenteral nutrition formula/solution inconsistent with evidence-based practice	NI-2.5	NI-2.9	FH-1.3	
Enteral or parenteral nutrition support intolerance history	NI-2.5	NI-2.10	FH-1.3	FH-2.1.2.1
	NI-2.9			
Long-term enteral or parenteral nutrition support	NI-2.9	NI-5.10.2	FH-1.3	FH-2.1.2.1
	NI-5.10.1			
Excess intake of parenteral or enteral nutrition or components of EN/PN	NI-1.3	NI-5.7.1	FH-1.3.1.1	FH-1.5.6
	NI-2.4	NC-3.3	FH-1.3.2.1	FH-1.6.1
	NI-5.6.3	NC-3.6	FH-1.5.1	FH-1.6.2
			FH-1.5.3	CS-1.1.1
			FH-1.5.4	CS-2
			FH-1.5.5	CS-4
Insufficient intake of fat, essential fatty acids	NI-5.5.1		FH-1.5.1.1	CS-2.1.1
			FH-1.5.1.8	CS-2.1.2
Insufficient intake of parenteral or enteral nutrition	NI-1.2	NI-2.7	FH-1.3.1.1	CS-1.1.1
	NI-2.3		FH-2.3.1	CS-2.2.1
Alcohol intake, excessive	NI-2.1	NC-3.4	FH-1.4.1	
	NI-4.3	NC-3.5		
	NI-5.2	NC-4.1.2		
	NC-1.2	NC-4.1.1		
Excess intake of alcohol and/or binge drinking	NI-4.3		FH-1.4.1	
Alcohol intake during pregnancy	NI-4.3	NC-3.5	FH-1.4.1	CH-2.1.6
	NC-3.4			

Parameter (not all-inclusive)	Nutrition Diagnostic Terminology		Nutrition Assessment and/or ME Code	
Excess intake of bioactive substances	NI-4.2		FH-1.4	
Insufficient intake of bioactive substances	NI-4.1		FH-1.4	
Excess intake of plant foods containing soluble fiber, β-glucan, or plant sterol and stanol esters	NI-4.2		FH-1.4.2.1 FH-1.4.2.3 FH-1.5.6.2	CS-2.4.1 CS-2.4.2
Insufficient intake of fiber, soy protein, β-glucan, or plant sterol and stanol esters	NI-4.1	NI-5.8.5	FH-1.4.2 FH-1.5.6	CS-2.4.1 CS-2.4.2
Ready access to available foods/products with bioactive substance	NI-4.2		FH-1.4.2 FH-6.1	FH-6.2
Excess intake of fiber	NI-5.3	NI-5.8.6	FH-1.5.6.1	CS-2.4.1
Excess intake of fat from high-risk lipids (saturated fat, trans fat, cholesterol)	NI-5.5.2	NI-5.5.3	FH-1.5.1.2 FH-1.5.1.3	FH-1.5.1.7 CS-2.1.2
Excess intake of fat and/or foods prepared with added fat	NI-5.3 NI-5.5.2	NI-5.5.3	FH-1.5.1.1	CS-2.1.1
Insufficient intake or incorrect ratio of fat, monounsaturated, polyunsaturated, DHA/ARA, omega 3, or fatty acid chain length desired	NI-5.5.3		FH-1.5.1.1 FH-1.5.1.4 FH-1.5.1.5	FH-1.5.1.6 CS-2.1.1
Excess intake of amino acids (specify)	NI-5.7.1		FH-1.5.4.5 CS-2.2.1	CS-2.2.2
Excess intake of protein	NI-5.3 NI-5.6.2	NC-2.2	FH-1.5.3	CS-2.2.1
Insufficient intake of protein	NI-2.1 NI-5.6.1 NC-4.1.1 NC-4.1.2	NC-4.1.3 NC-4.1.4 NC-4.1.5	FH-1.5.3 CS-2.2.1	
Insufficient intake of amino acids	NI-5.7.1			
Protein or other supplementation intake different from recommended	NI-5.6.2 NI-5.6.3	NI-5.7.1	FH-1.5.3 FH-1.5.4	CS-2.2.1 CS-2.2.2
Insufficient intake of carbohydrate	NI-5.8.1		FH-1.5.5	CS-2.3.1
Intake different from recommended carbohydrate	NI-5.8.2 NI-5.8.3	NI-5.8.4	FH-1.5.5 FH-5.1.1	FH-3.1.1.1
Intake different from recommended carbohydrate, protein, and/or fat intake from enteral and/or parenteral nutrients	NI-2.4 NI-2.5 NI-2.6	NI-2.8 NI-2.9	FH-1.3.1	FH-1.5

Parameter (not all-inclusive)	Nutrition Diagnostic Terminology		Nutrition Assessment and/or ME Code	
EN formula composition that is inconsistent with ability to digest and absorb nutrients	NI-2.5		FH-1.3.1.1	PD-1.1.5
Insufficient intake of vitamin D intake/sunlight exposure	NI-5.9.1		FH-1.6.1.3	CS-4.1.3
Insufficient intake of vitamins	NI-5.9.1	NC-2.2	FH-1.6.1	CS-4.1
Excess intake of iron	NI-5.4		FH-1.6.2.3	CS-4.2.3
Excess intake of manganese	NI-5.4		FH-1.6.2.14	CS-4.2.9
Excess intake of zinc	NI-5.4		FH-1.6.2.8	CS-4.2.8
Excess intake of minerals or vitamins	NI-5.9.2 NI-5.10.2	NI-5.11.2	FH-1.6.1 FH-1.6.2	CS-4.1 CS-4.2
Excess intake of phosphorus	NI-5.3	NC-2.2	FH-1.6.2.6	CS-4.2.6
Excess intake of potassium	NC-2.2		FH-1.6.2.7	CS-4.2.5
Excess intake of sodium	NI-3.2 NI-5.3	NC-2.2	FH-1.6.2.7	CS-4.2.7
Insufficient intake of minerals	NI-5.10.1	NC-2.2	FH-1.6.2	CS-4.2
Fasting	NB-1.5	NB-3.4	FH-1.1.1.1 FH-2.1.5	CS-1.1.1
Intake of nonfood item	NB-1.2		FH-1.4.2.7	
Food and nutrient administration				
Chronic dieting behavior	NI-5.10.1 NC-3.1	NB-1.5	FH-2.1.2.3	FH-2.1.2.4
Inability to lose weight through conventional weight loss intervention	NC-3.3		FH-2.1.2.2 AD-1.1.4.1	AD-1.1.6
Previous failures to effectively change target behavior	NB-1.3	NB-1.6	FH-2.1.2.4	FH-4.2.7
Lack of facilities or accommodations for breastfeeding in community or at work	NC-1.3		FH-2.1.3.4	
Excess intake of convenience foods, pre-prepared meals, and foods prepared away from home	NI-2.2 NB-2.4		FH-2.1.3.1 FH-1.2.2.2	
Previous diet changes due to food allergy or intolerance	NI-5.6.3		FH-2.1.2.5	FH-2.1.26
EN conflict with oral intake	NI-2.6		FH-2.1.1.1 FH-2.1.1.2,	FH-2.1.1.3

Parameter (not all-inclusive)	Nutrition Diagnostic Terminology		Nutrition Assessment and/or ME Code	
PN conflict with oral or enteral nutrition intake	NI-2.10		FH-2.1.1.1 FH-2.1.1.2,	FH-2.1.1.3 FH-2.1.1.4
EN administration conflict with medications, QOL, therapies	NI-2.6		FH-2.1.1.3 FH-3.1.1 FH-3.1.2	FH-8.1.1 CH-2.2.1
PN administration conflict with medications, QOL, therapies	NI-2.10		FH-2.1.1.4 FH-3.1.1 FH-3.1.2	FH-8.1.1 CH-2.2.1
Feeding tube in the wrong position or removed	NI-2.3	NI-2.6	FH-2.1.4.1	
Feeding tube access type that warrants modification	NI-2.3	NI-2.6	FH-2.1.4.1	
Venous access type that warrants modification	NI-2.7	NI-2.10	FH-2.1.4.2	
Venous access in the wrong position or removed	NI-2.7	NI-2.10	FH-2.1.4.2	
Venous access compromised	NI-2.7	NI-2.10	FH-2.1.4.2	
Feeding position, EN suboptimal	NI-2.3	NI-2.6	FH-2.1.4.3	
Medication and complementary/alternative medicine use				
Insulin or insulin secretagogues	NI-5.8.4		FH-3.1.1 FH-3.1.2	FH-3.1.3 FH-3.2.1
Medication associated with weight loss	NC-3.2 NI-1.4		FH-3.1 FH-3.2.1 AD-1.1.4.2	AD-1.1.4.7 AD-1.1.6 CS-5.1.4
Medication, lipid lowering	NI-5.5.2		FH-3.1.1 FH-3.1.2	FH-3.1.3 FH-3.2.1
Medications administered in large amounts of fluid	NI-3.2		FH-3.1.1 FH-1.2.1	CS-3.1.1
Medications containing proteins not recommended	NI-5.6.3		FH-3.1.1 FH-1.6.1 FH-2.1	CS-2.2.1 CS-3.1.1
Medications affecting absorption or metabolism	NI-5.1		FH-3.1 FH-3.2.1 BD-1.4	BD-1.8.1 PD-1.1.5 CH-2.1.3
Medications associated with increased appetite	NI-1.5 NC-3.4		FH-3.1 FH-3.2.1	PD-1.1.5

Parameter (not all-inclusive)	Nutrition Diagnostic Terminology		Nutrition Assessment and/or ME Code	
Medications that affect appetite	NI-1.2 NI-1.4	NC-3.1	FH-3.1 FH-3.2.1	PD-1.1.5
Medications that cause altered glucose levels	NI-5.8.2 NI-5.8.3	NI-5.8.4	FH-3.1 FH-3.2.1	BD-1.5
Medications that cause anorexia	NI-2.1 NI-5.11.1		FH-3.1 FH-3.2.1	PD-1.1.5
Medications that cause somnolence and decreased cognition	NB-2.1		FH-3.1 FH-3.2.1	PD-1.1.7
Medications that impact RMR	NC-3.3 NC-3.6		FH-3.1 FH-3.2.1	BD-1.8 CS-1.1.1
Medications that impair fluid excretion	NI-3.2		FH-3.1 FH-3.2.1	BD-1.12
Medications that increase energy expenditure	NI-1.1		FH-3.1 FH-3.2.1	BD-1.8 CS-1.1.1
Medications that reduce requirements or impair metabolism of energy, protein, fat, or fluid	NI-2.4 NI-2.8 NC-3.6		FH-3.1 FH-3.2.1 BD-1.8 CS-1.1.1	CS-2.1.1 CS-2.2.1 CS-3.1.1
Medications that reduce thirst	NI-3.1		FH-3.1 FH-3.2.1	BD-1.12 PD-1.1.5
Medications that require nutrient supplementation that cannot be accomplished with food intake	NC-2.3 NC-2.4		FH-3.1 FH-3.2.1 FH-1.7.1	FH-1.7.2 CS-4
Medications with known food-medication interactions	NC-2.3	NC-2.4	FH-3.1	FH-3.2.1
Misuse of laxatives, enemas, diuretics, stimulants, and/or metabolic enhancers	NB-1.5		FH-3.1.3	FH-3.2.1
Medications that affect appetite or are associated with weight loss	NI-1.2 NC-3.2 NC-3.5		FH-3.1 FH-3.2.1 AD-1.1.4.2	AD-1.1.4.7 AD-1.1.6 CS-5.1.4
Intake that does not support replacement or mitigation of OTC, prescribed drugs, herbals, botanicals, or dietary supplements	NC-2.3 NC-2.4		FH-3.1 FH-3.2.1 FH-1.7.1	FH-1.7.2 CS-4
Medication (over the counter or prescribed), herbal, botanical, or complementary/alternative medicine intake	NC-2.3 NC-2.4	NB-1.2	FH-3.1 FH-3.2.1	

Parameter (not all-inclusive)	Nutrition Diagnostic Terminology		Nutrition Assessment and/or ME Code	
Prolonged use of substances known to increase vitamin requirements or reduce vitamin absorption	NI-5.9.1		FH-3.1 FH-3.2.1	FH-1.7.1 CS-4.1
Drug intake, excessive	NI-2.1 NI-5.2	NC-3.4 NC-4.1.1	FH-3.1.3	
Knowledge/Beliefs/Attitudes				
Avoidance or limitation of estimated total intake or intake of specific food/food groups	NI-5.2 NC-1.4 NC-4.1.1	NC-4.1.4 NC-4.1.5 NB-1.5	FH-1.2.2 FH-5.2	
Uncertainty regarding appropriate foods to prepare based upon nutrition prescription	NB-2.4		FH- 4.1 FH-5.1.4	FH-5.1.5
Uncertainty as to how to consistently apply food/nutrition information	NB-1.6 NB-1.7		FH-4.1 FH-5.1.4	FH-5.1.5
Inability to select (e.g., access) or unwillingness to select or disinterest in selecting food consistent with guidelines	NB-1.7 NC-3.5		FH-4.1 FH-5.1.1	FH-6 CH-2.1.12
Uncertainty of how to complete monitoring records	NB-1.4		FH-4.1	FH-5.1.4
Uncertainty regarding changes that could/should be made in response to data in self-monitoring records	NB-1.4	NB-2.3	FH-4.1	FH-5.1.4
Mother has insufficient knowledge of breastfeeding or infant hunger/satiety signals	NC-1.3		FH-4.1	FH-6.1.4
Belief that aging can be slowed by dietary limitations	NB-3.2		FH-4.2.11	
Cultural or religious practices that affect intake	NI-5.5.1 NI-5.6.1 NI-5.8.2 NI-5.8.4	NI-5.10.1 NI-5.11.1 NB-1.4	FH-1.2 FH-1.5 FH-1.6	CH-1.1.3 CH-3.1.7
Defensiveness, hostility, or resistance to change	NB-1.3		FH-4.2.7	
Denial of need for food- and nutrition-related changes	NB-1.3		FH-4.2.7	FH-4.2.11
Emotional distress, anxiety, or frustration surrounding meal times	NB-2.6		FH-4.2	FH-5.4
Food faddism	NC-3.1	NB-1.2	FH-4.2.11	
Food preoccupation	NB-1.5		FH-4.2.5	
Excessive reliance on nutrition terming and preoccupation with nutrient content of food	NB-1.5		FH-4.2.5	FH-4.2.11
Fear of foods or dysfunctional thoughts regarding food or food groups	NB-1.5		FH-4.2.5	FH-4.2.11

Parameter (not all-inclusive)	Nutrition Diagnostic Terminology		Nutrition Assessment and/or ME Code	
Relates concerns about previous attempts to learn information	NB-1.1 NB-2.5		FH-2.1.2.2 FH-4.1	FH-8.1.1
Frustration over lack of control	NB-2.5		FH-4.2.7	FH-8.1.1
Unsupported beliefs and attitudes	NI-5.5.2 NI-5.6.2 NI-5.6.3 NI-5.8.6 NI-5.10.2	NB-3.2 NB-3.4 NB-3.3 NC-3.5	FH-4.2.11	
Inaccurate or incomplete knowledge	NI-1.4 NI-1.5 NI-2.5 NI-2.6 NI-2.9 NI-2.10 NI-4.1 NI-4.2 NI-5.1 NI-5.5.1 NI-5.6.1 NI-5.6.2 NI-5.6.3 NI-5.7.1 NI-5.8.1 NI-5.8.2 NI-5.8.3	NI-5.8.5 NI-5.8.6 NI-5.10.1 NI-5.10.2 NI-5.11.1 NI-5.11.2 NB-1.1 NB-1.4 NB-1.7 NB-2.5 NB-3.1 NB-3.3 NB-3.4 NC-2.2 NC-3.5 NC-3.6	FH-4.1	
Provides inaccurate or incomplete written response to questionnaire/ written tool or is unable to read written tool	NB-1.1		FH-4.1.1	CH-1.1.5
Irrational thoughts about food's effect on the body	NB-1.5		FH-4.2.5	FH-4.2.11
Lack of efficacy or lack of confidence to make changes or to overcome barriers to change	NB-1.3	NB-1.6	FH-4.2.8	
Mother with lack of confidence in ability to breastfeed	NC-1.3		FH-4.2.8	
Unrealistic expectations of weight gain or ideal weight	NI-2.4	NI-2.8	FH-4.2.10	CS-5.1.3
Unwillingness or disinterest in applying nutrition-related recommendations	NC-3.3 NB-1.7	NB-2.5	FH-4.2.7 FH-4.2.4	FH-5.1.1 FH-5.1.5
Verbalizes unwillingness/disinterest in learning	NB-1.1		FH-4.2.7	
Weight preoccupation	NB-1.5		FH-4.2.6	CS-5.1.3

Parameter (not all-inclusive)	Nutrition Diagnostic Terminology		Nutrition Assessment and/or ME Code	
Behavior				
Incomplete self-monitoring records	NB-1.4		FH-5.1.4	
Embarrassment or anger at need for self-monitoring	NB-1.4	NB-2.3	FH-5.1.4	FH-4.2.13
Failure to complete any agreed-upon homework	NB-1.6		FH-5.1.1	
Failure to keep appointments/schedule or engage in counseling	NB-1.3	NB-1.6	FH-5.1.2	
Inability to recall agreed-upon changes	NB-1.6		FH-5.1.3	
Lack of compliance or inconsistent compliance with plan	NB-1.6		FH-5.1.1	FH-5.1.5
Lack of social and familial support	NB-1.4 NB-1.6	NB-2.5	FH-5.5.1	
Inability to change food- or activity-related behavior	NB-2.5			
Mother is concerned about breastfeeding/lack of support	NC-1.3 NC-3.5		FH-5.5.1	
Avoidance of food or calorie-containing beverages	NB-1.5 NC-3.5		FH-5.2 FH-1.2.1	FH-1.2.2
Avoidance of foods of age-appropriate texture	NC-1.2 NC-3.5		FH-5.2 FH-5.5	CH-1.1.1
Avoidance of social events where food is served	NB-1.5	NB-2.5	FH-5.2	
Eating alone, feeling embarrassed by the amount of food eaten	NB-1.5		FH-5.3.1 FH-2.1.3	FH-4.2.13
Eating much more rapidly than normal, eating until feeling uncomfortably full, consuming large amounts of food when not feeling hungry	NB-1.5		FH-5.3.1	
Excess intake of food in a defined time period	NB-1.5		FH-5.3.1	
Feeling disgusted with oneself, depressed, or guilty after overeating	NB-1.5		FH-5.3.1	FH-4.2.13
Less-than-optimal reliance on foods, food groups, supplements, EN/PN	NI-2.1	NI-2.11	FH-5.4	
Sense of lack of control of overeating during the episode	NB-1.5		FH-5.3.1	
Lack of developmental readiness	NC-1.2		FH-5.4	
Prolonged chewing, feeding time, spitting food out	NC-1.1 NC-1.2	NB-2.6	FH-5.4	

Parameter (not all-inclusive)	Nutrition Diagnostic Terminology		Nutrition Assessment and/or ME Code	
Factors Affecting Access to Food and Food-/Nutrition-Related Supplies				
Economic or transportation constraints that limit availability of food or supplies	NI-2.1	NB-2.4	FH-6.1	
	NI-5.2	NB-3.3	FH-6.4	
	NI-5.8.2	NB-3.4	CH-3.1.1	
	NI-5.8.3	NB-3.2		
	NI-5.8.4	NC-3.1		
	NI-5.11.1	NC-3.5		
Excess intake of mercury	NB-3.1		FH-6.2.2	
Food insecurity/unwillingness/uncertainty how to use available resources	NB-2.5		FH-6.1	
	NB-3.2		FH-6.4	
	NC-3.5			
Unsafe food procurement	NB-3.1		FH-6.2.2	
Unsafe food identification	NB-3.1		FH-6.2.6	
Mislabeled or unlabeled food	NB-3.1		FH-6.2.6	
Hunger	NI-5.2	NC-3.5	FH-6.1	
	NB-3.2			
Lack of suitable support system to access food, water, or supplies	NB-3.2	NB-3.3	FH-6.1	FH-6.4
	NB-3.5	NC-3.4	FH-6.3	
No self-management equipment	NB-1.4		FH-6.4.1	
Lack of access to assistive eating devices	NB-2.6		FH-6.4.2	
Ready access to available foods/products with bioactive substance	NI-4.2		FH-6.1	FH-1.4.2
Lack of access to appropriate food storage or preparation facility	NB-3.1		FH-6.2.3	FH-6.2.5
			FH-6.2.4	
Lack of access to potable water	NB-3.4		FH-6.3.1	
Physical Activity and Function				
Breastfeeding issues, low duration, crying, latch issues, lethargy, feeding resistance	NC-1.3	NC-3.5	FH-7.1	
Remembers to eat	NB-2.6		FH-7.2.7	
Recalls eating	NB-2.6		FH-7.2.8	
Decreased or sedentary activity level (due to barriers or other reasons)	NI-1.5	NC-3.6	FH-7.3	
	NC-3.3	NB-2.1		

Parameter (not all-inclusive)	Nutrition Diagnostic Terminology		Nutrition Assessment and/or ME Code	
Increased physical activity	NI-1.1 NC-3.1 NI-1.4	NC-3.5 NI-5.1 NB-2.2	FH-7.3	
Low level of nonexercise activity thermogenesis (NEAT)	NB-2.1		FH-7.3.11	
Excessive physical activity (ignoring family, job; exercising without rest/rehabilitation days or while injured or sick)	NB-1.5 NB-2.2		FH-7.3.2 FH-7.3.3 FH-7.3.4	FH-7.3.5 FH-7.3.6
Overtraining	NB-2.2		FH-7.3	
Low cardiorespiratory fitness and/or low muscle strength	NB-2.1		FH-7.3 PD-1.1.3	PD-1.1.4
Factors affecting physical activity access	NC-3.3 NB-1.3	NB-2.1	FH-7.4	
Lack of ability to shop, prepare meals	NI-1.4 NI-1.5	NI-5.2 NI-5.11.1	FH-7.2.1 FH-7.2.6	FH-7.2.10
Physical activity, easy fatigue with increased activity; unable to achieve desired levels	NI-2.3 NI-2.7		FH-7.3	
Change in functional indicators, eg, handgrip strength or others	NC-4.1.1 NC-4.1.2 NC-4.1.3	NC-4.1.4 NC-4.1.5	FH-7.3	
Change in physical activity	NI-1.5		FH-7.3	
Utensil biting	NB-2.6		FH-7.2.10	FH-5.4.4
Food, less than optimal use of	NB-2.6		FH-7.2	FH-5.4
Foods provided not conducive to self-feeding	NB-2.6		FH-6.2.2	FH-6.2.3
Dropping foods, utensils; lack of strength for feeding	NB-2.6		FH-7.2.2	FH-7.2.3
Nutrition-Related Patient/Client-Centered Measures				
Unfavorable QOL or other quality of life rating	NB-2.5		FH-8.1.1	
Frustration or dissatisfaction with MNT recommendations	NB-1.6	NB-2.5	FH-8.1.1	

Nutrition Assessment Matrix

Anthropometric Data and Related Diagnostic Terminology

Parameter (not all-inclusive)	Findings	Nutrition Diagnostic Terminology			Nutrition Assessment and/or ME Code	
Height						
Height/length	loss	NI-5.10.1			AD-1.1.1 (adults)	AD-1.1.6 (peds)
Weight change						
Weight	change, rapid	NC-2.2	NC-3.6	NB-1.5	AD-1.1.4 (adults)	AD-1.1.6 (peds)
	gain	NI-1.3	NI-1.5	NI-2.2	AD-1.1.4.1 (adults)	AD-1.1.6 (peds)
		NI-2.11	NI-3.2	NC-2.3		
		NC-3.3	NC-3.4	NC-3.6		
	in excess of lean tissue accretion	NI-2.4	NI-2.5	NI-2.6	AD-1.1.4.1 (adults)	AD-1.1.6 (peds)
		NI-2.8	NI-2.9			
	interdialytic	NI-5.3			AD-1.1.4.4	AD-1.1.4.5
	loss	NI-1.2	NI-1.4	NI-2.1	AD-1.1.4.2 (adults)	AD-1.1.6 (peds)
		NI-2.3	NI-2.5	NI-2.6		
		NI-2.7	NI-2.9	NI-2.11		
		NI-3.1	NI-4.1	NI-4.2		
		NC-5.1	NI-5.2	NI-5.5.1		
		NI-5.7.1	NI-5.8.3	NC-1.3		
		NC-1.4	NC-2.1	NC-3.2		
		NC-3.5	NB-2.2	NB-2.6		
		NB-3.2	NB-3.3	NB-3.4		
	unintentional	NI-1.1	NI-1.4	NI-2.3	AD-1.1.4.8	
		NI-2.7	NI-5.1	NC-3.2		
		NC-3.5	NC-4.1	NB-3.3		
	decreased	NI-1.4	NC-3.1	NC-3.2	AD-1.1.4.2 (adults)	AD-1.1.6 (peds)
		NC-3.5	NB-2.2	NB-3.3		
	failure to gain as planned	NI-1.4	NI-2.3	NI-2.7	AD-1.1.4 (adults)	AD-1.1.6 (peds)
		NI-5.2	NI-5.8.3	NC-1.3		
		NC-3.2	NC-3.5	NC-4.1		
		NB-1.6	NB-2.2	NB-3.3		

Parameter (not all-inclusive)	Findings	Nutrition Diagnostic Terminology			Nutrition Assessment and/or ME Code	
Body Mass						
BMI	increased	NI-1.3	NI-1.5	NC-3.3	AD-1.1.5.1 (adults)	AD-1.1.6 (peds)
		NB-1.5	NB-2.1	NB-3.2		
	decreased	NI-1.4	NI-2.3	NI-2.7	AD-1.1.5.1 (adults)	AD-1.1.6 (peds)
		NI-5.1	NC-4.1	NC-3.1		
		NC-3.5	NB-1.5	NB-3.2		
		NB-3.3				
	normal	NC-4.1			AD-1.1.5.1 (adults)	AD-1.1.6.1
						AD-1.1.6.2 (peds)
Growth Pattern Indices						
Growth pattern indices	delayed	NI-1.1	NI-1.4	NI-2.1	AD-1.1.6	
		NI-2.3	NI-2.7	NI-2.11		
		NI-5.1	NI-5.2	NI-5.5.1		
		NI-5.6.1	NI-5.6.2	NI-5.7.1		
		NI-5.8.3	NI-5.9.2	NI-5.11.2		
		NC-1.4	NC-2.1	NC-3.1		
		NC-3.2	NC-3.5	NC-4.1		
		NB-2.2	NB-3.2	NB-3.3		
	increased more than expected	NC-3.6			AD-1.1.6	
Body Compartment Estimates						
Body fat percentage	increased	NI-1.3			AD-1.1.7	
Body fat percentage	decreased	NI-5.1	NC-3.5		AD-1.1.7	
Bone mineral density	decreased	NI-5.10.1	NI-5.11.1	NC-1.4	AD-1.1.7	
		NC-2.1				
Mid-arm muscle circumference	decreased	NI-5.1	NC-3.1	NC-3.5	AD-1.1.7	
Triceps skinfold	increased	NC-3.3			AD-1.1.7	
	decreased	NI-5.1	NC-3.1	NC-3.5	AD-1.1.7	
Waist circumference	increased	NC-3.3			AD-1.1.7	

Nutrition Assessment Matrix

Biochemical Data, Medical Tests and Procedures and Related Diagnostic Terminology

Parameter (not all-inclusive)	Findings	Nutrition Diagnostic Terminology		Nutrition Assessment and/or ME Code
Biochemical data				
Acid-base balance				
pCO_2	abnormal	NI-2.4 NI-2.8	NC-2.2	BD-1.1.3
pO_2	abnormal	NC-2.2		BD-1.1.4
Electrolyte and renal profile				
BUN	increased	NI-3.1 NI-5.6.3 NI-5.3	NC-2.2 NI-5.6.2 NB-1.5	BD-1.2.1
Creatinine	elevated	NI-5.3	NC-2.2	BD-1.2.2
BUN:creatinine ratio	increased	NI-2.4 NI-2.8	NC-2.2	BD-1.2.3
GFR, glomerular filtration rate	decreased	NI-5.3 NC-2.2	NI-5.6.2 NI-5.6.3	BD-1.2.4
Sodium, serum	decreased	NI-3.2 NC-3.4	NB-1.5	BD-1.2.5
	increased	NI-3.1		BD-1.2.5
Chloride, serum	decreased	NB-1.5		BD-1.2.6
Potassium, serum	decreased	NI-2.5 NI-5.1 NB-1.5 NI-2.6	NI-5.4 NI-2.9 NC-2.2	BD-1.2.7
	increased	NI-5.1 NI-5.3	NC-2.2	BD-1.2.7
Magnesium, serum	decreased	NI-5.1 NI-5.4	NI-5.10.1	BD-1.2.8
	increased	NI-5.10.2	NI-5.11.2	BD-1.2.8
Calcium, serum	decreased	NI-2.3 NI-2.7	NI-5.10.1	BD-1.2.9

Parameter (not all-inclusive)	Findings	Nutrition Diagnostic Terminology		Nutrition Assessment and/or ME Code	
Calcium, serum ionized	decreased	NI-5.9.1		BD-1.2.10	
	increased	NI-5.9.2		BD-1.2.10	
Phosphorus, serum	decreased	NI-5.1 NI-5.10.1	NI-5.4 NI-5.9.1	BD-1.2.11	
	increased	NI-2.5 NI-5.3 NI-2.6	NI-5.10.2 NI-2.8 NI-5.11.2	BD-1.2.11	
Osmolality, serum or plasma	decreased	NI-3.2		BD-1.2.12	
	increased	NI-3.1		BD-1.2.12	
Parathyroid hormone	increased	NI-5.9.1 NC-2.1	NI-5.9.2 NC-1.4	BD-1.2.13	
Essential fatty acid profile					
Triene:tetraene ratio	increased	NI-5.5.1		BD-1.3.1	
Gastrointestinal profile					
ALT, alanine aminotransferase	increased	NC-2.1	NC-2.2	BD-1.4.2	
AST, aspartate aminotransferase	increased	NI-4.3 NB-2.2	NC-2.1 NC-2.2	BD-1.4.3	
GGT, gamma-glutamyl transferase	elevated	NI-4.3	NC-2.1	BD-1.4.4	
Gastric residual volume, specify	increased	NI-2.6		BD-1.4.5	
Liver enzymes	elevated	NI-1.3 NI-2.10 NI-5.5.2 NB-2.2 NI-2.8	NI-4.2 NI-5.5.3 NI-2.9 NI-5.3 NC-2.2	BD-1.4.1 BD-1.4.2 BD-1.4.3	BD-1.4.4 BD-1.4.15
Bilirubin, total serum	increased	NI-5.5.2 NI-5.5.3	NC-2.2	BD-1.4.6	
Ammonia, serum	increased	NI-5.6.3 NI-5.7.1	NC-2.2	BD-1.4.7	
Toxicology reports (including alcohol)	positive	NI-4.3	NB-3.1	BD-1.4.8	
PT, PTT, INR	abnormal	NI-2.3 NI-5.9.2	NI-2.7 NI-5.9.1	BD-1.4.9 BD-1.4.10	BD-1.4.11

Parameter (not all-inclusive)	Findings	Nutrition Diagnostic Terminology		Nutrition Assessment and/or ME Code	
Fat, fecal	increased	NI-5.1 NI-5.5.2	NC-1.4	BD-1.4.12	
Amylase, serum	increased	NI-5.5.2	NI-5.5.3	BD-1.4.13	
Lipase	increased	NI-5.5.2	NI-5.5.3	BD-1.4.14	
Digestive enzymes	altered	NC-1.4		BD-1.4.15	
D-xylose	abnormal	NI-5.1	NC-1.4	BD-1.4.16	
Breath test	abnormal	NC-1.4		BD-1.4.22 BD-1.4.23 BD-1.4.24	BD-1.4.25 BD-1.4.26
Intestinal biopsy	abnormal	NC-1.4		BD-1.4.18	
Stool culture	positive	NC-1.4 NB-3.1	NB-3.4	BD-1.4.19	
Gastric emptying study	abnormal	NC-1.4		BD-1.4.20	
Small bowel transit time	abnormal	NC-1.4		BD-1.4.21	
Scan results (e.g., abdominal/pelvic X-ray, CT, ultrasound)	abnormal	NC-1.4		BD-1.4.31 BD-1.4.32 BD-1.4.33 BD-1.4.34 BD-1.4.35	BD-1.4.36 BD-1.4.37 BD-1.4.38 BD-1.4.39
pH	abnormal	NC-1.4		BD-1.4.42	
Sphincter	abnormal	NC-1.4		BD-1.4.44	
Motility	abnormal	NC-1.4		BD-1.4.36 BD-1.4.37 BD-1.4.38	BD-1.4.39 BD-1.4.40 BD-1.4.41
Reflux	abnormal	NC-1.4		BD-1.4.43	

Parameter (not all-inclusive)	Findings	Nutrition Diagnostic Terminology		Nutrition Assessment and/or ME Code	
Glucose/endocrine profile					
Glucose, blood	decreased	NI-5.8.3 NC-2.1 NI-5.8.4	NC-3.4 NC-2.2 NB-1.5	BD-1.5.1	BD-1.5.2
	increased	NI-2.4 NI-5.8.2 NC-2.1 NC-3.5 NI-2.8	NI-5.8.3 NC-2.2 NI-3.1 NI-5.8.4 NC-3.4	BD-1.5.1	BD-1.5.2
Hemoglobin A1c	increased	NI-5.8.2	NC-2.2	BD-1.5.3	
GTT (glucose tolerance test)	abnormal	NI-5.8.2		BD-1.5.6	
Cortisol levels	abnormal	NB-2.2 NC-3.4	NC-3.5	BD-1.5.7	
IGF binding protein	abnormal	NB-2.2		BD-1.5.8	
Thyroid function tests (TSH, T4, T3)	abnormal	NI-5.10.2 NC-3.5	NB-1.5 NC-3.4	BD-1.5.9 BD-1.5.10	BD-1.5.11
Pituitary hormones (GH, ACTH, LH, FSH)	abnormal	NC-2.1 NC-3.4	NC-3.5	BD-1.5.12 BD-1.5.13	BD-1.5.14 BD-1.5.15
Inflammatory profile					
C-reactive protein	elevated	NI-5.1	NI-5.5.3	BD-1.6.1	
Lipid profile					
Cholesterol, serum	decreased	NI-4.2	NI-5.1	BD-1.7.1	
	increased	NI-4.1 NI-5.5.3 NI-5.3	NB-1.5 NI-5.5.2	BD-1.7.1	
Cholesterol, HDL	decreased	NI-5.3 NI-5.10.2	NI-5.5.2 NI-5.5.3	BD-1.7.2	
Cholesterol, LDL	increased	NI-5.3 NI-5.5.2	NI-5.5.3	BD-1.7.3	
Triglycerides	increased	NI-5.3 NI-5.5.2	NI-5.5.3	BD-1.7.7	
Lipid profile, serum	abnormal	NC-2.2 NB-1.7	NC-3.4 NB-1.5	BD-1.7	

Parameter (not all-inclusive)	Findings	Nutrition Diagnostic Terminology		Nutrition Assessment and/or ME Code
Metabolic rate profile				
Resting metabolic rate	increased	NI-1.1	NC-3.1	BD-1.8.1
Respiratory quotient, measured	abnormal	NI-1.3	NI-2.7	BD-1.8.2
		NI-2.3		
Mineral profile				
Copper, serum	decreased	NI-2.3	NC-1.4	BD-1.9.1
		NI-5.10.2	NI-5.10.1	
		NB-3.3	NI-5.11.1	
		NI-2.7		
Boron, serum or plasma	decreased	NI-2.1	NI-5.10.1	BD-1.9.4
		NI-2.3		
	increased	NI-5.10.2		
Fluoride, plasma	decreased	NI-2.1	NI-5.10.1	BD-1.9.6
		NI-2.3		
	increased	NI-5.10.2		
Manganese, blood, plasma	decreased	NI-2.3	NI-5.10.1	BD-1.9.7
		NI-2.7		
	increased	NI-5.10.2		
Molybdenum, serum	decreased	NI-2.3	NI-5.10.1	BD-1.9.8
		NI-2.7		
	increased	NI-5.10.2		
Selenium, serum	decreased	NI-2.3	NI-5.10.1	BD-1.9.9
		NI-2.7		
	increased	NI-5.10.2		
Iodine, urinary	decreased	NI-5.10.1	NI-5.11.1	BD-1.9.2
		NB-3.3	NC-1.4	
Zinc, plasma	decreased	NI-2.3	NC-3.5	BD-1.9.3
		NC-1.4	NI-5.11.1	
		NB-3.3	NB-2.2	
		NI-2.7		

Parameter (not all-inclusive)	Findings	Nutrition Diagnostic Terminology		Nutrition Assessment and/or ME Code
Nutritional anemia profile				
Hemoglobin	decreased	NI-5.10.1	NC-2.1	BD-1.10.1
Hematocrit	increased	NC-2.1	NB-2.2	BD-1.10.2
Mean corpuscular volume	increased	NI-4.3	NC-2.1	BD-1.10.3
Folate, RBC	decreased	NI-5.9.1 NB-3.3	NI-5.11.1 NC-2.1	BD-1.10.4
Folic acid, serum	decreased	NI-5.9.1 NC-2.1 NI-5.11.1	NB-3.3 NC-1.4	BD-1.10.8
Vitamin B12, serum	decreased	NI-5.9.1 NC-2.1 NI-5.11.1	NB-3.3 NC-1.4	BD-1.10.6
Homocysteine, serum	increased	NI-5.9.1 NC-1.4	NC-2.1	BD-1.10.9
Ferritin, serum	decreased	NB-2.2 NB-3.3 NC-1.4	NC-3.5 NC-2.1	BD-1.10.10
	increased	NI-5.10.2	NI-5.11.1	BD-1.10.10
Iron	decreased	NI-2.3 NC-1.4 NB-3.3 NI-2.7	NC-2.1 NI-5.11.1 NC-3.5	BD-1.10.11
Iron binding capacity	decreased	NI-2.3 NC-1.4 NI-2.7	NC-2.1 NI-5.11.1 NB-3.3	BD-1.10.12
Protein profile				
Albumin, serum	decreased	NI-5.1	NC-3.4	BD-1.11.1
Prealbumin	decreased	NI-5.1		BD-1.11.2
Transferrin	increased	NI-4.3 NI-5.10.2	NI-5.11.1	BD-1.11.3

Parameter (not all-inclusive)	Findings	Nutrition Diagnostic Terminology		Nutrition Assessment and/or ME Code	
Amino acids	abnormal	NI-5.6.3		BD-1.11.6	BD-1.11.31
		NC-2.2		BD-1.11.7	BD-1.11.32
		NI-5.7.1		BD-1.11.8	BD-1.11.33
		NC-3.5		BD-1.11.9	BD-1.11.34
		NC-2.1		BD-1.11.10	BD-1.11.35
				BD-1.11.11	BD-1.11.36
				BD-1.11.12	BD-1.11.37
				BD-1.11.13	BD-1.11.38
				BD-1.11.14	BD-1.11.39
				BD-1.11.15	BD-1.11.40
				BD-1.11.16	BD-1.11.41
				BD-1.11.17	BD-1.11.42
				BD-1.11.18	BD-1.11.43
				BD-1.11.19	BD-1.11.44
				BD-1.11.20	BD-1.11.45
				BD-1.11.21	BD-1.11.46
				BD-1.11.22	BD-1.11.47
				BD-1.11.23	BD-1.11.48
				BD-1.11.24	BD-1.11.49
				BD-1.11.25	BD-1.11.50
				BD-1.11.26	BD-1.11.51
				BD-1.11.27	BD-1.11.52
				BD-1.11.28	BD-1.11.53
				BD-1.11.29	BD-1.11.54
				BD-1.11.30	
Tissue transglutaminase antibodies	abnormal	NC-1.4		BD-1.11.56	BD-1.11.57
Carbohydrate deficient transferrin	increased	NI-4.3		BD-1.11.60	
Urine profile					
Urine volume, specify	decreased	NI-3.1	NB-3.4	BD-1.12.5	
	fewer diapers than reference standard in 24 hours	NC-1.3		BD-1.12.5	
Urine calcium	decreased	NI-5.10.1	NI-5.11.1	BD-1.12.5	
Urine ketones	present	NB-1.5	NC-3.5	BD-1.12.8	
Urine specific gravity	increased	NI-3.1	NB-3.4	BD-1.12.3	
	decreased	NI-3.1		BD-1.12.3	
Urine microalbumin	increased	NC-2.2		BD-1.12.10	
Urine porphyrins	positive	NC-2.1		BD-1.12.27	

Parameter (not all-inclusive)	Findings	Nutrition Diagnostic Terminology		Nutrition Assessment and/or ME Code
Vitamin profile				
Retinol, serum	decreased	NI-5.9.1	NI-5.11.1	BD-1.13.1
	increased	NI-5.9.2	NI-5.11.2	BD-1.13.1
Vitamin C, plasma	decreased	NI-5.9.1	NI-5.11.1	BD-1.13.2
Alpha tocopherol, plasma	decreased	NI-5.9.1	NI-5.11.1	BD-1.13.4
Erythrocyte transketolase activity	increased	NI-5.9.1	NI-5.11.1	BD-1.13.5
Erythrocyte glutathione reductase	increased	NI-5.9.1	NI-5.11.1	BD-1.13.6
N'methyl-nicotanimide	decreased	NI-5.9.1	NI-5.11.1	BD-1.13.7
	increased	NI-5.9.2	NI-5.11.2	BD-1.13.7
Pyridoxal 5'phosphate, plasma	decreased	NI-5.9.1	NI-5.11.1	BD-1.13.8
	increased	NI-5.9.2	NI-5.11.2	BD-1.13.8
Pantothenic acid, plasma	decreased	NI-5.9.1	NI-5.11.1	BD-1.13.9
	increased	NI-5.9.2	NI-5.11.2	BD-1.13.9
Biotin, serum	decreased	NI-5.9.1	NI-5.11.1	BD-1.13.10
	increased	NI-5.9.2	NI-5.11.2	BD-1.13.10
Carbohydrate metabolism profile				
Galactose-1-phosphate in RBCs	abnormal	NI-5.8.3 NC-3.5	NC-2.1 NC-2.2	BD-1.14.1
Galactose-1-phosphate uridyl transferase	abnormal	NI-5.8.3 NC-3.5	NC-2.1 NC-2.2	BD-1.14.2
Fructose	abnormal	NI-5.8.3 NC-3.5	NC-2.1 NC-2.2	BD-1.14.3
Fatty acid profile				
Acylcarnitine, carnitine, and other measures of fatty acid metabolism	abnormal	NI-5.5.3 NC-3.5	NC-2.1 NC-2.2	BD-1.15

Nutrition Assessment Matrix

Nutrition-Focused Physical Findings Data and Related Nutrition Diagnostic Terminology

Parameter (not all-inclusive)	Findings	Nutrition Diagnostic Terminology		Nutrition Assessment and/or ME Code	
Overall findings					
Thin, wasted	present	NC-1.4	NC-2.1	PD-1.1.1.3	
Adipose					
Fat, subcutaneous	decreased	NI-1.4	NC-4.1.3	PD-1.1.2.1	PD-1.1.2.3
		NI-2.9	NB-1.5		
		NC-4.1.2	NB-3.3		
		NC-4.1.5	NI-2.7		
		NB-2.2	NC-4.1.1		
		NI-2.5	NC-4.1.4		
		NC-3.2	NB-2.1		
	increased	NI-1.5	NC-3.3	PD-1.1.2.2	PD-1.1.2.6
		NB-3.2	NB-1.5	PD-1.1.2.4	PD-1.1.2.7
				PD-1.1.2.5	
Bones					
Rachitic rosary	present	NI-5.9.1	NI-5.11.1	PD-1.1.3.4	
Rickets	present	NI-5.9.1	NI-5.11.1	PD-1.1.3.5	
Cardiovascular-pulmonary system					
Edema, pulmonary	crackles or rales	NI-3.2		PD-1.1.4.10	
Dyspnea (shortness of breath)	present	NI-3.2	NB-2.6	PD-1.1.4.5	
		NC-2.2			
Digestive system					
Abdominal distention, belching, bloating, cramping, pain, gas	present	NI-4.2	NC-1.4	PD-1.1.5.1	PD-1.1.5.4
		NI-5.8.3	NB-3.4	PD-1.1.5.2	PD-1.1.5.15
		NI-5.10.2	NI-5.5.3	PD-1.1.5.3	PD-1.1.5.16
		NB-3.1	NI-5.9.2		
		NI-5.5.2	NB-1.5		
		NI-5.8.6			
Self-induced vomiting, diarrhea, constipation, flatulence	present	NB-1.5		PD-1.1.5.9	PD-1.1.5.16
				PD-1.1.5.11	PD-1.1.5.27

Parameter (not all-inclusive)	Findings	Nutrition Diagnostic Terminology		Nutrition Assessment and/or ME Code	
Appetite, specify	hunger	NI-5.2	NC-3.4	PD-1.1.5.21	
		NC-2.3	NC-3.1		
		NB-3.3	NB-3.2		
		NC-1.3			
	anorexia	NI-1.2	NC-1.4	PD-1.1.5.6	
		NI-5.10.2	NI-3.2		
		NC-2.3	NC-2.2		
		NI-2.1			
Ascites	present	NI-3.2	NC-2.2	PD-1.1.5.7	
Bowel function	constipation	NI-4.2	NC-1.4	PD-1.1.5.9	
		NI-5.8.5	NI-5.8.3		
		NI-5.4	NB-1.5		
	diarrhea	NI-2.3	NI-5.8.2	PD-1.1.5.11	
		NI-2.7	NC-1.3		
		NI-5.2	NB-3.1		
		NI-5.5.3	NI-2.6		
		NI-5.8.6	NI-4.2		
		NB-1.5	NI-5.5.2		
		NI-2.5	NI-5.8.3		
		NI-3.1	NC-1.4		
		NI-5.4	NB-3.4		
	steatorrhea	NI-5.2	NI-5.5.2	PD-1.1.5.17	
		NC-1.4	NI-5.5.3		
	flatus	NI-5.8.6	NB-1.5	PD-1.1.5.16	
		NC-1.4			
	volume/frequency increased	NI-5.8.6		PD-1.1.5	
	incontinence	NC-1.4		PD-1.1.5	
Bowel sounds	abnormal	NC-1.4		PD-1.1.5.19	PD-1.1.5.20
Epigastric pain	present	NI-5.4	NI-5.5.3	PD-1.1.5.13	
		NI-5.5.2			
Reflux, GERD	present	NI-5.8.3		PD-1.1.5	

Parameter (not all-inclusive)	Findings	Nutrition Diagnostic Terminology		Nutrition Assessment and/or ME Code
Nausea	present	NI-2.1	NI-4.2	PD-1.1.5.24
		NI-2.7	NI-5.9.2	
		NI-3.2	NC-2.2	
		NI-5.8.6	NI-2.6	
		NC-1.4	NI-2.10	
		NI-2.3	NI-5.4	
		NI-2.9	NB-3.1	
Vomiting	present	NI-2.1	NC-1.4	PD-1.1.5.27
		NI-2.7	NB-3.1	
		NI-5.7.1	NI-2.6	
		NC-1.3	NI-5.4	
		NB-1.5	NI-5.9.2	
		NI-2.3	NC-2.2	
		NI-3.2	NB-3.4	
		NI-5.8.6		
Edema				
Edema, peripheral , generalized	present	NI-2.4	NC-2.2	PD-1.1.4
		NI-2.9	NC-4.1.3	
		NI-5.6.1	NB-1.5	
		NC-4.1.2	NI-2.8	
		NC-4.1.5	NI-5.3	
		NI-2.5	NC-4.1.1	
		NI-3.2	NC-4.1.4	
Mucosa (mouth and pharynx)	edema	NI-5.9.1	NI-5.11.1	PD-1.1.6.14
Extremities				
Joint, arthralgia, effusions, mobility changes	present	NI-1.2	NI-5.9.1	PD-1.1.7
		NI-5.8.1		
Peripheral cyanosis	present	NB-1.5		PD-1.1.7.23
Eyes				
Bitot's spots	present	NI-5.9.1		PD-1.1.8.3
Night blindness	present	NI-5.9.1		PD-1.1.8.12
Vision, specify	decreased	NC-3.2	NB-3.1	PD-1.1.8
		NB-2.4		
Xeropthalmia	present	NI-5.9.1	NI-5.9.2	PD-1.1.8.15

Parameter (not all-inclusive)	Findings	Nutrition Diagnostic Terminology		Nutrition Assessment and/or ME Code	
Genitourinary system					
Hair					
Hair (specify, eg, brittle, lifeless, loss)	present	NI-2.3	NI-5.10.2	PD-1.1.10.3	PD-1.1.10.11
		NI-5.1	NB-1.5	PD-1.1.10.5	PD-1.1.10.14
		NI-5.9.2	NI-2.11	PD-1.1.10.9	
		NC-1.4	NI-5.9.1		
		NI-2.7	NI-5.11.1		
		NI-5.6.1			
Lanugo hair formation on face and trunk	present	NB-1.5		PD-1.1.10.15	
Follicular hyperkeratosis	present	NI-5.9.1		PD-1.1.10.7	
Head					
Fontanelle, bulging or sunken (in infants)	bulging	NI-5.9.2		PD-1.1.11.3	
Headache	present	NI-3.2	NI-5.9.2	PD-1.1.11.5	
Nasal mucosa dry	present	NI-5.9.2		PD-1.1.11.9	
Altered olfactory sense	decreased	NC-3.2		PD-1.1.11.1	
Hand and nails					
Nail changes	blue, clubbing	NI-5.10.2	NC-2.2	PD-1.1.12	
		NI-5.11.1			
Mouth					
Taste	alteration	NI-2.1	NC-2.3	PD-1.1.13.1	PD-1.1.13.21
		NB-1.5	NC-3.2	PD-1.1.13.14	
Cheilosis	present	NI-5.9.1	NC-2.1	PD-1.1.13.9	
		NC-1.4			
Dry mucous membranes	present	NI-2.3	NB-2.6	PD-1.1.13.13	
		NI-3.1	NB-3.4		
		NC-1.4	NI-5.9.2		
		NB-3.3	NC-1.2		
		NI-2.7	NB-3.1		
		NC-1.1			
Retains food in mouth	present	NC-1.1		PD-1.1.13.29	
Gums, gingivitis, bleeding	present	NI-2.3	NI-5.11.1	PD-1.1.13.17	PD-1.1.13.20
		NI-5.9.1	NI-2.11	PD-1.1.13.18	PD-1.1.13.32
		NI-2.7	NI-5.1		
Ketotic breath	present	NI-5.8.1		PD-1.1.13.22	
Lips, dry or cracked	present	NI-5.9.2		PD-1.1.13.2	PD-1.1.13.11

Parameter (not all-inclusive)	Findings	Nutrition Diagnostic Terminology		Nutrition Assessment and/or ME Code	
Drooling	present	NC-1.1	NB-2.6	PD-1.1.13.12	
Oral lesion	present	NC-1.2	NC-2.1	PD-1.1.13.26	
		NC-1.4			
Parotid swelling	present	NB-1.5		PD-1.1.13.27	
Stomatitis	present	NI-5.9.1	NI-5.11.1	PD-1.1.13.2	
Muscles					
Muscle atrophy	present	NI-1.4	NC-4.1.1	PD-1.1.14.1	PD-1.1.14.10
		NI-2.7	NC-4.1.4	PD-1.1.14.6	PD-1.1.14.11
		NI-5.1	NB-2.1	PD-1.1.14.7	PD-1.1.14.12
		NC-3.5	NI-2.5	PD-1.1.14.8	PD-1.1.14.13
		NC-4.1.3	NI-5.6.1	PD-1.1.14.9	
		NB-1.5	NC-3.2		
		NB-3.3	NC-4.1.2		
		NI-2.3	NC-4.1.5		
		NI-2.9	NB-2.2		
		NC-3.1			
Muscle soreness, weakness	present	NI-3.2	NB-2.2	PD-1.1.14.4	PD-1.1.14.5
		NB-1.5	NC-3.4		
		NC-1.1			
Nerves, cognition, and feelings					
Abnormal gait	present	NI-5.9.1		PD-1.1.16.1	
Confusion, loss of concentration	present	NI-5.9.1	NB-1.5	PD-1.1.16.5	PD-1.1.16.11
Cranial nerve finding	altered	NC-1.1	NC-1.2	PD-1.1.16.6	
Dizziness	present	NB-3.1		PD-1.1.16.12	
Neurological changes	present	NI-2.3	NI-2.7	PD-1.1.16	
		NI-4.2	NI-2.11		
Decreased vibratory sense	present	NI-5.9.1		PD-1.1.16.7	
Hands and feet	tingling, numbness	NI-5.9.1		PD-1.1.16.19	PD-1.1.16.23
				PD-1.1.16.20	PD-1.1.16.24
Feels cold	present	NB-1.5		PD-1.1.16.13	
Skin					
Calcinosis	present	NI-5.9.2	NI-5.10.2	PD-1.1.17.2	
Ecchymosis	present	NI-5.9.1		PD-1.1.17.9	

Parameter (not all-inclusive)	Findings	Nutrition Diagnostic Terminology		Nutrition Assessment and/or ME Code	
Skin, specify	changes consistent with nutrient deficiency/excess	NI-5.5.1	NB-1.7	PD-1.1.17	
		NC-1.4	NI-5.11.1		
		NI-5.9.1	NB-3.4		
	dermatitis	NC-1.4	NI-5.5.3	PD-1.1.17.6	
		NI-5.5.1			
	dry	NI-2.1	NI-3.1	PD-1.1.17.8	
		NB-1.5	NI-5.5.1		
	erythema, scaling, and peeling	NI-5.9.2		PD-1.1.17.10	PD-1.1.17.40
				PD-1.1.17.19	
	Flushing, skin rash	NI-5.9.1	NI-5.9.2	PD-1.1.17.12	PD-1.1.17.48
		NC-1.4	NI-4.2	PD-1.1.17.42	
Impaired skin integrity	decreased	NI-2.1	NI-5.1	PD-1.1.17.15	
		NI-3.1	NI-2.7		
		NB-3.3	NC-1.1		
		NI-2.3			
Jaundice	present	NC-2.2		PD-1.1.17.16	
Teeth					
Teeth	missing, caries, damaged enamel, poorly fitting dentures	NI-1.2	NB-1.5	PD-1.1.18	
		NC-1.2	NI-5.8.2		
		NI-2.11			
Throat and swallowing					
Pain, coughing, choking, swallow impairment	present	NI-3.1	NC-1.3	PD-1.1.19.1	PD-1.1.19.9
		NC-1.1		PD-1.1.19.2	PD-1.1.19.10
Food sticks on swallowing	present	NC-1.1		PD-1.1.19.5	
Hoarse voice	present	NC-1.1	NB-2.6	PD-1.1.19.7	
Tongue					
Red, glossitis	present	NI-5.9.1	NI-5.11.1	PD-1.1.20.2	PD-1.1.20.15
		NC-2.1	NC-1.4	PD-1.1.20.5	
Impaired tongue movement, extrusion	present	NC-1.2	NB-2.6	PD-1.1.20.3	
		NC-1.1			
Short or split frenulum (infants)	present	NC-1.3		PD-1.1.20.11,	PD-1.1.20.12
Vital signs					

Nutrition Assessment Matrix

Client History Data and Related Diagnostic Terminology

Parameter (not all-inclusive)	Nutrition Diagnostic Terminology		Nutrition Assessment and/or ME Code
Personal history			
Literacy factors	NB-1.1		CH-1.1.5
Ethnic- and cultural-related issues	NB-2.5		CH-1.1.3
Physical disability, developmental disability or limitation	NI-2.11	NB-3.2	CH-1.1.9
	NB-2.6	NC-3.3	
	NB-3.4	NB-3.3	
	NC-3.1		
Patient/client/family Medical/Health history			
Cardiovascular			CH-2.1.2 P or F
Angina	NI-5.5.2		CH-2.1.2 P or F
Arrythmias	NI-4.2	NB-1.5	CH-2.1.2 P or F
Atherosclerosis	NI-5.5.2	NI-5.5.3	CH-2.1.2 P or F
Cardiovascular/heart disease	NI-3.2	NI-5.10.2	CH-2.1.2 P or F
	NI-5.2	NC-4.1.5	
	NI-5.9.2	NI-4.2	
	NC-4.1.2	NI-5.5.3	
	NB-2.3	NC-2.2	
	NI-4.1	NB-1.2	
	NI-5.3		
Cardiac changes	NB-3.1		CH-2.1.2 P or F
Hyperlipidemia	NI-5.5.2	NI-5.5.3	CH-2.1.2 P or F
Hypertension	NI-4.2	NI-5.3	CH-2.1.2 P or F
	NI-4.3		
Hypertriglyceridemia	NI-4.3		CH-2.1.2 P or F
Endocrine/metabolism			
Cushing's syndrome	NC-3.4	NC-3.6	CH-2.1.3 P or F

Parameter (not all-inclusive)	Nutrition Diagnostic Terminology		Nutrition Assessment and/or ME Code
Diabetes mellitus	NI-3.1	NC-4.1.2	CH-2.1.3 P or F
	NI-5.8.4	NB-1.4	
	NC-3.5	NI-5.8.2	
	NB-1.2	NC-2.2	
	NI-5.5.3	NC-4.1.5	
	NC-1.2	NB-2.3	
Giantism	NC-3.6		CH-2.1.3 P or F
Hyperthyroidism (pre- or untreated)	NC-3.2	NC-3.5	CH-2.1.3 P or F
Hypoglycemia	NI-5.8.3	NI-5.8.4	CH-2.1.3 P or F
Hypothyroidism	NC-3.3	NC-3.4	CH-2.1.3 P or F
	NC-3.6	NC-3.5	
Inborn errors of metabolism	NI-5.6.3	NC-2.1	CH-2.1.3 P or F
	NI-5.8.3	NI-5.8.2	
	NC-3.5	NC-2.2	
	NI-5.7.1		
Metabolic syndrome	NI-2.2	NI-5.8.4	CH-2.1.3 P or F
Obesity, childhood	NC-3.3		CH-2.1.3 P or F
Obesity, overweight	NI-2.2	NI-5.10.1	CH-2.1.3 P or F
	NI-5.8.4	NB-1.4	
	NC-4.1	NI-5.8.2	
	NI-5.5.3	NC-3.3	
Obesity, morbid	NB-2.1		CH-2.1.3 P or F
Other endocrine, pituitary disorders	NC-2.1	NC-3.6	CH-2.1.3 P or F
	NC-3.4		
Poisoning from foodstuffs or poisonous plants	NB-3.1		CH-2.1.5 P or F
Poisoning by drugs, medicinals, or biological substances	NB-3.1		CH-2.1.3 P or F
Refeeding syndrome	NI-5.4		CH-2.1.3 P or F
Excretory			
Kidney stones	NI-5.10.1		CH-2.1.4 P or F
Nephrotic syndrome	NI-3.2		CH-2.1.4 P or F

Parameter (not all-inclusive)	Nutrition Diagnostic Terminology		Nutrition Assessment and/or ME Code
Kidney disease	NI-3.2	NI-5.10.2	CH-2.1.4 P or F
	NI-5.6.3	NB-2.3	
	NI-5.9.2	NI-5.6.2	
	NC-2.2	NI-5.9.1	
	NI-5.3	NC-2.1	
	NI-5.7.1		
SIADH	NI-3.2		CH-2.1.4 P or F
Gastrointestinal			
Achalasia	NC-1.1		CH-2.1.5 P or F
Biliary disease	NI-5.5.2	NI-5.5.3	CH-2.1.5 P or F
Candidiasis	NC-1.2	NC-1.3	CH-2.1.5 P or F
Celiac disease	NI-5.6.3	NC-1.4	CH-2.1.5 P or F
	NI-5.10.1	NI-5.9.1	
	NC-3.5	NC-2.1	
	NI-5.8.1		
Crohn's disease	NI-2.3	NC-1.2	CH-2.1.5 P or F
	NI-5.3	NC-3.5	
	NC-2.1	NI-5.1	
	NI-2.7	NC-1.4	
Diverticulitis	NI-5.8.6	NC-1.4	CH-2.1.5 P or F
Dysphasia	NC-1.1	NC-3.2	CH-2.1.5 P or F
	NB-2.6	NC-3.5	
Encephalopathy, hepatic	NI-5.3		CH-2.1.5 P or F
Foodborne illness, e.g., bacterial, viral, and parasitic infection	NB-3.1		CH-2.1.5 P or F
Gastrointestinal stricture, obstruction	NI-5.8.6	NC-1.4	CH-2.1.5 P or F
	NC-4.1.5	NC-4.1.2	
Thrush	NC-1.3		CH-2.1.5 P or F
Inflammatory bowel disease	NI-5.8.5	NI-5.8.6	CH-2.1.5 P or F
	NC-1.4	NI-5.10.1	
Irritable bowel syndrome	NI-5.3	NI-5.8.6	CH-2.1.5 P or F
	NC-4.1.5	NC-1.4	
Lactase deficiency	NI-5.8.2		CH-2.1.5 P or F
Leukoplakia, oral	NC-1.2		CH-2.1.5 P or F

Parameter (not all-inclusive)	Nutrition Diagnostic Terminology		Nutrition Assessment and/or ME Code
Liver disease	NI-2.9	NI-5.8.1	CH-2.1.5 P or F
	NI-4.3	NI-5.10.2	
	NI-5.5.2	NC-3.5	
	NI-5.7.1	NI-3.2	
	NI-5.10.1	NI-5.5.1	
	NC-2.2	NI-5.6.2	
	NI-2.10	NI-5.9.2	
	NI-5.3	NC-2.1	
	NI-5.5.3	NB-2.3	
Malabsorption	NI-2.1	NC-1.4	CH-2.1.5 P or F
	NI-5.5.1	NC-4.1.2	
	NI-5.9.1	NI-5.2	
	NC-4.1.1	NI-5.8.1	
	NC-4.1.5	NC-3.5	
	NI-5.6.1	NC-4.1.3	
Maldigestion	NC-1.4	NC-4.1.3	CH-2.1.5 P or F
	NC-4.1.2	NC-4.1.1	
	NC-3.5	NC-4.1.5	
Malnutrition	NI-2.3	NC-4.1.4	CH-2.1.5 P or F
	NI-5.2	NB-3.4	
	NC-3.5	NI-5.1	
	NC-4.1.3	NC-3.1	
	NB-3.3	NC-4.1.2	
	NI-2.7	NC-4.1.5	
	NC-1.4	NB-3.2	
	NC-4.1.1		
Other, GI function	NI-2.5	NI-2.6	CH-2.1.5 P or F
	NC-1.4	NI-2.9	
Pancreatitis	NI-5.5.2	NI-5.5.3	CH-2.1.5 P or F
Pancreatic disease, insufficiency	NI-4.3	NI-5.8.2	CH-2.1.5 P or F
	NI-5.8.1	NI-5.5.2	
	NI-5.5.1	NC-3.5	
Pellagra	NI-5.9.1		CH-2.1.5 P or F
Phytobezoar	NI-5.8.6		CH-2.1.5 P or F
Polyps, colon	NI-5.10.1		CH-2.1.5 P or F
Prolapsing hemorrhoids	NI-5.8.6		CH-2.1.5 P or F

Parameter (not all-inclusive)	Nutrition Diagnostic Terminology		Nutrition Assessment and/or ME Code	
Short bowel syndrome	NI-5.8.6 NC-2.1 NI-5.9.1	NC-3.5 NI-5.10.1	CH-2.1.5 P or F	
Ulcer disease	NI-5.8.5	NI-5.8.6	CH-2.1.5 P or F	
Vagotomy	NC-1.4		CH-2.1.5 P or F	
Wired jaw	NC-1.2		CH-2.1.5 P or F	
Gynecological				
Amenorrhea	NB-2.2		CH-2.1.6 P or F	
Giving birth to an infant with fetal alcohol syndrome	NI-4.3		CH-2.1.6 P or F FH-1.4.1.1	FH-1.4.1.2 FH-1.4.1.3
Engorgement	NC-1.3		CH-2.1.6 P or F FH-6.1.4	
Mastitis	NC-1.3		CH-2.1.6 P or F FH-6.1.4	
Polycystic ovary disease	NI-5.10.1		CH-2.1.6 P or F	
Postmenopausal without estrogen supplementation	NI-5.10.1		CH-2.1.6 P or F	
Premature birth	NI-2.3 NI-5.9.1 NI-2.7	NC-1.3 NI-5.1 NC-3.5	CH-2.1.6 P or F	
Premenstrual syndrome	NI-5.10.1		CH-2.1.6 P or F	
Hematology/oncology				
Anemia	NI-5.9.1 NI-5.10.1	NB-1.5	CH-2.1.7 P or F	
Cancer, head, neck, or pharyngeal	NI-2.5 NI-2.10 NC-4.1.5 NI-2.6	NC-1.2 NI-2.9 NC-4.1.2	CH-2.1.7 P or F	
Cancer (other)	NI-5.9.2 NC-4.1.2 NC-3.2	NC-4.1.5 NC-3.5 NC-1.2	CH-2.1.7 P or F	
Hyperemia	NI-5.9.1		CH-2.1.7 P or F	

Parameter (not all-inclusive)	Nutrition Diagnostic Terminology		Nutrition Assessment and/or ME Code
Immune			
AIDS/HIV	NI-2.1	NI-5.5.1	CH-2.1.8 P or F
	NI-5.1	NC-3.5	
	NC-3.2	NI-2.7	
	NI-2.3	NC-1.2	
Allergies	NI-5.6.3	NI-5.8.3	CH-2.1.8 P or F
	NI-5.7.1		
Arthritis	NB-2.1		CH-2.1.8 P or F
Infection	NI-2.1	NI-5.2	CH-2.1.8 P or F
	NI-3.1	NI-5.8.2	
	NC-3.5	NB-3.1	
Sepsis or severe infection	NI-2.1	NC-4.1.3	CH-2.1.8 P or F
	NC-3.5	NI-5.8.2	
	NI-5.5.1	NC-4.1.5	
Integumentary			
Burns	NI-2.3	NC-3.5	CH-2.1.9 P or F
	NI-2.7	NI-2.6	
	NC-3.2	NI-5.1	
	NC-4.1.5	NC-4.1.3	
	NI-2.5		
	NI-2.8		
Musculoskeletal			
Cleft lip/palate, oral malformation	NC-1.2	NC-3.5	CH-2.1.10 P or F
	NC-1.3		
Fractures, stress	NB-2.2		CH-2.1.10 P or F
Fluorosis	NI-5.10.2		CH-2.1.10 P or F
Osteomalacia	NI-5.9.1		CH-2.1.10 P or F
Rachitic rosary in children	NI-5.9.1		CH-2.1.10 P or F
Rickets	NI-5.9.1		CH-2.1.10 P or F
Rheumatic conditions	NC-1.2	NC-3.4	CH-2.1.10 P or F
Neurological			
Alzheimer's disease	NI-1.1	NB-2.6	CH-2.1.11 P or F
	NC-1.2		

Parameter (not all-inclusive)	Nutrition Diagnostic Terminology		Nutrition Assessment and/or ME Code
Cerebral palsy	NI-1.1	NC-1.2	CH-2.1.11 P or F
	NB-2.4	NC-3.5	
Cognitive impairment	NB-2.3	NB-2.4	CH-2.1.11 P or F
Dementia	NI-1.2	NB-3.2	CH-2.1.11 P or F
	NB-3.1	NB-2.6	
	NI-3.1	NB-3.3	
Headache	NI-4.2	NB-3.1	CH-2.1.11 P or F
Head injury	NC-3.5	NC-4.1.5	CH-2.1.11 P or F
	NC-4.1.3		
Multiple sclerosis	NB-2.6		CH-2.1.11 P or F
Neurologic changes	NB-3.1		CH-2.1.11 P or F
Neurological disorders	NI-2.11	NB-2.6	CH-2.1.11 P or F
	NC-3.6		
Parkinson's disease	NI-1.1	NB-2.6	CH-2.1.11 P or F
Paralysis	NB-2.6		CH-2.1.11 P or F
Paraplegia	NB-2.4		CH-2.1.11 P or F
Porphyria	NC-2.1		CH-2.1.11 P or F
Seizure disorder	NI-5.8.1		CH-2.1.11 P or F
Sensory processing issues	NI-2.11		CH-2.1.11 P or F
Spina bifida	NC-3.4	NC-3.6	CH-2.1.11 P or F
Stroke	NB-2.6		CH-2.1.11 P or F
Tardive dyskinesia	NB-2.6		CH-2.1.11 P or F
Tremors	NB-2.6		CH-2.1.11 P or F
Psychological			
Addictive, obsessive, or compulsive tendencies	NB-2.2		CH-2.1.12 P or F
Alcohol, drug abuse	NI-1.2	NC-2.1	CH-2.1.12 P or F
	NC-3.5	NC-2.2	FH-3.1.3
Anxiety disorder	NI-2.2	NB-2.1	CH-2.1.12 P or F
Binge eating	NB-2.2		CH-2.1.12 P or F
Bulimia nervosa	NB-2.2		CH-2.1.12 P or F

Parameter (not all-inclusive)	Nutrition Diagnostic Terminology		Nutrition Assessment and/or ME Code
Depression	NI-2.1	NC-3.3	CH-2.1.12 P or F
	NC-3.2	NB-2.1	
	NB-1.5	NI-4.3	
	NI-2.2	NC-3.5	
Emotional impairment	NB-2.3		CH-2.1.12 P or F
Mental illness	NI-1.2	NB-1.1	CH-2.1.12 P or F
	NC-3.1	NB-3.1	
	NB-1.7	NI-5.8.6	
	NB-3.3	NB-1.2	
	NI-2.11	NB-3.2	
Personality disorder	NB-1.5		CH-2.1.12 P or F
Pica	NC-3.1	NB-1.2	CH-2.1.12 P or F
Psychiatric illness	NC-3.4		CH-2.1.12 P or F
Eating disorders, depression, obsessive–compulsive disorders, anxiety disorders	NI-1.2	NC-4.1.4	CH-2.1.12 P or F
	NI-5.8.6	NB-2.2	
	NC-4.1.1	NI-5.5.1	
	NB-1.5	NC-3.5	
	NI-2.1	NC-4.1.5	
	NC-3.2		
Respiratory			
Asthma	NI-4.2	NC-3.4	CH-2.1.13 P or F
	NI-5.9.2		
Chronic obstructive pulmonary disease	NI-1.1	NC-4.1.5	CH-2.1.13 P or F
	NC-4.1.3	NC-3.5	
	NC-3.2		
Cystic fibrosis	NI-1.1	NC-3.5	CH-2.1.13 P or F
	NC-2.1	NC-1.4	
	NC-4.1.5	NC-4.1.3	
	NI-5.5.2		
Lung injury, ARDS	NI-2.5	NC-4.1.3	CH-2.1.13 P or F
	NI-2.6	NI-2.9	
	NI-2.10		
Pulmonary failure	NI-5.2	NC-3.5	CH-2.1.13 P or F
Respiratory changes	NB-3.1		CH-2.1.13 P or F
Tuberculosis	NI-2.1	NI-5.5.1	CH-2.1.13 P or F

Parameter (not all-inclusive)	Nutrition Diagnostic Terminology		Nutrition Assessment and/or ME Code
Upper respiratory infections or pneumonia	NC-1.1 NC-4.1.3	NC-4.1.5	CH-2.1.13 P or F
Other			
Autism	NI-2.11		CH-2.1.14 P or F
Change in level of care or transfer of care	NI-2.5 NI-2.10	NI-2.6 NI-2.9	CH-2.1.14 P or F
Chronic fatigue syndrome	NB-2.1		CH-2.1.14 P or F
Chronic or acute disease, trauma, organ failure	NI-2.5 NI-5.2 NC-3.1 NC-4.1.2 NB-3.2 NI-2.6 NI-5.5.1	NC-3.2 NC-4.1.3 NB-3.3 NI-2.9 NI-5.10.1 NC-3.5 NC-4.1.5	CH-2.1.14 P or F
Chyle fluid leak	NI-5.5.2		CH-2.1.14 P or F
Critical illness	NI-2.5 NI-2.6 NI-2.10	NC-3.5 NI-2.9	CH-2.1.14 P or F
Down syndrome, Prader–Willi syndrome	NC-3.4	NC-3.6	CH-2.1.14 P or F
Injuries, frequent and prolonged	NB-2.2		CH-2.1.14 P or F
Transplantation	NI-5.5.2		CH-2.1.14 P or F
Pain, acute or chronic	NI-1.2	NI-2.1	CH-2.1.14 P or F
Conditions altering energy/nutrient needs or affecting ability to meet needs	NI-1.4 NI-5.11.2 NI-1.5	NC-3.5 NI-5.11.1 NC-3.6	CH-2.1.14 P or F
Treatments/therapy			
Medical treatment/therapy			
Chemotherapy	NC-1.2 NC-3.2	NC-3.5	CH-2.2.1
Esophageal dilatation	NC-1.4		CH-2.2.1
Radiation therapy	NC-1.2 NC-2.1	NC-3.5	CH-2.2.1
Rigorous therapy regimen	NC-3.5	NB-2.4	CH-2.2.1

Parameter (not all-inclusive)	Nutrition Diagnostic Terminology		Nutrition Assessment and/or ME Code
Medical therapy/treatment altering energy/nutrient needs or affecting ability to meet needs	NI-1.4 NI-5.11.2 NI-1.5	NC-3.5 NI-5.11.1	CH-2.2.1
Surgical treatment			
Bowel, intestinal resection	NI-2.3 NI-5.5.1 NI-2.7	NI-5.6.1 NI-5.1 NC-1.4	CH-2.2.2
Breast surgery	NC-1.3		CH-2.2.2
Esophagostomy	NC-1.4		CH-2.2.2
Gastric bypass, bariatric surgery	NI-5.10.1	NC-1.4	CH-2.2.2
Gastrectomy	NC-1.4		CH-2.2.2
Knee surgery	NB-2.1		CH-2.2.2
Oral surgery, recent major	NC-1.2		CH-2.2.2
Ostomy, new	NB-1.4		CH-2.2.2
Surgery	NI-2.5 NI-2.10 NC-3.5 NB-2.4 NI-2.6	NI-5.2 NC-4.1.3 NI-2.9 NC-3.2 NC-4.1.5	CH-2.2.2
Surgery requiring recumbent position	NB-2.6		CH-2.2.2
Surgery altering energy/nutrient needs or affecting ability to meet needs	NI-1.4 NI-5.11.2 NI-1.5	NC-3.5 NI-5.11.1	CH-2.2.2
Palliative/end-of-life care	NI-2.5 NO 1.1	NI-2.6 NI-2.9	CH-2.2.4
Social history			
Socioeconomic status associated with altered nutrient intake	NI-5.6.1 NC-4.1.1	NC-4.1.4	CH-3.1.1
Change in living environment/independence/isolation	NI-5.10.1	NI-5.11.1	CH-3.1.2
Domestic issues—abuse, physical, sexual, or emotional	NC-3.3		CH-3.1.3
Lack of suitable support system to access food or water	NC-3.5 NB-3.2	NB-3.4	CH-3.1.4

Parameter (not all-inclusive)	Nutrition Diagnostic Terminology		Nutrition Assessment and/or ME Code
Geographic location low sunlight exposure/sunscreen use	NI-5.9.1	NI-5.10.1	CH-3.1.5
Geographic location associated with altered nutrient intake	NC-4.1.1		CH-3.1.5
Geographic location associated with risk of environmental emergency/disaster	NI-5.11.1	NB-3.4	CH-3.1.5
Occupation of athlete, dancer, gymnast	NC-3.1		CH-3.1.6
Recent other lifestyle or life changes, e.g., quit smoking, initiated exercise, work change, home relocation	NI-1.4	NB-2.5	CH-3.1.9
History of recent crisis, new medical diagnosis, or change in existing diagnosis or condition	NI-1.4 NB-1.4 NI-4.3	NB-2.3 NB-1.1 NB-2.5	CH-3.1.8

Nutrition Diagnosis Etiology Matrix

Below are the etiology categories and their definitions. Etiologies are grouped by the type of cause or contributing risk factor. In two specific instances, Access and Behavior etiologies, these alone may be the cause or contributing risk factor of the nutrition diagnosis, or the practitioner may determine a more specific root cause, eg, the beliefs and attitudes of the problem.

Etiology Category	Definition
Beliefs–Attitudes Etiologies	Cause or contributing risk factors related to the conviction of the truth of some nutrition-related statement or phenomenon; feelings or emotions toward that truth or phenomenon and activities
Cultural Etiologies	Cause or contributing risk factors related to the patient/client's values, social norms, customs, religious beliefs, and/or political systems
Knowledge Etiologies	Cause or contributing risk factors impacting the level of understanding about food, nutrition, and health or nutrition-related information and guidelines
Physical Function Etiologies	Cause or contributing risk factors related to physical ability to engage in specific tasks; may be cognitive in nature
Physiologic–Metabolic Etiologies	Cause or contributing risk factors related to medical/health status that may have a nutritional impact (excludes psychological etiologies—see separate category)
Psychological Etiologies	Cause or contributing risk factors related to a diagnosed or suspected mental health/psychological problem (*Diagnostic and Statistical Manual of Mental Disorders* [*DSM*])
Social–Personal Etiologies	Cause or contributing risk factors associated with the patient/client's personal and/or social history
Treatment Etiologies	Cause or contributing risk factors related to medical or surgical treatment or other therapies and management or care
Access Etiologies	Cause or contributing risk factors that affect intake and the availability of safe, healthful food, water, and food-/nutrition-related supplies. A more specific root cause of Access Etiologies may not be known but may eventually reveal Beliefs–Attitudes, Cultural, Knowledge, Physical Function, Psychological, Social–Personal, or Treatment Etiologies
Behavior Etiologies	Cause or contributing risk factors related to actions which influence achievement of nutrition-related goals. A more specific root cause of Behavior Etiologies may not be known but may eventually reveal Beliefs–Attitudes, Cultural, Knowledge, Physical Function, Psychological, Social–Personal, or Treatment Etiologies

Category	Etiology	Diagnosis
Beliefs–Attitudes	Altered body image	Poor nutrition quality of life (NB-2.5)
Beliefs–Attitudes	Food preference	Limited food acceptance (NI-2.11), Excessive fat intake (NI-5.5.2), Intake of types of fats inconsistent with needs (specify) (NI-5.5.3), Undesirable food choices (NB-1.7)
Beliefs–Attitudes	Denial of need to change	Not ready for diet/lifestyle change (NB-1.3)
Beliefs–Attitudes	Desire for a cure for a chronic disease through the use of alternative therapy	Unsupported beliefs/attitudes about food- or nutrition-related topics (NB-1.2)
Beliefs–Attitudes	Disbelief in science-based food and nutrition information	Unsupported beliefs/attitudes about food- or nutrition-related topics (NB-1.2)
Beliefs–Attitudes	End-of-life care if patient/client or family does not desire nutrition support	Enteral nutrition composition inconsistent with needs (NI-2.5), Enteral nutrition administration inconsistent with needs (NI-2.6), Parenteral nutrition composition inconsistent with needs (NI-2.9), Parenteral nutrition administration inconsistent with needs (NI-2.10)
Beliefs–Attitudes	Familial, societal, biological/genetic, and/or environmental related obsessive desire to be thin	Disordered eating pattern (NB-1.5)
Beliefs–Attitudes	Food faddism	Imbalance of nutrients (NI-5.4), Excessive protein intake (NI-5.6.2), Intake of types of proteins inconsistent with needs (specify) (NI-5.6.3), Excessive mineral intake (specify) (NI-5.10.2)
Beliefs–Attitudes	Limited food acceptance due to food aversion	Inadequate oral intake (NI-2.1), Limited food acceptance (NI-2.11)
Beliefs–Attitudes	Unsupported beliefs/attitudes about food, nutrition, and nutrition-related information	Excessive energy intake (NI-1.3), Inadequate oral intake (NI-2.1), Excessive oral intake (NI-2.2), Limited food acceptance (NI-2.11), Excessive alcohol intake (NI-4.3), Imbalance of nutrients (NI-5.4), Excessive fat intake (NI-5.5.2), Intake of types of fats inconsistent with needs (specify) (NI-5.5.3), Excessive protein intake (NI-5.6.2), Intake of types of proteins inconsistent with needs (specify) (NI-5.6.3), Intake of types of amino acids inconsistent with needs (specify) (NI-5.7.1), Excessive fiber intake (NI-5.8.6), Excessive mineral intake (specify) (NI-5.10.2), Predicted breastfeeding difficulty (NC-1.5), Underweight (NC-3.1), Growth rate below expected (NC-3.5), Food- and nutrition-related knowledge deficit (NB-1.1), Not ready for diet/lifestyle change (NB-1.3), Limited adherence to nutrition-related recommendations (NB-1.6), Physical inactivity (NB-2.1), Excessive physical activity (NB-2.2), Limited access to food (NB-3.2), Limited access to potable water (NB-3.4)
Beliefs–Attitudes	Irritability	Breastfeeding difficulty (NC-1.3)
Beliefs–Attitudes	Lack of self-efficacy for making change or demoralization from previous failures at change	Not ready for diet/lifestyle change (NB-1.3), Limited adherence to nutrition-related recommendations (NB-1.6), Poor nutrition quality of life (NB-2.5)
Beliefs–Attitudes	Lack of confidence in ability to change	Limited adherence to nutrition-related recommendations (NB-1.6)
Beliefs–Attitudes	Lack of value for behavior change or competing values	Excessive energy intake (NI-1.3), Excessive oral intake (NI-2.2), Excessive alcohol intake (NI-4.3), Excessive fat intake (NI-5.5.2), Intake of types of fats inconsistent with needs (specify) (NI-5.5.3), Self-monitoring deficit (NB-1.4), Limited adherence to nutrition-related recommendations (NB-1.6), Physical inactivity (NB-2.1), Inability to manage self-care (NB-2.3)

Category	Etiology	Diagnosis
Beliefs—Attitudes	Lacks motivation and/or readiness to apply or support systems change	Undesirable food choices (NB-1.7)
Beliefs—Attitudes	Negative impact of current or previous medical nutrition therapy (MNT)	Poor nutrition quality of life (NB-2.5)
Beliefs—Attitudes	Not ready for diet/lifestyle change	Overweight, adult or pediatric (NC-3.3.1); Obese, pediatric (NC-3.3.2); Obese, Class I (NC-3.3.3); Obese, Class II (NC-3.3.4); Obese, Class III (NC-3.3.5); Unintended weight gain (NC-3.4); Excessive growth rate (NC-3.6); Self-monitoring deficit (NB-1.4); Inability to manage self-care (NB-2.3); Poor nutrition quality of life (NB-2.5)
Beliefs—Attitudes	Perception of inadequate milk supply	Breastfeeding difficulty (NC-1.3), Predicted breastfeeding difficulty (NC-1.5)
Beliefs—Attitudes	Perception that lack of resources (eg, time, financial, or interpersonal) prevent:	
	Selection/food choices consistent with recommendations	Undesirable food choices (NB-1.7)
	Changes	Not ready for diet/lifestyle change (NB-1.3), Limited adherence to nutrition-related recommendations (NB-1.6)
	Sufficient level of activity	Physical inactivity (NB-2.1)
	Self-monitoring	Self-monitoring deficit (NB-1.4), Inability to manage self-care (NB-2.3)
Beliefs—Attitudes	Unwilling or disinterested in:	
	Learning/applying information	Food- and nutrition-related knowledge deficit (NB-1.1), Not ready for diet/lifestyle change (NB-1.3), Limited adherence to nutrition-related recommendations (NB-1.6), Undesirable food choices (NB-1.7), Inability to manage self-care (NB-2.3)
	Reducing energy intake	Excessive energy intake (NI-1.3)
	Reducing intake	Excessive oral intake (NI-2.2)
	Modify protein or amino acid intake	Intake of types of proteins inconsistent with needs (specify) (NI-5.6.3), Intake of types of amino acids inconsistent with needs (specify) (NI-5.7.1)
	Tracking progress	Self-monitoring deficit (NB-1.4)
	Unwillingness to purchase or consume fiber-containing foods	Inadequate fiber intake (NI-5.8.5)
	Weight regulation/preoccupation significantly influences self-esteem	Disordered eating pattern (NB-1.5)
Cultural	Culture of overeating	Predicted excessive energy intake (NI-1.5)
Cultural	Practices that affect nutrient intake	Predicted inadequate nutrient intake (specify) (NI-5.11.1)

Category	Etiology	Diagnosis
Cultural	Cultural practices that affect ability to:	
	Access to food, fluid, nutrients	Inadequate energy intake (NI-1.2), Inadequate oral intake (NI-2.1), Inadequate fluid intake (NI-3.1), Starvation Related Malnutrition (undernutrition) (NC-4.1.1), Inadequate protein-energy intake (NI-5.2), Inadequate protein intake (NI-5.6.1), Inadequate carbohydrate intake (NI-5.8.1), Inadequate vitamin intake (specify) (NI-5.9.1), Inadequate mineral intake (specify) (NI-5.10.1), Unintended weight loss (NC-3.2), Limited access to food (NB-3.2), Limited access to potable water (NB-3.4)
	Make appropriate food choices	Inadequate fat intake (NI-5.5.1)
	Breastfeed	Breastfeeding difficulty (NC-1.3), Predicted breastfeeding difficulty (NC-1.5)
	Learn/apply information	Food- and nutrition-related knowledge deficit (NB-1.1), Undesirable food choices (NB-1.7)
	Manage self-care	Inability to manage self-care (NB-2.3)
	Reduce carbohydrate intake	Excessive carbohydrate intake (NI-5.8.2)
	Regulate types of protein or amino acids consumed	Intake of types of proteins inconsistent with needs (specify) (NI-5.6.3), Intake of types of amino acids inconsistent with needs (specify) (NI-5.7.1)
	Regulate timing of carbohydrate consumption	Inconsistent carbohydrate intake (NI-5.8.4)
	Regulate types of carbohydrate consumed	Intake of types of carbohydrate inconsistent with needs (specify) (NI-5.8.3)
	Track personal progress	Self-monitoring deficit (NB-1.4)
Knowledge	Food and nutrition knowledge deficit	Inadequate energy intake (NI-1.2); Excessive energy intake (NI-1.3); Excessive oral intake (NI-2.2); Inadequate fluid intake (NI-3.1); Excessive fluid intake (NI-3.2); Inadequate bioactive substance intake (specify) (NI-4.1); Excessive bioactive substance intake (specify) (NI-4.2); Excessive alcohol intake (NI-4.3); Starvation related malnutrition (undernutrition) (NC-4.1.1); Acute disease or injury related malnutrition (undernutrition) (NC-4.1.3); Inadequate protein-energy intake (NI-5.2); Imbalance of nutrients (NI-5.4); Excessive fat intake (NI-5.5.2); Inadequate protein intake (NI-5.6.1); Excessive protein intake (NI-5.6.2); Inadequate carbohydrate intake (NI-5.8.1); Inadequate fiber intake (NI-5.8.5); Excessive mineral intake (specify) (NI-5.10.2); Predicted breastfeeding difficulty (NC-1.5); Overweight, adult or pediatric (NC-3.3.1); Obese, pediatric (NC-3.3.2); Obese, Class I (NC-3.3.3); Obese, Class II (NC-3.3.4); Obese, Class III (NC-3.3.5); Excessive growth rate (NC-3.6); Self-monitoring deficit (NB-1.4); Inability to manage self-care (NB-2.3); Poor nutrition quality of life (NB-2.5); Limited access to food (NB-3.2); Limited access to nutrition-related supplies (NB-3.3); Limited access to potable water (NB-3.4)

Category	Etiology	Diagnosis
Knowledge	**Food and nutrition knowledge deficit concerning:**	
	• Sufficient oral food/beverage intake	Inadequate oral intake (NI-2.1)
	• Consumption of an appropriate variety of foods	Excessive mineral intake (specify) (NI-5.10.2)
	• Potentially unsafe food	Intake of unsafe food (NB-3.1)
	• Proper infant feeding, food/feeding preparation and storage	Intake of unsafe food (NB-3.1)
	• Adequate energy intake	Underweight (NC-3.1)
	• Appropriate amount or types of dietary protein or amino acids	Non illness related pediatric malnutrition (undernutrition) (NC-4.1.4), Inadequate protein-energy intake (NI-5.2), Inadequate protein intake (NI-5.6.1), Intake of types of proteins inconsistent with needs (specify) (NI-5.6.3), Intake of types of amino acids inconsistent with needs (specify) (NI-5.7.1)
	• Appropriate amount or types of dietary fat	Inadequate protein-energy intake (NI-5.2), Inadequate fat intake (NI-5.5.1), Excessive fat intake (NI-5.5.2), Intake of types of fats inconsistent with needs (specify) (NI-5.5.3)
	• Appropriate amount or types of dietary carbohydrate	Excessive carbohydrate intake (NI-5.8.2), Intake of types of carbohydrate inconsistent with needs (specify) (NI-5.8.3)
	• Appropriate timing of carbohydrate intake	Inconsistent carbohydrate intake (NI-5.8.4)
	• Physiological causes requiring careful timing and consistency in the amount of carbohydrate	Inconsistent carbohydrate intake (NI-5.8.4)
	• Physiological causes altering carbohydrate digestion or metabolism	Intake of types of carbohydrate inconsistent with needs (specify) (NI-5.8.3)
	• Physiological causes requiring use of modified carbohydrate intake	Excessive carbohydrate intake (NI-5.8.2)
	• Desirable quantities of fiber	Inadequate fiber intake (NI-5.8.5), Excessive fiber intake (NI-5.8.6)
	• Correct enteral formula needed	Inadequate enteral nutrition infusion (NI-2.3)
	• Food and supplemental sources of vitamins	Inadequate vitamin intake (specify) (NI-5.9.1), Excessive vitamin intake (specify) (NI-5.9.2)
	• Food and supplemental sources of minerals	Inadequate mineral intake (specify) (NI-5.10.1)
	• Recommended dose of vitamin and mineral supplements	Imbalance of nutrients (NI-5.4)
	• Management of diagnosis requiring mineral restriction	Excessive mineral intake (specify) (NI-5.10.2)
	• Management of diagnosed genetic disorder altering mineral homeostasis	Excessive mineral intake (specify) (NI-5.10.2)

Category	Etiology	Diagnosis
	• Correct amount of enteral/parenteral formula	Excessive energy intake (NI-1.3), Excessive parenteral nutrition infusion (NI-2.8)
	• Correct parenteral nutrition components or administration	Inadequate parenteral nutrition infusion (NI-2.7), Parenteral nutrition composition inconsistent with needs (NI-2.9), Parenteral nutrition administration inconsistent with needs (NI-2.10)
	• Appropriate/correct access for delivering EN/PN	Inadequate enteral nutrition infusion (NI-2.3), Inadequate parenteral nutrition infusion (NI-2.7), Parenteral nutrition administration inconsistent with needs (NI-2.10)
	• Health benefits of physical activity	Physical inactivity (NB-2.1)
	• How to make nutrition-related changes	Limited adherence to nutrition-related recommendations (NB-1.6)
	• Food–drug interactions	Food–medication interaction (NC-2.3), Predicted food–medication interaction (NC-2.4)
	• The part of the caregiver	Excessive enteral nutrition infusion (NI-2.4), Excessive parenteral nutrition infusion (NI-2.8), Enteral nutrition composition inconsistent with needs (NI-2.5), Enteral nutrition administration inconsistent with needs (NI-2.6), Parenteral nutrition composition inconsistent with needs (NI-2.9), Parenteral nutrition administration inconsistent with needs (NI-2.10)
	• Consumption of high-dose nutrient supplements	Imbalance of nutrients (NI-5.4)
	• Infant/child hunger cues	Food- and nutrition-related knowledge deficit (NB-1.1)
Knowledge	Lack of prior exposure or exposure to inaccurate nutrition-related information	Food- and nutrition-related knowledge deficit (NB-1.1), Unsupported beliefs/attitudes about food or nutrition-related topics (NB-1.2), Self-monitoring deficit (NB-1.4), Undesirable food choices (NB-1.7), Inability to manage self-care (NB-2.3)
Knowledge	Lack of prior exposure to accurate information regarding physical activity	Physical inactivity (NB-2.1)
Knowledge	Failure to adjust for lifestyle changes or restricted mobility and decreased metabolism	Excessive energy intake (NI-1.3)
Physical function	Irritability	Breastfeeding difficulty (NC-1.3)
Physical function	Inability to physically: • Bend elbow at wrist • Grasp cups and utensils • Sit with hips square and back straight • Support neck and/or control head and neck • Coordinate hand movement to mouth	Self-feeding difficulty (NB-2.6)
Physical function	Lack of self-feeding ability	Unintended weight loss (NC-3.2)
Physical function	Diminished ability to shop	Limited access to food (NB-3.2), Limited access to nutrition-related supplies (NB-3.3), Limited access to potable water (NB-3.4)
Physical function	Limited physical strength or range of motion	Self-feeding difficulty (NB-2.6)
Physical function	Physical inactivity	Overweight, adult or pediatric (NC-3.3.1); Obese, pediatric (NC-3.3.2); Obese, Class I (NC-3.3.3); Obese, Class II (NC-3.3.4); Obese, Class III (NC-3.3.5); Excessive growth rate (NC-3.6)

Category	Etiology	Diagnosis
Physical function	Change in physical activity anticipated	Predicted inadequate energy intake (NI-1.4), Predicted excessive energy intake (NI-1.5)
Physical function	Voluntary or involuntary physical activity/movement	Increased energy expenditure (NI-1.1)
Physiologic–Metabolic	Age-related demands	Inadequate protein intake (NI-5.6.1), Growth rate below expected (NC-3.5)
Physiologic–Metabolic	Alteration in gastrointestinal tract:	
	• Decreased functional length of GI tract	Increased nutrient needs (specify) (NI-5.1), Starvation related malnutrition (undernutrition) (NC-4.1.1), Chronic disease or condition related malnutrition (undernutrition) (NC-4.1.2), Acute disease or injury related malnutrition (undernutrition) (NC-4.1.3), Illness related pediatric malnutrition (undernutrition) (NC-4.1.5), Altered GI function (NC-1.4), Growth rate below expected (NC-3.5)
	• Alteration in GI anatomical structure	Increased nutrient needs (specify) (NI-5.1), Starvation related malnutrition (undernutrition) (NC-4.1.1), Chronic disease or condition related malnutrition (undernutrition) (NC-4.1.2), Acute disease or injury related malnutrition (undernutrition) (NC-4.1.3), Illness related pediatric malnutrition (undernutrition) (NC-4.1.5), Altered GI function (NC-1.4), Inadequate fat intake (NI-5.5.1), Growth rate below expected (NC-3.5)
	• Alteration in GI function	Limited food acceptance (NI-2.11), Inadequate bioactive substance intake (specify) (NI-4.1), Excessive bioactive substance intake (specify) (NI-4.2), Increased nutrient needs (specify) (NI-5.1), Starvation related malnutrition (undernutrition) (NC-4.1.1), Chronic disease or condition related malnutrition (undernutrition) (NC-4.1.2), Acute disease or injury related malnutrition (undernutrition) (NC-4.1.3), Illness related pediatric malnutrition (undernutrition) (NC-4.1.5), Inadequate fat intake (NI-5.5.1), Altered GI function (NC-1.4), Growth rate below expected (NC-3.5)
	• Change in GI tract motility	Altered GI function (NC-1.4)
	• Change in GI-related organ function	Increased nutrient needs (specify) (NI-5.1), Altered GI function (NC-1.4), Growth rate below expected (NC-3.5)
	• Compromised endocrine function	Impaired nutrient utilization (NC-2.1), Growth rate below expected (NC-3.5)
Physiologic–Metabolic	Altered cholesterol metabolism/regulation	Decreased nutrient needs (specify) (NI-5.3)
Physiologic–Metabolic	Breast or nipple abnormality	Breastfeeding difficulty (NC-1.3), Predicted breastfeeding difficulty (NC-1.5)
Physiologic–Metabolic	Changes in taste, appetite	Excessive fat intake (NI-5.5.2), Intake of types of fats inconsistent with needs (specify) (NI-5.5.3)
Physiologic–Metabolic	Conditions leading to excess fluid loss	Inadequate fluid intake (NI-3.1)
Physiologic–Metabolic	Craniofacial malformations	Biting/chewing (masticatory) difficulty (NC-1.2)
Physiologic–Metabolic	Decreased energy needs	Overweight, adult or pediatric (NC-3.3.1); Obese, pediatric (NC-3.3.2); Obese, Class I (NC-3.3.3); Obese, Class II (NC-3.3.4); Obese, Class III (NC-3.3.5); Excessive growth rate (NC-3.6)
Physiologic–Metabolic	Decreased ability to consume sufficient energy, nutrients	Inadequate energy intake (NI-1.2), Inadequate oral intake (NI-2.1), Inadequate protein-energy intake (NI-5.2), Inadequate protein intake (NI-5.6.1), Inadequate vitamin intake (specify) (NI-5.9.1), Inadequate mineral intake (specify) (NI-5.10.1), Unintended weight loss (NC-3.2), Growth rate below expected (NC-3.5)

Category	Etiology	Diagnosis
Physiologic–Metabolic	Decreased nutrient needs related to low activity levels due to chronic disease or organ failure	Excessive enteral nutrition infusion (NI-2.4), Excessive parenteral nutrition infusion (NI-2.8), Excessive vitamin intake (specify) (NI-5.9.2)
Physiologic–Metabolic	Decreased total fat need or recommendation	Excessive fat intake (NI-5.5.2)
Physiologic–Metabolic	Altered fatty acid need or recommendation	Intake of types of fats inconsistent with needs (specify) (NI-5.5.3)
Physiologic–Metabolic	Developmental delay	Limited food acceptance (NI-2.11)
Physiologic–Metabolic	Difficulty chewing or swallowing high-fiber foods	Inadequate fiber intake (NI-5.8.5)
Physiologic–Metabolic	Difficulty latching on	Breastfeeding difficulty (NC-1.3)
Physiologic–Metabolic	Excessive energy intake	Overweight, adult or pediatric (NC-3.3.1); Obese, pediatric (NC-3.3.2); Obese, Class I (NC-3.3.3); Obese, Class II (NC-3.3.4); Obese, Class III (NC-3.3.5); Excessive growth rate (NC-3.6)
Physiologic–Metabolic	Food allergies and aversions impeding food choices consistent with guidelines	Undesirable food choices (NB-1.7)
Physiologic–Metabolic	Food intolerances	Decreased nutrient needs (specify) (NI-5.3)
Physiologic–Metabolic	Genetic predisposition to overweight/obesity	Predicted excessive energy intake (NI-1.5)
Physiologic–Metabolic	Heart failure	Decreased nutrient needs (specify) (NI-5.3)
Physiologic–Metabolic	Illness causing unexpected weight gain because of head trauma, immobility, paralysis, or related condition	Unintended weight gain (NC-3.4)
Physiologic–Metabolic	Impaired cognitive ability, including learning disabilities, neurological or sensory impairment, and dementia	Inadequate fluid intake (NI-3.1), Starvation related malnutrition (undernutrition) (NC-4.1.1), Food- and nutrition-related knowledge deficit (NB-1.1), Not ready for diet/lifestyle change (NB-1.3), Self-monitoring deficit (NB-1.4), Undesirable food choices (NB-1.7), Inability to manage self-care (NB-2.3), Impaired ability to prepare foods/meals (NB-2.4), Self-feeding difficulty (NB-2.6), Limited access to food (NB-3.2)
Physiologic–Metabolic	Inadequate energy intake	Underweight (NC-3.1)
Physiologic–Metabolic	Inadequate milk supply	Breastfeeding difficulty (NC-1.3), Chronic disease or condition related malnutrition (undernutrition) (NC-4.1.2), Acute disease or injury related malnutrition (undernutrition) (NC-4.1.3)
Physiologic–Metabolic	Increased energy needs	Underweight (NC-3.1)
Physiologic–Metabolic	Injury, condition, physical disability, or limitation that reduces physical activity or activities of daily living	Illness related pediatric malnutrition (undernutrition) (NC-4.1.5), Physical inactivity (NB-2.1)
Physiologic–Metabolic	Intolerance of EN/PN	Inadequate enteral nutrition infusion (NI-2.3), Inadequate parenteral nutrition infusion (NI-2.7)
Physiologic–Metabolic	Kidney, liver, cardiac, endocrine, neurologic, and/or pulmonary dysfunction	Limited food acceptance (NI-2.11), Excessive fluid intake (NI-3.2), Biting/chewing (masticatory) difficulty (NC-1.2), Altered nutrition-related laboratory values (specify) (NC-2.2), Growth rate below expected (NC-3.5), Non illness related pediatric malnutrition (undernutrition) (NC-4.1.4), Illness related pediatric malnutrition (undernutrition) (NC-4.1.5)

Category	Etiology	Diagnosis
Physiologic–Metabolic	Lack of developmental readiness to perform self-management tasks	Inability to manage self-care (NB-2.3)
Physiologic–Metabolic	Lethargy, sleepiness	Breastfeeding difficulty (NC-1.3)
Physiologic–Metabolic	Limited vision	Self-feeding difficulty (NB-2.6)
Physiologic–Metabolic	Limited food acceptance	Inadequate oral intake (NI-2.1), Growth rate below expected (NC-3.5)
Physiologic–Metabolic	Liver dysfunction	Decreased nutrient needs (specify) (NI-5.3), Excessive protein intake (NI-5.6.2), Intake of types of proteins inconsistent with needs (specify) (NI-5.6.3), Intake of types of amino acids inconsistent with needs (specify) (NI-5.7.1)
Physiologic–Metabolic	Loss of appetite awareness	Excessive oral intake (NI-2.2)
Physiologic–Metabolic	Malnutrition/malabsorption	Increased nutrient needs (specify) (NI-5.1), Breastfeeding difficulty (NC-1.3), Predicted breastfeeding difficulty (NC-1.5), Growth rate below expected (NC-3.5)
Physiologic–Metabolic	Mastitis and/or painful breasts, nipples	Breastfeeding difficulty (NC-1.3), Predicted breastfeeding difficulty (NC-1.5)
Physiologic–Metabolic	Mechanical issues such as inflammation; surgery; stricture; oral, pharyngeal, and esophageal tumors; mechanical ventilation	Swallowing difficulty (NC-1.1), Biting/chewing (masticatory) difficulty (NC-1.2)
Physiologic–Metabolic	Inborn errors of metabolism	Intake of types of proteins inconsistent with needs (specify) (NI-5.6.3), Intake of types of amino acids inconsistent with needs (specify) (NI-5.7.1), Altered nutrition-related laboratory values (specify) (NC-2.2), Illness related pediatric malnutrition (undernutrition) (NC-4.1.5)
Physiologic–Metabolic	Metabolic abnormality	Excessive protein intake (NI-5.6.2), Intake of types of proteins inconsistent with needs (specify) (NI-5.6.3), Intake of types of amino acids inconsistent with needs (specify) (NI-5.7.1), Illness related pediatric malnutrition (undernutrition) (NC-4.1.5)
Physiologic–Metabolic	Metabolic disorders	Impaired nutrient utilization (NC-2.1), Intake of types of amino acids inconsistent with needs (specify) (NI-5.7.1), Illness related pediatric malnutrition (undernutrition) (NC-4.1.5)
Physiologic–Metabolic	Motor causes related to neurological or muscular disorders	Swallowing difficulty (NC-1.1)
Physiologic–Metabolic	Oral pain	Breastfeeding difficulty (NC-1.3)
Physiologic–Metabolic	Other organ dysfunction that leads to biochemical changes	Altered nutrition-related laboratory values (specify) (NC-2.2)
Physiologic–Metabolic	Partial or complete edentulism	Biting/chewing (masticatory) difficulty (NC-1.2)
Physiologic–Metabolic	Physical disability	Impaired ability to prepare foods/meals (NB-2.4), Limited access to food (NB-3.2), Limited access to potable water (NB-3.4)
Physiologic–Metabolic	Physiologic causes requiring modified amount or timing of carbohydrate intake	Excessive carbohydrate intake (NI-5.8.2), Intake of types of carbohydrate inconsistent with needs (specify) (NI-5.8.3), Inconsistent carbohydrate intake (NI-5.8.4)

Category	Etiology	Diagnosis
Physiologic–Metabolic	Physiological causes increasing nutrient needs due to:	
	• Accelerated growth or anabolism	Increased energy expenditure (NI-1.1), Inadequate enteral nutrition infusion (NI-2.3), Inadequate parenteral nutrition infusion (NI-2.7), Increased nutrient needs (specify) (NI-5.1), Inadequate mineral intake (specify) (NI-5.10.1), Growth rate below expected (NC-3.5)
	• Altered absorption or metabolism	Inadequate fluid intake (NI-3.1), Increased nutrient needs (specify) (NI-5.1), Inadequate protein intake (NI-5.6.1), Inadequate carbohydrate intake (NI-5.8.1), Inadequate vitamin intake (specify) (NI-5.9.1), Inadequate mineral intake (specify) (NI-5.10.1), Predicted inadequate nutrient intake (specify) (NI-5.11.1), Chronic disease or condition related malnutrition (undernutrition) (NC-4.1.2), Illness related pediatric malnutrition (undernutrition) (NC-4.1.5), Inadequate protein-energy intake (NI-5.2), Unintended weight loss (NC-3.2), Growth rate below expected (NC-3.5)
	• Disease/condition	Inadequate enteral nutrition infusion (NI-2.3), Inadequate parenteral nutrition infusion (NI-2.7), Inadequate fluid intake (NI-3.1), Increased nutrient needs (specify) (NI-5.1), Chronic disease or condition related malnutrition (undernutrition) (NC-4.1.2), Illness related pediatric malnutrition (undernutrition) (NC-4.1.5), Inadequate protein-energy intake (NI-5.2), Inadequate protein intake (NI-5.6.1), Intake of types of proteins inconsistent with needs (specify) (NI-5.6.3), Intake of types of amino acids inconsistent with needs (specify) (NI-5.7.1), Inadequate vitamin intake (specify) (NI-5.9.1), Unintended weight loss (NC-3.2), Growth rate below expected (NC-3.5)
	• Maintenance of body temperature	Increased energy expenditure (NI-1.1), Inadequate fluid intake (NI-3.1), Growth rate below expected (NC-3.5)
	• Prolonged catabolic illness	Inadequate energy intake (NI-1.2), Inadequate oral intake (NI-2.1), Inadequate fluid intake (NI-3.1), Chronic disease or condition related malnutrition (undernutrition) (NC-4.1.2), Illness related pediatric malnutrition (undernutrition) (NC-4.1.5), Inadequate protein-energy intake (NI-5.2), Inadequate protein intake (NI-5.6.1), Inadequate vitamin intake (specify) (NI-5.9.1), Inadequate mineral intake (specify) (NI-5.10.1), Unintended weight loss (NC-3.2), Growth rate below expected (NC-3.5)
Physiologic–Metabolic	Altered metabolism	Predicted excessive energy intake (NI-1.5), Predicted excessive nutrient intake (NI-5.11.2)
Physiologic–Metabolic	Poor sucking ability	Breastfeeding difficulty (NC-1.3), Predicted breastfeeding difficulty (NC-1.5), Growth rate below expected (NC-3.5)
Physiologic–Metabolic	Prematurity	Altered nutrition-related laboratory values (NC-2.2), Growth rate below expected (NC-3.5), Illness related pediatric malnutrition (undernutrition) (NC-4.1.5)
Physiologic–Metabolic	Renal dysfunction	Decreased nutrient needs (specify) (NI-5.3), Excessive protein intake (NI-5.6.2), Intake of types of proteins inconsistent with needs (specify) (NI-5.6.3), Intake of types of amino acids inconsistent with needs (specify) (NI-5.7.1)
Physiologic–Metabolic	Small for gestational age, intrauterine growth retardation/restriction, and/or lack of progress/ appropriate weight gain per day	Underweight (NC-3.1), Growth rate below expected (NC-3.5)
Physiologic–Metabolic	Soft tissue disease (primary or oral manifestations of a systemic disease)	Biting/chewing (masticatory) difficulty (NC-1.2), Starvation related malnutrition (undernutrition) (NC-4.1.1)

Category	Etiology	Diagnosis
Physiologic–Metabolic	Swallowing difficulty and altered suck and breathing patterns in infants	Swallowing difficulty (NC-1.1), Breastfeeding difficulty (NC-1.3), Predicted breast-feeding difficulty (NC-1.5)
Physiologic–Metabolic	Xerostomia	Biting/chewing (masticatory) difficulty (NC-1.2)
Psychological	Alcohol or drug addiction	Excessive alcohol intake (NI-4.3), Impaired nutrient utilization (NC-2.1)
Psychological	Addictive personality	Excessive physical activity (NB-2.2)
Psychological	Mental illness, confusion, or altered awareness	Intake of unsafe food (NB-3.1), Excessive oral intake (NI-2.2)
Psychological	Psychological causes such as depression or disordered eating	Inadequate energy intake (NI-1.2), Inadequate oral intake (NI-2.1), Inadequate fluid intake (NI-3.1), Excessive fluid intake (NI-3.2), Starvation related malnutrition (under-nutrition) (NC-4.1.1), Non illness related pediatric malnutrition (undernutrition) (NC-4.1.4), Illness related pediatric malnutrition (undernutrition) (NC-4.1.5), Inadequate protein-energy intake (NI-5.2), Inadequate fat intake (NI-5.5.1), Inadequate protein intake (NI-5.6.1), Inadequate carbohydrate intake (NI-5.8.1), Excessive carbohydrate intake (NI-5.8.2), Intake of types of carbohydrate inconsistent with needs (specify) (NI-5.8.3), Inconsistent carbohydrate intake (NI-5.8.4), Inadequate fiber intake (NI-5.8.5), Inadequate vitamin intake (specify) (NI-5.9.1), Excessive vitamin intake (specify) (NI-5.9.2), Inadequate mineral intake (specify) (NI-5.10.1), Unintended weight loss (NC-3.2), Growth rate below expected (NC-3.5), Undesirable food choices (NB-1.7), Excessive physical activity (NB-2.2), Limited access to food (NB-3.2), Limited access to nutrition-related supplies (NB-3.3)
Social–Personal	Lack of role models	Breastfeeding difficulty (NC-1.3), Physical inactivity (NB-2.1)
Social–Personal	Lack of social support for implementing changes	Breastfeeding difficulty (NC-1.3), Predicted breastfeeding difficulty (NC-1.5), Non illness related pediatric malnutrition (undernutrition) (NC-4.1.4), Not ready for diet/lifestyle change (NB-1.3), Self-monitoring deficit (NB-1.4), Limited adherence to nutrition-related recommendations (NB-1.6), Physical inactivity (NB-2.1), Inability to manage self-care (NB-2.3), Poor nutrition quality of life (NB-2.5)
Social–Personal	Family or social history of overeating	Predicted excessive energy intake (NI-1.5)
Social–Personal	Increased psychological/life stress	Predicted breastfeeding difficulty (NC-1.5); Overweight, adult or pediatric (NC-3.3.1); Obese, pediatric (NC-3.3.2); Obese, Class I (NC-3.3.3); Obese, Class II (NC-3.3.4); Obese, Class III (NC-3.3.5); Predicted inadequate energy intake (NI-1.4); Predicted excessive energy intake (NI-1.5)
Social–Personal	Change in living situation	Predicted inadequate energy intake (NI-1.4), Predicted excessive energy intake (NI-1.5), Predicted inadequate nutrient intake (specify) (NI-5.11.1), Predicted breast-feeding difficulty (NC-1.5)
Social–Personal	Living in a geographic location with danger for environmental emergency	Predicted inadequate nutrient intake (specify) (NI-5.11.1)
Treatment	Accidental vitamin and/or mineral overdose from oral, enteral, or parenteral sources	Excessive vitamin intake (specify) (NI-5.9.2), Excessive mineral intake (specify) (NI-5.10.2)
Treatment	Calories/kcal/kJ unaccounted for from IV infusion and/or medications	Excessive energy intake (NI-1.3)
Treatment	Changes in taste, appetite	Excessive fat intake (NI-5.5.2), Intake of types of fats inconsistent with needs (specify) (NI-5.5.3)

Category	Etiology	Diagnosis
Treatment	Changes in GI tract motility	Altered GI function (NC-1.4)
Treatment	Chronic use of medications known to cause weight gain, such as use of certain antidepressants, antipsychotics, corticosteroids, certain HIV medications	Unintended weight gain (NC-3.4), Excessive growth rate (NC-3.6)
Treatment	Difficulty chewing or swallowing high-fiber foods	Inadequate fiber intake (NI-5.8.5)
Treatment	Excessive energy intake	Overweight, adult or pediatric (NC-3.3.1); Obese, pediatric (NC-3.3.2); Obese, Class I (NC-3.3.3); Obese, Class II (NC-3.3.4); Obese, Class III (NC-3.3.5)
Treatment	Food intolerances	Decreased nutrient needs (specify) (NI-5.3)
Treatment	High level of fatigue or other side effect of therapy	Undesirable food choices (NB-1.7), Impaired ability to prepare foods/meals (NB-2.4)
Treatment	Improvement in patient/client status, allowing return to total or partial oral diet; changes in the course of disease resulting in changes in nutrient requirements	Enteral nutrition composition inconsistent with needs (NI-2.5), Enteral nutrition administration inconsistent with needs (NI-2.6), Parenteral nutrition composition inconsistent with needs (NI-2.9), Parenteral nutrition administration inconsistent with needs (NI-2.10)
Treatment	Inadequate energy intake	Underweight (NC-3.1)
Treatment	Infusion volume not reached or schedule for infusion interrupted	Inadequate enteral nutrition infusion (NI-2.3), Inadequate parenteral nutrition infusion (NI-2.7)
Treatment	Insufficient electrolyte replacement when initiating feeding (PN/EN, including oral)	Imbalance of nutrients (NI-5.4)
Treatment	Lack of, compromised, or incorrect access for delivering EN/PN	Inadequate enteral nutrition infusion (NI-2.3), Inadequate parenteral nutrition infusion (NI-2.7)
Treatment	Mechanical issues such as inflammation; surgery; stricture; oral, pharyngeal, and esophageal tumors; mechanical ventilation	Swallowing difficulty (NC-1.1), Biting/chewing (masticatory) difficulty (NC-1.2)
Treatment	Medications that increase appetite	Excessive energy intake (NI-1.3), Excessive oral intake (NI-2.2),
Treatment	Medications that increase nutrient needs	Increased nutrient needs (specify) (NI-5.1)
Treatment	Medications that affect nutrient metabolism	Impaired nutrient utilization (NC-2.1)
Treatment	Medications that increase fluid needs or decrease thirst	Inadequate fluid intake (NI-3.1)
Treatment	Misused specialized protein products	Intake of types of proteins inconsistent with needs (specify) (NI-5.6.3)
Treatment	Misused specialized amino acid products	Intake of types of amino acids inconsistent with needs (specify) (NI-5.7.1)
Treatment	Misdiagnosis of lactose intolerance/lactase deficiency	Inadequate mineral intake (specify) (NI-5.10.1)
Treatment	Nutrient–nutrient interaction and/or drug–nutrient interaction	Inadequate enteral nutrition infusion (NI-2.3), Inadequate parenteral nutrition infusion (NI-2.7), Inadequate vitamin intake (specify) (NI-5.9.1), Inadequate mineral intake (specify) (NI-5.10.1), Food-Medication Interaction (NC-2.3), Predicted food-medication interaction (NC-2.4)

Category	Etiology	Diagnosis
Treatment	Overfeeding of parenteral/enteral nutrition (PN/EN)	Excessive energy intake (NI-1.3)
Treatment	Planned procedure, therapy, or medication predicted to increase energy expenditure or nutrient need	Predicted inadequate energy intake (NI-1.4), Predicted inadequate nutrient intake (specify) (NI-5.11.1)
Treatment	Planned therapy or medication predicted to reduce energy/nutrient need or metabolic rate/metabolism	Predicted excessive energy intake (NI-1.5), Predicted excessive nutrient intake (NI-5.11.2)
Treatment	Planned procedure, therapy, or medication predicted to hinder breastfeeding	Predicted breastfeeding difficulty (NC-1.5)
Treatment	Planned procedure, therapy, or medication predicted to decrease ability to consume sufficient energy or nutrients	Predicted inadequate energy intake (NI-1.4), Predicted inadequate nutrient intake (specify) (NI-5.11.1)
Treatment	Prolonged adherence to a low-fiber or low-residue diet	Inadequate fiber intake (NI-5.8.5)
Treatment	Prolonged hospitalization	Unintended weight loss (NC-3.2)
Treatment	Renal dysfunction	Decreased nutrient needs (specify) (NI-5.3), Excessive protein intake (NI-5.6.2), Intake of types of proteins inconsistent with needs (specify) (NI-5.6.3), Intake of types of amino acids inconsistent with needs (specify) (NI-5.7.1)
Treatment	Xerostomia	Biting/chewing (masticatory) difficulty (NC-1.2)
Access	Access to foods and supplements in excess of needs	Excessive vitamin intake (specify) (NI-5.9.2)
Access	Caregiver intentionally or unintentionally not providing access to food or nutrition-related supplies	Limited access to food (NB-3.2), Limited access to nutrition-related supplies (NB-3.3), Limited access to potable water (NB-3.4)
Access	Community and geographical constraints	Inadequate vitamin intake (specify) (NI-5.9.1), Limited access to food (NB-3.2), Limited access to nutrition-related supplies (NB-3.3), Limited access to potable water (NB-3.4)
Access	Environmental causes, eg, inadequately tested nutrient bioavailability of fortified foods, beverages, and supplements; marketing of fortified foods, beverages, and supplements as a substitute for natural food source of nutrient(s)	Inadequate vitamin intake (NI-5.9.1), Inadequate mineral intake (specify) (NI-5.10.1)
Access	Exposure to contaminated water or food, eg, community outbreak of illness documented by surveillance and/or response agency	Intake of unsafe food (NB-3.1), Limited access to food (NB-3.2), Limited access to potable water (NB-3.4)
Access	Failure to participate in federal food programs such as WIC, National School Breakfast/Lunch Program, food stamps	Limited access to food (NB-3.2), Limited access to potable water (NB-3.4)
Access	Financial constraints that may prevent sufficient level of activity (eg, to address cost of equipment, shoes, or club membership to gain access)	Physical inactivity (NB-2.1)

Category	Etiology	Diagnosis
Access	Lack of or limited access to:	
	• Adaptive foods or eating devices conducive to self-feeding	Self-feeding difficulty (NB-2.6)
	• Available and safe exercise environment and/or equipment	Physical inactivity (NB-2.1)
	• Fluid	Inadequate fluid intake (NI-3.1), Inadequate fiber intake (NI-5.8.5)
	• Fortified foods and beverages	Inadequate mineral intake (specify) (NI-5.10.1)
	• Specialized protein products	Excessive protein intake (NI-5.6.2)
	• Food or artificial nutrition	Inadequate energy intake (NI-1.2), Inadequate oral intake (NI-2.1), Starvation related malnutrition (undernutrition) (NC-4.1.1), Non illness related pediatric malnutrition (undernutrition) (NC-4.1.4), Inadequate protein-energy intake (NI-5.2), Inadequate fat intake (NI-5.5.1), Inadequate protein intake (NI-5.6.1), Intake of types of proteins inconsistent with needs (NI-5.6.3), Intake of types of amino acids inconsistent with needs (NI-5.7.2), Inadequate carbohydrate intake (NI-5.8.1), Inadequate vitamin intake (specify) (NI-5.9.1), Inadequate mineral intake (specify) (NI-5.10.1), Underweight (NC-3.1), Unintended weight loss (NC-3.2), Growth rate below expected (NC-3.5), Poor nutrition quality of life (NB-2.5)
	• Fiber-containing foods	Inadequate fiber intake (NI-5.8.5)
	• Food that contains a bioactive substance	Inadequate bioactive substance intake (NI-4.1)
	• Healthy food choices	Excessive energy intake (NI-1.3), Excessive oral intake (NI-2.2), Excessive fat intake (NI-5.5.2), Intake of types of fats inconsistent with needs (specify) (NI-5.5.3)
	• Recommended foods	Undesirable food choices (NB-1.7)
	• Sufficient quantity or variety of culturally appropriate healthful food or water	Limited access to food (NB-3.2), Limited access to potable water (NB-3.4)
	• Safe and/or clear and accurately labeled food supply	Excessive bioactive substance intake (NI-4.2)
	• Food storage equipment/facilities	Intake of unsafe food (NB-3.1)
	• Self-management tools or decision guides or other nutrition-related supplies	Inability to manage self-care (NB-2.3), Limited access to nutrition-related supplies (NB-3.3)
Access	Limited, absent, or failure to participate in community supplemental food programs such as food pantries, emergency kitchens, or shelters, with a sufficient variety of culturally appropriate healthful foods or nutrition-related supplies	Limited access to food (NB-3.2), Limited access to nutrition-related supplies (NB-3.3), Limited access to potable water (NB-3.4)
Access	Schools lacking nutrition/wellness policies or application of policies ensuring convenient, appetizing, competitively priced, culturally appropriate healthful foods at meals, snacks, and school-sponsored activities	Limited access to food (NB-3.2), Limited access to potable water (NB-3.4)

Category	Etiology	Diagnosis
Behavior	Addictive behavior	Excessive physical activity (NB-2.2)
Behavior	Consumption of high-dose nutrient supplements	Imbalance of nutrients (NI-5.4)
Behavior	Eating behavior serves a purpose other than nourishment (e.g., pica)	Unsupported beliefs/attitudes about food or nutrition-related topics (NB-1.2), Limited food acceptance (NI-2.11)
Behavior	Excessive energy intake	Overweight, adult or pediatric (NC-3.3.1); Obese, pediatric (NC-3.3.2); Obese, Class I (NC-3.3.3); Obese, Class II (NC-3.3.4); Obese, Class III (NC-3.3.5)
Behavior	Excessive physical activity	Underweight (NC-3.1)
Behavior	Food and nutrition compliance limitations	Excessive carbohydrate intake (NI-5.8.2), Intake of types of carbohydrate inconsistent with needs (specify) (NI-5.8.3), Inconsistent carbohydrate intake (NI-5.8.4)
Behavior	Food or activity behavior-related difficulty	Poor nutrition quality of life (NB-2.5)
Behavior	Food preparation or eating patterns that involve only high-fiber foods to the exclusion of other nutrient-dense foods	Excessive fiber intake (NI-5.8.6)
Behavior	Disordered eating pattern	Excessive physical activity (NB-2.2); Underweight (NC-3.1); Overweight, adult or pediatric (NC-3.3.1); Obese, pediatric (NC-3.3.2); Obese, Class I (NC-3.3.3); Obese, Class II (NC-3.3.4); Obese, Class III (NC-3.3.5); Non illness related pediatric malnutrition (undernutrition) (NC-4.1.4); Illness related pediatric malnutrition (undernutrition) (NC-4.1.5)
Behavior	Feeding via bottle or other route that may affect breastfeeding	Breastfeeding difficulty (NC-1.3), Predicted breastfeeding difficulty (NC-1.5)
Behavior	Frequent intake of foods containing bioactive substances	Excessive bioactive substance intake (NI-4.2)
Behavior	Limited food acceptance due to behavioral issues	Inadequate oral intake (NI-2.1), Growth rate below expected (NC-3.5)
Behavior	Inability to limit or refuse offered foods	Excessive oral intake (NI-2.2)
Behavior	Inadequate energy intake	Underweight (NC-3.1)
Behavior	Lack of focus and attention to detail, difficulty with time management and/or organization	Self-monitoring deficit (NB-1.4)
Behavior	Lifestyle change that reduces physical activity or activities of daily living	Physical inactivity (NB-2.1)
Behavior	Overconsumption of a limited variety of foods	Excessive mineral intake (specify) (NI-5.10.2)
Behavior	Poor food planning, purchasing, and preparation practices	Excessive oral intake (NI-2.2), Inadequate fiber intake (NI-5.8.5), Limited access to food (NB-3.2)
Behavior	Reluctance or avoidance of self-feeding	Self-feeding difficulty (NB-2.6)

Terminology Index

Nutrition Diagnostic Terminology

Intake (NI)

Coordination of Nutrition Care
by a Nutrition Professional (RC)

Collaboration and Referral of Nutrition Care (1), *353–354*

Team meeting (RC-1.1)

Referral to RDN with different expertise (RC-1.2)

Collaboration with other providers (RC-1.4)

Discharge and Transfer of Nutrition Care to a New Setting or Provider (2), *355–356*

Discharge and transfer to other providers (RC-2.1)

Discharge and transfer to community agencies/ programs (RC-2.2)

Discharge and transfer to another nutrition professional (RC-2.3)